CONTEMPORARY ISSUES
IN INTELLECTUAL DISABILITIES

D1338705

DISABILITY STUDIES

Series Editor: Joav Merrick

National Institute of Child Health and Human Development,
Ministry of Social Affairs, Jerusalem

Additional books in this series can be found on Nova's website at:

https://www.novapublishers.com/catalog/index.php?cPath=23_29&seriesp=Disability+St
udies+%28Joav+Merrick+-+Series+Editor+-
+National+Institute+of+Child+Health+and+Human+
Development%2C+Ministry+of+Social+Affairs%2C+Jerusalem

This book is due for return on or before the last date shown below.

DISABILITY STUDIES

CONTEMPORARY ISSUES IN INTELLECTUAL DISABILITIES

V.P. PRASHER
EDITOR

Nova Science Publishers, Inc.
New York

For permission to use material from this book please contact us:
Telephone 631-231-7269; Fax 631-231-8175
Web Site: http://www.novapublishers.com

NOTICE TO THE READER

The Publisher has taken reasonable care in the preparation of this book, but makes no expressed or implied warranty of any kind and assumes no responsibility for any errors or omissions. No liability is assumed for incidental or consequential damages in connection with or arising out of information contained in this book. The Publisher shall not be liable for any special, consequential, or exemplary damages resulting, in whole or in part, from the readers' use of, or reliance upon, this material. Any parts of this book based on government reports are so indicated and copyright is claimed for those parts to the extent applicable to compilations of such works.

Independent verification should be sought for any data, advice or recommendations contained in this book. In addition, no responsibility is assumed by the publisher for any injury and/or damage to persons or property arising from any methods, products, instructions, ideas or otherwise contained in this publication.

This publication is designed to provide accurate and authoritative information with regard to the subject matter covered herein. It is sold with the clear understanding that the Publisher is not engaged in rendering legal or any other professional services. If legal or any other expert assistance is required, the services of a competent person should be sought. FROM A DECLARATION OF PARTICIPANTS JOINTLY ADOPTED BY A COMMITTEE OF THE AMERICAN BAR ASSOCIATION AND A COMMITTEE OF PUBLISHERS.

Library of Congress Cataloging-in-Publication Data

Contemporary issues in intellectual disabilities / [edited by] V.P. Prasher.
    p. ; cm.
  ISBN 978-1-61668-023-7 (hardcover)
 1. Mental retardation. I. Prasher, Vee P.
 [DNLM: 1. Mental Retardation. 2. Autistic Disorder. 3. Learning
Disorders. WM 300 C761 2010]
  RC570.C66 2010
  616.85'88--dc22
                            2010001747

Published by Nova Science Publishers, Inc. † New York

To Pattie Saunders

CONTENTS

PREFACE

The International Association for the Scientific Studies of Intellectual Disabilities is an established international organization with links to the World Health Organization, that promotes better social and healthcare for individuals with intellectual disabilities[*]. It is a multi-professional organization involved in a number of diverse activities which are brought together at quadrennial international conferences. These international meetings are an opportunity for researchers and clinicians to present contemporary issues and to be able to high light advances in the biological, behavioral, and social science fields of intellectual disabilities.

The International Association for the Scientific Studies of Intellectual Disabilities held their 13th World Congress Meeting in August 2008 in Cape Town, South Africa. Following the 13th World Congress, participants were invited to contribute to this book. I am eternally grateful for their contribution and their support in this venture, which we hope will improve the lives of individuals with intellectual disabilities in the different parts of the world.

Vee Prasher

---

[*] The term 'intellectual disabilities' is used in this text to be synonymous with 'mental retardation', 'learning disabilities', 'mental handicap' and 'intellectual handicap.'

EDITOR'S CONTACT INFORMATION

Professor Vee Prasher MBChB, MedSc, MRCPsych,MD, PhD, F.IASSID
Professor of Neuropsychiatry
c/o The Greenfields
Monyhull
30 Brookfield Road
Kings Norton
Birmingham
B30 3QY
UK
Tel no 0044 (0) 121 465 8762
Fax no 0044 (0) 121 449 2293
Pager 07623 984619
Email vprasher@compuserve.com

PART I. MENTAL HEALTH

It is now well established that children and adults with intellectual disabilities (ID) suffer from a higher prevalence rate of both challenging behavior and mental health problems as compared to individuals without ID. *Furniss* highlights a number of issues in the investigation of an association between challenging behavior and underlying mental disorders. The use of categorical criteria remains controversial. *Barnhill* discusses the newly published 'Diagnostic Manual-Intellectual Disability'. Although this new diagnostic criteria is a welcome addition to improving the accuracy of psychiatric diagnosis in persons with ID, further field testing is required. A particular area of diagnostic concern is that of detecting a psychotic illness in a person with ID. *Friedlander and colleagues* highlight the under researched area of early onset psychosis in children and adolescents. The authors highlight that psychosis is an umbrella term for other more specific diagnostic groups of schizophrenia and mood disorders with psychotic features.

The clinical management and treatment of mental health in persons with ID is still in its infancy. This is highlighted by *Voss and colleagues*, who in their 10 year review, demonstrate the high rates of prescribing of typical antipsychotics along with the frequent use of anxiolytic and sedating drugs. Polypharmacy remains an ongoing issue.

Mental health can be gender specific with particular disorders being exclusive to females (for example premenstrual syndrome) or predominantly associated with males (for example paedophilia). *Mason* reports findings from her study of premenstrual syndrome (PMS) in women with Down syndrome. The hypothesis that PMS would be higher in this population was not supported. *Taggart* reviews the literature of mental health in women with ID and goes on to discuss staffs' knowledge and perception of working women with ID and mental health. Gender-sensitive psychiatric services are required. The need for such services are further demonstrated by *Curen* in his case discussion of a young male with ID and paedophila.

Chapter 1

PSYCHIATRIC SYMPTOMATOLOGY AND FUNCTION OF CHALLENGING BEHAVIOR IN CHILDREN WITH INTELLECTUAL DISABILITIES

F. Furniss

The Hesley Group Doncaster and University of Leicester, U.K.

INTRODUCTION

Children with intellectual disabilities (ID) experience higher rates of both problematic behaviors and specific mental health difficulties as compared to children without ID. Prevalence rates of up to 25% for problematic behavior and 22% for anxiety disorders have been reported for children with ID, although prevalence figures vary substantially across studies, possibly due to differences in sampling, definitions of ID, and methods for ascertainment of mental health difficulties (Whitaker & Read, 2006).

A number of studies involving adults with ID have investigated the possibility that there may be a specific association between presentation of challenging behavior and experiencing mental health difficulties (Holden & Gitlesen, 2003; Rojahn et al, 2004). Myrbakk and von Tetzchner (2008) for example asked carers to complete various well-established checklists designed to screen for mental health problems for 71 adults with ID reported to present at least one moderate or severe problem behavior and a comparison group not presenting any moderate or severe problem and found that even when checklist items referring to problem behaviors were discounted, the group presenting challenging behaviors scored higher than the comparison group on global psychopathology scores and on subscales measuring features of possible psychosis, depression, anxiety, mania, and obsessive-compulsive disorder.

A number of possible explanations have been offered for this association between presentation of challenging behaviors and presence of mental health difficulties. The apparent association may result from carers reporting challenging behaviors as indicators of mental health difficulties (Holden & Gitlesen, 2009). Alternatively, challenging behaviors, especially in people with ID, may be "atypical symptoms" of mental health problems (Marston et al, 1997; Tsiouris et al, 2003). Two further possibilities are that psychiatric symptoms and challenging behaviors may be caused by a common third variable, or that challenging behaviors may lead to social consequences (e.g. relative social isolation) which lead to the development of mental health problems (Ross & Oliver, 2002).

An additional possibility is that mental health problems may act as motivating operations for challenging behavior (Holden & Gitlesen, 2008). For example, depression may increase the aversiveness of requests to engage in activities, motivating challenging behavior which is socially reinforced by avoidance of participation in those activities, whereas mania may enhance the reinforcing value of social interaction and activities, motivating positively socially reinforced challenging behavior. Holden & Gitlesen (2008) investigated this possibility in a study of 119 adults with ID presenting challenging behaviors. In 21% the main challenging behavior was self-injury, in 30% aggression, in 8% property destruction, and in 40% other challenging behavior. Staff who knew participants completed the Psychiatric-Assessment-Schedule-for-Adults-with-Developmental-Disability (PAS-ADD) checklist (revised) (Moss, 2002) and completed the Motivation Assessment Scale (MAS) (Durand & Crimmins, 1988) concerning the participant's most severe challenging behavior. On the PAS-ADD checklist, 10% of participants scored above the threshold indicating a possible organic condition, 24% had scores exceeding threshold for possible affective/neurotic disorder, and 18% had scores exceeding threshold for possible psychotic disorder. With respect to the motivation of challenging behavior, the MAS indicated a primary function of automatic (non-social) reinforcement in 28% of participants, escape from demands for 34%, positive social reinforcement in 20%, and positive tangible reinforcement in 32%. No associations were found between PAS-ADD scores above threshold for organic, affective/neurotic, or psychotic disorder and primary function of challenging behavior, and few specific symptoms were associated with specific functions.

Since children with ID appear to be at elevated risk for mental health difficulties (including anxiety) and challenging behavior (Emerson, 2003; Whitaker & Read, 2006; Kaptein et al, 2007), investigation of the possible relationship between mental health difficulties and motivation of challenging behavior in children also seems warranted. Additionally, any such relationship may be clearer in children than in adults with long histories of emotional and behavioral difficulties. The work reported here was undertaken as a pilot study to explore the feasibility of investigating whether motivation of challenging behavior differs in children according to the severity of two specific mental health difficulties (anxiety and mood disorder); it was predicted that children with higher levels of anxiety or more depressed mood would be more likely to show escape from demands or social interaction as a primary function for challenging behavior.

METHODOLOGY

Participants were 20 students from two residential schools, 18 male and 2 female, aged 15 or under (mean age 13 years 5 months), with severe ID and challenging behavior, whose parents agreed to data from clinical assessments being used for research purposes. This was a retrospective "casenote" study using data from assessments already completed for clinical purposes. The Diagnostic Assessment for the Severely Handicapped II (DASH-II) (Matson et al, 1996) and the Questions About Behavioral Function (QABF) scale (Vollmer & Matson,

1995) or the Functional Assessment for Multiple Causality (FACT) (Matson et al., 2003), were completed for each participant on the basis of information from a carer who knew the person well. The QABF or FACT were completed for the young person's primary challenging behavior. In 12 cases this was aggression to others, in 5 cases self-injury, and in 3 cases other challenging behavior. For analysis, participants were divided into two groups, those scoring above and below the clinical cut-off point on the DASH-II anxiety and mood disorder subscales. It was predicted that in each case participants in the "above clinical cut-off" group would show significantly higher scores on the "escape" subscale of the QABF or FACT (when used to assess the function of their primary challenging behavior) than the participants in the "below clinical cut-off" group.

RESULTS

The 13 participants scoring above the clinical cut-off on the DASH-II anxiety subscale had a mean QABF/FACT escape subscale score of 9.2, while the 7 participants with anxiety scores below the clinical cut-off had a mean QABF/FACT escape subscale score of 5.4 (t (18) = 1.67, p (one-tailed) = 0.07). The 10 participants scoring above the clinical cut-off on the DASH-II mood subscale had a mean QABF/FACT escape subscale score of 8.3, while the 10 participants with mood scores below the clinical cut-off had a mean QABF/FACT escape subscale score not significantly different at 7.4. Participants' DASH-II anxiety and mood subscale scores were highly correlated (r = 0.72).

DISCUSSION

The present pilot study presents multiple methodological weaknesses including small sample size and use of a mental health screening assessment (the DASH-II) with cut-offs derived from an adult sample. No evidence was found for a relationship between lowered mood and the function of challenging behavior. Suggestive evidence was however found for a relationship between elevated anxiety and an escape function for challenging behavior. However, the high correlation between DASH-II anxiety and mood disorder subscale scores throws into question the utility of investigating relationships between behavioral function and measures structured according to diagnostic categories. The conditions defined by current categorical psychiatric diagnostic systems may well not map uniquely on to underlying pathological processes, and investigation of relationships between behavioral function and endophenotypes more directly related to physiological processes (Bearden et al, 2008) may represent a more fruitful approach to understanding interactions between biological and social processes in the development and maintenance of challenging behavior.

REFERENCES

Bearden, C.E., Glahn, D.C., Lee, A.D., Chiang, M-C., van Erp, T.G.M., Cannon, T.D., Reiss, A.L., Toga, A.W & Thompson, P.M.(2008). Neural phenotypes of common and rare genetic variants. *Biological Psychology, 79,* 43-57.

Durand, V. M., & Crimmins, D. B. (1988). Identifying the variables maintaining self-injurious behavior. *Journal of Autism and Developmental Disorders, 18*(1), 99-117.

Emerson, E. (2003). Prevalence of psychiatric disorders in children and adolescents with and without intellectual disability. *Journal of Intellectual Disability Research, 47,* 51-58.

Holden, B. & Gitlesen, J.P. (2003). Prevalence of psychiatric symptoms in adults with mental retardation and challenging behavior. *Research in Developmental Disabilities, 24,* 323-332.

Holden, B. & Gitlesen, J.P. (2008). The relationship between psychiatric symptomatology and motivation of challenging behavior: a preliminary study. *Research in Developmental Disabilities, 29,* 408-413.

Holden, B. & Gitlesen, J.P. (2009). The overlap between psychiatric symptoms and challenging behavior: a preliminary study. *Research in Developmental Disabilities, 30,* 210-218.

Kaptein, S., Jansen, D.E.M.C., Vogels, A.G.C. & Reijneveld, S.A. (2007). Mental health problems in children with intellectual disability: use of the strengths and difficulties questionnaire. *Journal of Intellectual Disability Research, 52,* 125-131.

Marston, G.M., Perry, D.W. & Roy, A. (1997). Manifestations of depression in people with intellectual disability. *Journal of Intellectual Disability Research, 41,* 476-480.

Matson, J. L., Baglio, C. S., Smiroldo, B. B., Hamilton, M., Paclawskyj, T., Williams, D. & Kirkpatrick-Sanchez, S. (1996). Characteristics of autism as assessed by the Diagnostic Assessment for the Severely Handicapped-II (DASH-II). *Research in Developmental Disabilities, 17,* 135-143.

Matson, J. L., Kuhn, D. E., Dixon, D. R., Mayville, S. B., Laud, R. B., Cooper, C. L., et al. (2003). The development and factor structure of the functional assessment for multiple causality (FACT). *Research in Developmental Disabilities, 24*(6), 485-495.

Moss, S. (2002). *The PAS-ADD Checklist.* Brighton, U.K.; Pavilion Publishing.

Myrbakk, E. & von Tetzchner, S. (2008). Psychiatric disorders and behavior problems in people with intellectual disability. *Research in Developmental Disabilities, 29,* 316-332.

Rojahn, J., Matson, J.L., Naglieri, J.A. & Mayville, E. (2004). Relationships between psychiatric conditions and behavior problems among adults with mental retardation. *American Journal on Mental Retardation, 109,* 21-33.

Ross, E. & Oliver, C. (2002). The relationship between levels of mood, interest, and pleasure and "challenging behavior" in adults with severe and profound intellectual disability. *Journal of Intellectual Disability Research, 46,* 191-197.

Tsiouris, J.A., Mann, R., Patti, P.J. & Sturmey, P. (2003). Challenging behaviors should not be considered as depressive equivalents in individuals with intellectual disability. *Journal of Intellectual Disability Research, 47,* 14-21.

Vollmer, T.R. & Matson, J.L. (1995). *User's guide: Questions About Behavioral Function (QABF).* Scientific Publishers, Inc., Baton Rouge, LA.

Whitaker, S. & Read, S. (2006). The prevalence of psychiatric disorders among people with intellectual disabilities: an analysis of the literature. *Journal of Applied Research in Intellectual Disabilities, 19,* 330-345.

Chapter 2

DIAGNOSTIC MANUAL-INTELLECTUAL DISABILITY: DIFFERENTIAL DIAGNOSIS OF CHILDREN WITH INTELLECTUAL DISABILITIES

J. Barnhill

University of North Carolina School of Medicine, USA

INTRODUCTION

This paper focuses on several problems that complicate the diagnosis of psychiatric disorders among children with intellectual disabilities (ID). These difficulties relate in large part to problems we have fitting children with ID into many of the categories outlined in the Diagnostic and Statistical Manual (DSM-IV-TR; American Psychiatric Association, 2000). The recently published Diagnostic Manual-Intellectual Disability (DM-ID; Fletcher et al, 2007) offers some relief by providing modified diagnostic criteria that better suit the clinical realities of ID individuals with mental illness while preserving the multi-axial descriptive format of the DSM. Although judged quite helpful by a modest sample of clinicians in the field, the DM-ID currently lacks statistical validation through extensive field trials (Fletcher et al in press).

DIAGNOSTIC CRITERIA AND MI-ID

The diagnosis of psychiatric disorders requires defining specific syndromes based on the presence of co-occurring cognitive, emotional and behavioral symptoms (Royal College of Psychiatrists, 2001; Hurley et al 2007, Ursano et al 2008). Lacking definable biological correlates (lab tests, definitive neuroimaging) we must rely on data derived from self-reports, psychological testing and direct observation (Sovenr, 1986; Barnhill, 2003: Harris, 2006). Historically, psychiatric diagnosis involved either descriptive approaches (Kraeplin's and others) or etiologically grounded nomenclatures based in part on psychodynamic models. The Research Diagnostic Criteria (RDC) and subsequent iterations of the Diagnostic and

Statistical Manual changed the focus of psychiatric diagnosis in the United States by adapting Kraeplin's model of categorical diagnoses (descriptive psychiatric syndromes) based on observable/measurable symptoms (Barnhill, 2003).

Although this change represents a major advance in psychiatry, less emphasis was placed on the diagnosis of mental disorders among individuals with ID (Sovner, 1986; LaMalfa et al 1997, Fletcher et al 2007). Problems emerged as it became apparent that the use of descriptive-categorical criteria (symptoms of depression) did not resolve the many diagnostic problems inherent to the ID population, especially those growing out of developmental deficits in language, cognition, emotional expression and capacity to report internal states to the clinician (Royal College of Psychiatrists, 2001; Fletcher et al 2007).

DIAGNOSTIC CONUNDRUMS AMONG CHILDREN WITH MI-ID

The diagnosis of childhood psychopathology requires additional modifications in order to accommodate the ongoing effects of brain maturation on the expression and course of mental disorders (Giedd, 1997; Ursano et al, 2008). Children with ID present an additional set of problems, namely how to integrate the effects of ID, genetic, metabolic and neurological deficits, differences in the trajectory of development and learning experiences with risks for psychopathology (Harris, 1995; Ursano et al, 2008). Accommodating these factors to existing diagnostic criteria, even after considering recent modifications for children in the DSM-IV-TR (American Psychiatric Association, 1994), remains a major challenge for researchers and clinicians.

It also became apparent that the existing diagnostic criteria never fully captured the spectrum of risks, vulnerability and resiliency factors among ID children with mental illness (Othmer et al 1998; Maser et al 2002; Perugi et al 2002). In part this limitation minimizes etiological factors and the multi-directional affects of each of these factors across the spectrum of ID (level of adaptive and measurable intellectual deficits) and associated neurodevelopmental disorders (Ratey et al, 1996; Willemsen-Swinkels et al 2002; Harris 2006). These limitations made it difficult to readily differentiate and categorize stress-related symptoms, chronic impulse dyscontrol, externalizing-disruptive behaviors, and aggressive behaviors from primary mental disorders (Harris, 1995, Barnhill 2003; Kim-Cohen 2007). Other factors such as comorbid autism and related syndromes, disorders of learning, communication and motor coordination, syndromes linked to medical and neurological conditions exert powerful influences (Skuster et al, 1992: Pulsifer, 1996; Ratey et al, 1996). Failing to account for these during the assessment and differential diagnosis increases the risk for misattribution and inappropriate diagnosis of some syndromes (e.g. schizophrenias), while overshadowing other more common disorders such as tic, mood and anxiety disorders (Cadenhead, 2002; Barnhill 2003).

A second set of problems arise due to our rethinking of adult onset psychiatric disorders in terms of neurodevelopmental disorders (Cloninger et al, 1993; Cloninger 1998; Cadenhead, 2002; Fletcher et al, 2007). This model assumes disorders like schizophrenia represent a possible combination of disrupted fetal neuronal migration and maturation setting the stage for over exuberant synaptic pruning during late adolescence in the etiology of schizophrenia (two hit model). This suggests that schizophrenia is the culmination of these developmental risk factors and other multi-dimensional, environmental insults (Cadenhead, 2002). Such multi-hit, transactional models may also partly explain the relationship between low measured levels of intelligence and other mental disorders (Sovner, 1986; Skuster et al, 1993; Barnhill 2003).

Many additional issues complicate diagnosis in ID children with mental illness. Firstly there is considerable phenomenological and biological heterogeneity found among individuals with most psychiatric disorders (Judd et al, 2002; Maser, 2002; Perugi et al, 2002; Barnhill 2003). Using schizophrenia as an example, there are subtypes (early onset, paranoid, disorganized, etc) as well as a spectrum of severity that can include some personality disorders (subsyndromal disorders) and childhood disorders that are probable prodromal conditions for adult onset syndromes (Ratey et al 1996; Skuster et al, 1992; Ursano et al 2008).

Our incomplete understanding also applies to some mood and anxiety disorders, especially the relationship between mood instability, impulsivity and bipolar disorder (Boyce et al 1992; Perugi et al, 2002; Rapee, 2002). For example many children with attention deficit hyperactivity disorder persist in modified form into adulthood, while others morph into mood and anxiety, antisocial personality or substance dependency disorders (Ursano et al 2008). Unfortunately we do not fully understand the forces that lead to the progression of these prodromal phenotypes and subsyndromal disorders towards the expression on the full syndrome (Modavsky et al, 2001; Cloninger, 1998; Cadenhead, 2002; Wilemsen-Swinkels et al, 2002; Perugi et al, 2002). The complex interaction between level of ID and this progression or metamorphoses requires ongoing attention and research (Rapee, 2002).

This form of developmental heterogeneity also contaminates existing diagnostic criteria, especially when similar symptoms appear in different diagnostic categories. For example, the relationship between attention deficit hyperactivity disorder and prepubertal bipolar disorders can be problematic since both disorders share similar symptoms during development. The problem is more confusing for children with severe-profound ID (Perugi et al, 2002; Ursano et al 2008). Some of this uncertainty arises from problems defining the boundary between psychiatric and neurologically based (organic) disorders (Hurley, 1996; Skuster et al 1992; Ratey et al 1996; Barnhill 2003).

Lastly, the boundary between behavioral phenotype and developmental psychiatric disorders is less certain (Chess et al 1984; La Malfa et al 1997; Modavsky et al 2001). Part of our current dilemma is due to our limited understanding of the developmental trajectories of behavioral phenotypes and what factors may push development in the direction of psychopathology. Resolving these issues may eventually force clinicians to think dimensionally rather than categorically; shift focus to sophisticated genetic analysis and endophenotyping, or both (Barnhill, 2003).

DM-ID AND CHILDREN

The DM-ID culminates an attempt to modify diagnostic criteria for children with ID. Reviewing the criteria it remains abundantly clear that the DM-ID has a better evidence base for children mild/moderate ID than severe-profound ID. The most likely cause of this discrepancy involves establishing appropriate boundaries between diagnostic categories and psychopathology resulting from an interaction between multiple genetic, temperamental, and psychosocial developmental influences (Fletcher et al, 2007). Several neuro-genetic disorders have associated behavioral phenotypes that may resemble subsyndromal forms of primary psychiatric disorders (Royal College of Psychiatrists, 2001; Barnhill, 2003; Hurley et al, 2007). In many clinical situations a solution requires the extrapolation of data from retrospective studies of adult patients. Retrospectively are useful, especially when there is evidence vulnerability factors (positive family history), secondary insults (puberty or mild head trauma) and prodromal symptoms (Lewis, 1992; Skuster et al, 1992; Ratey et al, 1996; Barnhill, 2003). But we also need prospective studies in order to understand the developmental trajectory of these syndromes and determine how protective and vulnerability factors play out. In short, we need more data on the developmental course of children with ID who are at risk for major psychiatric disorders.

We continue to face challenges integrating neurobiological data, molecular genetics and behavioral pharmacology with data from functional behavioral analysis (Barnhill, 2003; Harris, 2006). In general behavioral data includes quantitative measures of nonspecific challenging behaviors and less emphasis on the role played by genetic or neuropsychiatric disorders. These factors influence the sensitivity, intensity and patterns of responding to antecedent conditions ; typology or topography of target behaviors; responses to reinforcement and/or desensitization to associative conditioning (Sturmey et al, 2004; Gardner et al, 2004; Bostic et al, 2006). Expanding our models to include these observations requires stepping beyond the usual concept of baseline exaggeration (Sovner, 1986; Judd et al, 2002). For example the baseline exaggeration of aggression during an episode of depression may need to include affective state, sensitivity to new environmental cues, efficacy of differential reinforcement strategies as well as the typology of aggressive behavior (Gardner et al 2004; Sturmey, 2004).

Addressing these issues adds not only complexity to the diagnostic process; it forces clinicians to reconsider etiology in the process of differential diagnosis. Etiological subtype analysis (endophenotypes) becomes more relevant because children with severe ID bring an additional burden of metabolic insults, treatment refractory seizure disorders, and both structural and developmental brain dysfunction to the table (Barnhill, 2003; Harris, 2006). Because children with severe-profound ID also display greater sensitivity to adverse environmental factors, excessive reliance on categorical-descriptive and even multi-axial nomenclatures may fail to capture subtle differences in phenomenology, clinical course and treatment response (Royal College of Psychiatrists, 2001; Kim-Cohen, 2007).

CONCLUSION

It is apparent that psychiatric diagnosis remains within the art of hypothesis testing and that we should continue to exercise caution when using categorical diagnostic criteria to diagnoses psychiatric disorders in ID children with mental illness (Fletcher et al, in press). We continue to face problems with competing heterogeneities while working and a paucity of research into the diagnosis of psychiatric disorders in children with severe-profound ID (Barnhill, 2003; Harris, 2006). As a result the DM-ID remains a work in progress and subject to future revision, especially balancing a categorical descriptive model with one that includes the wealth of data from the neurosciences regarding genetic risk and vulnerability factors (etiology). In the meantime these issues remain (Fletcher et al, in press):

1. The field-testing and validation of the DM-ID must move beyond a consensus-based model towards one based on statistical analysis and validation studies of the criteria modifications.

2. We must expand our sparse evidenced based literature for children with severe-profound ID. To be successful need to integrate data about endophenotypes, developmental aspects of behavioral phenotypes, subsyndromal and spectrum disorders and molecular neurosciences. This synthesis might move us beyond current categorical diagnoses towards subtyping syndromes etiologically. This shift may result in a shift towards a greater use of dimensional approaches to classification (Fletcher et al, in press).

3. The DM-ID retains the multi-axial format but we may need to revise our current Axes IV and V. We may need to shift emphasis to formulation and synthesis that includes attempts to define the relationship between adaptation and psychosocial stressors and data from functional behavioral analysis and biological research (Barnhill, 2003).

REFERENCES

American Psychiatric Association. *Diagnostic and Statistical Manual of Mental Disorders, Fourth Edition, Revised*. Washington, DC: American Psychiatric Association, 1994.

Barnhill J (2003) Can the DSM-IV-TR Be Salvaged for Individuals with Severe Intellectual Disability. *Mental Health Aspects Developmental Disorders*, 6, 85-98.

Bostic JQ, Rho Y (2006). Target Symptom Psychopharmacology: Between the Forest and the Trees, *Child Adol Psychiatric Clin of North America,* 15, 289-302

Boyce WT, Barr RG, Zeltzer LK (1992). Temperament and psychobiology of childhood stress. *Pediatrics,* 90, 483-486.

Cadenhead KS (2002). Vulnerability markers in the schizophrenia spectrum: Implications for phenomenology, genetics, and the identification of the schizophrenia prodrome. *Psychiatric Clin North America,* 25, 837-853.

Chess S, Thomas A. *Origins and Evolution of Behavior Disorders: From Infancy to Early Adult Life*. New York, NY: Brunner-Mazel, 1984.

Cloninger CR, Svrakic DM, Przybeck TR (1993). A psychobiological model of temperament and character. *Arch Gen Psychiatry,* 50, 975-990.

Cloninger CR. The genetics and psychobiology of the seven-factor model of personality. In: Silk KR (Ed), *Biology of Personality Disorders.* Washington, DC: American Psychiatric Press Inc, 1998, p63-67.

Fletcher RL, Havercamp, S, Ruedrich S, Benson B, Barnhill LJ, Cooper SA, Stavralakaki C (in press) Field Study of the Clinical Usefulness of a Diagnostic Manual for Mental Disorders in Persons with Intellectual Disability. *J Clin Psychiatry*.

Fletcher R, Loeschen E, Stavralakaki C, First M. *Diagnostic Manual: Intellectual Disabilities*. Kinston NY: NADD Press, 2007.

Gardner WI, Griffiths DM. Treatment of Aggression and Related Disruptive Behaviors in Persons with Intellectual Disabilities and Mental Health Issues. In Matson, JL, Land RB, Matson ML (Eds) *Behavioral Modification for Persons with Developmental Disabilities*. Baton Rouge, LSU Press, 2004, 279-308.

Giedd JN. Normal development (1997). *Child Adol Psychiatric Clin N Am*. 6, 265-282.

Harris J. Emotional expression and regulation. In: Harris JC (Ed), *Developmental Neuropsychiatry: Assessment, Diagnosis & Treatment of Developmental Disorders*. New York, NY: Oxford University Press, Inc., 1995, 203-218.

Harris J. *Intellectual Disability: Understanding its Development, Cause Classification Education and Treatment*. New York, Oxford University Press, 2006.

Hurley AD, Levitas A, Lecavalier L, Kates WK. Assessment and Diagnostic Procedures. In Fletcher R, Loeschen E, Stavralakaki C, First M (eds) the *Diagnostic Manual-Intellectual Disability*, Kingston, NADD Press, 2007, pp9-24.

Judd LL, Schettler PJ, Akiskal HS (2002). The prevalence, clinical relevance, and public health significance of subthreshold depressions. *Psychiatr Clin North Am*. 25, 685-698.

Kim-Cohen J (2007). Resilience and Developmental Psychopathology. *Child Adol Psychiatric Clin North America*, 16, p271-84

La Malfa G, Campigli M, Bertelli M, et al (1997). The psychopathological model of mental retardation: Theoretical and therapeutic considerations. *Research Dev Disability*, 18, 407-413.

Lewis M (1992). Individual differences in response to stress. *Pediatrics*, 90, 487-490.

Maser JD, Patterson T (2002). Spectrum and nosology: Implications for the DSM-V. *Psychiatr Clin North Am*. 25, 855-885.

Moldavsky M, Lev D, Lerman-Sagie T (2001). Behavioral phenotypes of genetic syndromes: A reference guide for psychiatrists *J Am Acad Child Adolescent Psychiatry*, 40, 749-761.

Othmer E, Othmer JP, Othmer SC (1998). Brain Functions and Psychiatric Disorders. A Clinical Review. *Psychiatric Clinical North Am*. 21, 517-566.

Perugi G, Akiskal HS (2002). The soft bipolar spectrum redefined: Focus on cyclothymic, anxious-sensitive, impulse-dyscontrol, and binge-eating connection in bipolar II and related conditions. *Psychiatr Clin North Am*. 25, 713-737.

Pulsifer MB (1996). The Nneuropsychology of mental retardation. *J International Neuropsychol Soc*. 2, 59-176.

Rapee RM (2002). The development and modification of temperamental risk for anxiety disorders: Prevention of a lifetime of anxiety? *Biol Psychiatry*, 52, 947-957.

Ratey JJ, Dynek MP. Neuropsychiatry of mental retardation and cerebral palsy. In: Fogel BS, Schaffer RB, Rao SM (Eds), *Neuropsychiatry: A Comprehensive Textbook*, 1996. Baltimore: Williams and Wilkins, pp549-569.

Skuster DZ, Digre KB, Corbett JJ (1992). Neurologic conditions presenting as psychiatric disorders. *Psychiatric Clin North Am*. 5, 311-333.

Sovner R (1986). Limiting factors in the use of the DSM-III criteria with mentally ill/mentally retarded persons. *Psychopharmacol Bull*. 22, 1055-1059.

Sturmey P, Bernstein H. Functional Analysis of Maladaptive Behaviors. In Matson, JL, Land RB, Matson ML (Eds) *Behavioral Modification for Persons with Developmental Disabilities*. Baton Rouge, LSU Press, 2004, 101-29.

Royal College of Psychiatrists: DC-LD (Diagnostic Criteria of Psychiatric Disorders for Use in Adults with Learning Disabilities/Mental Retardation). Occasional Paper (OP) 48. London: Gaskell 2001.

Ursano Am, Katheiser PM, Barnhill LJ. Disorders Usually Appearing in Infancy, Childhood and Adolescence. In Hales RM, Yudovsky SE, Gabbard GO (Eds), Textbook of Psychiatry 5th Edition 2008, Washington: American Psychiatric Association Press, pp 861-920.

Willemsen-Swinkels SH, Buitelaar JK (2002). The autistic spectrum: Subgroups, boundaries, and treatment. *Psychiatric Clin North Am.* 25, 811-836.

Chapter 3

EARLY ONSET PSYCHOSIS IN YOUTH WITH INTELLECTUAL DISABILITIES

R. Friedlander[1], J. Klancnik[1] and T. Donnelly[2]
[1] BC Childrens Hospital, Vancouver, B.C. Canada.
[2] Douglas College Coquitlam, B.C. Canada

INTRODUCTION

Individuals with intellectual disabilities (ID) may be more susceptible to psychotic illness (Bouras et al, 2004). There are, however, only a limited number of reports on the presentation and course of psychosis in adults with ID (Clarke, 1999; Fraser & Nolan, 1994; Reid, 1972). Less still is known about individuals with ID who develop psychosis in childhood and adolescence, so called "Early Onset Psychosis (EOP)". Approximately 20% of those with EOP, have been reported to have an IQ <80 (Werry et al, 1994; McClellan & McCurry, 1999), ID is often used as an exclusion criterion in research (Gordon et al, 1994; McKenna et al, 1994; Russell, 1994). There is, therefore, few published research studies of individuals with both ID and EOP.

Although current research indicates that schizophrenia can be reliably diagnosed in adults with mild ID (Meadows et al, 1991; Reid, 1989), verbal limitations in those with more severe ID make diagnosis much more difficult (Clarke, 1999; Reid, 1989; Tyrer & Dunstan, 1997), and clinicians have been therefore advised to be particularly cautious in diagnosing schizophrenia or other psychotic illnesses in the presence of ID (Feinstein & Reiss, 1996). Psychosis may be difficult to differentiate from imaginatory worlds of childhood extending past expected age; the significance of fixed and unusual beliefs may be difficult to clarify in youth with developmental delays and hallucinations may be challenging to accurately elicit and differentiate from self talk and dissociative phenomena. Even in the non-ID population, the diagnosis of EOP may be confused with other conditions (McClellan et al, 1999; McClellan & Werry, 2001; Thomsen, 1996).

In our earlier studies (Lee et al, 2003; Friedlander & Donnelly, 2004), we developed a protocol for consensual diagnosis of EOP in ID, based on multidisciplinary assessment, extensive review and follow-up. In the first publication (Lee et al, 2003) we demostrated that it is possible to make reliable diagnoses of schizophrenia in youth with ID and that the symptoms remained stable over a 2 year period. In the subsequent paper (Friedlander & Donnelly, 2004), we described characteristics of youth with ID, presenting with a broader spectrum of apparent psychosis, not just schizophrenia (Friedlander & Donnelly, 2004).

METHODOLOGY

In this chapter we present data collected on 51 individuals with ID with presentation of apparent psychotic symptoms prior to age 19 years. The individuals are from our cohort of patients seen by the Developmental Disability Mental Health Service, a specialized multidisciplinary team serving individuals with both ID and mental illness in the Lower Mainland of British Columbia, a population of two and a half million people.

FINDINGS

The patients fell into 4 broad diagnostic groups: schizophrenia or schizoaffective disorder (52.9%); Mood Disorder with Psychotic features (17.6%); Psychosis NOS (Not otherwise specified),(17.6%); Non psychotic (11.8%).

The average age of onset of active psychotic symptoms was 14.7 years for the shcizophrenic/ schizoaffective group (SZ/SA), 14.5 years for the mood disorder patients and 13.5 years for the Psychosis NOS group.

The average age of onset of the psychotic symptoms in all groups was strikingly young, considering that psychotic disorders are considered rare before the age of 14 years (Thomsen, 1996). The duration of untreated psychotic symptoms (DUP) is considered an independent marker of prognosis, with DUP of under 3 months associated with a better prognosis (Harris et al, 2005).

In our study, the DUP was 5 months for the SZ/SA group, 7 months for the Mood Disorder group and 1 month for the Psychosis NOS group. The DUP in our cohort was longer than 3 months (except in the Psychosis NOS group), which indicated that the need for earlier identification and intervention of psychosis in this population.

CONCLUSION

Clinically, it can be very difficult deciding whether the psychotic symptoms are real or not. This could lead to delay in diagnosis and treatment, because families are naturally reluctant to deal with the implications and risks of antipsychotic medications, in the absence of a defintive diagnosis.

The Early Psychosis Intervention Model developed in Australia, however, provides a framework for support and intervention for high risk youth, when the diagnosis is still evolving and unclear (McGorry et al, 2007). This makes sense as we found our families were more open to benign supportive interventions such as psychoeducation and stress management, in the earlier stages of the disorder.

REFERENCES

Bouras, N., Martin, G., Leese, M., et al. Schizophrenia-spectrum psychoses in people with and without intellectual disabilitiies, *Journal of Intellectual Disability Research,* 2004; 48:548-555.

Clarke D. Functional psychoses in people with mental retardation. In Psychotic and Behavioral Disorders in Developmental Disabilities and Mental retardation. (ed. N. Bouras). 1999; Cambridge:Cambridge University Press.

Feinstein C. and Reiss A.L. Psychiatric disorders in mentally retarded children and adolescents. The challenges of meaningful diagnosis. In: Child and Adolescent Psychiatric Clinics of North America. (ed. F. Volkmar). 1996: 827 - 852. Philadelphia: W. B. Saunders.

Fraser W., Nolan M. Psychiatric disorders in mental retardation. In Mental health in mental retardation. (ed. N. Bouras). 1994; 79 - 92. Cambridge: Cambridge University Press.

Friedlander, R, and Donnelly, T. Early onset psychosis in youth with intellectual disability. *Journal of Intellectual Disability Research,* 2004; 48:540-547.

Gordon C.T., Frazier J.A., McKenna K. et al. Childhood-onset schizophrenia : an NIMH study in progress. *Schizophrenia Bulletin,* 1994; 20: 697 - 712.

Harris MG, Henry LP, Harrigan SM et al. The relationships between duration of untreated psychosis and outcome: an eight year prosepective study. *Schizophrenia Res.* 2005;79 (1): 85-93.

Hurley A.D.The misdiagnosis of hallucinations and delusions in persons with mental retardation : A neurodevelopmental perspective. *Seminars in Clinical Neuropsychiatry,* 1996; 12: 122 - 133.

Lee P., Moss S., Friedlander R. et al. Early onset schizophrenia in children with mental retardation : diagnostic reliability and stability of clinical features. *Journal of the American Academy of Child and Adolescent Psychiatry,* 2003;42, 162-169.

McClellan J. McCurry C. (1999) Early onset psychotic disorders : Diagnostic stability and clinical characteristics. *European Child and Adolescent Psychiatry,* 1999; 8: 13 - 19.

McClellan J., McCurry C., Snell J.et al. Early onset psychotic disorders. Course and outcome over a 2 year period. *Journal of the American Academy of Child and Adolescent Psychiatry,* 1999; 38:1380 - 1388.

McClellan, J., Werry, J. Practice parameters for the assessment and treatment of children and adolescents with schizophrenia. *Journal of the American Academy of Child and Adolescent Psychiatry,* 2001; 40 (Supp.): 7.

McGorry PD, Killackey E, Yung AR. Early intervention in psychotic disorders: detection and treatment of the first episode and the critical early stages. *Med J Aust.* 2007; 87: S 8-10.

McKenna K., Gordon C.T., Lenane M. et al. Looking for childhood - onset of schizophrenia : the first 71 cases screened. *Journal of the American Academy of Child and Adolescent Psychiatry,* 1994; 33: 636 - 644.

Meadows G., Turner T., Campbell L.. et al. Assessing schizophrenia in adults with mental retardation. *British Journal of Psychiatry,* 1991;158 : 103 -105.

Reid A.H. Psychoses in adult mental defectives II : schizophrenia and paranoid psychoses. *British Journal of Psychiatry,* 1972; 120: 213 - 218.

Reid A.H. Schizophrenia in mental retardation : clinical features. *Research in Developmental Disabilities,* 1989; 10: 241 - 249.

Russell A.T. The clinical presentation of childhood-onset schizophrenia. *Schizophrenia Bulletin,* 1994; 20: 631 - 46.

Thomsen P.H. Schizophrenia with childhood and adolescent onset : a nationwide register based study. *Acta Psychiatr Scan.* 1996; 94:187 - 193.

Tyrer S.P., Dunstan J.A. Schizophrenia in those with learning disability. In : Psychiatry in learning disability. (ed. S. G. Read). 1997; 185 - 215. London:W. B. Saunders.

Werry J.S., McClellan J.M., Andrews L.K. et al. Clinical features and outcome of child and adolescent schizophrenia. *Schizophrenia Bulletin,* 1994; 20: 619 - 30.

Chapter 4

PSYCHOPHARMACOTHERAPY IN ADULTS WITH INTELLECTUAL DISABILITIES – A REVIEW OVER A TEN YEAR PERIOD

T. Voss[1]., B. Schmidt[1], R. Grohmann[2]., C. Schade[1]., and A. Diefenbacher[1]

[1]Department of Psychiatry, Koenigin Elisabeth Herzbergeev. hospital, Berlin, Germany
[2]Department of Psychiatry, Ludwig-Maximilians University Munich, Germany

INTRODUCTION

People with intellectual disabilities (ID) show a 3 to 4 times higher prevalence to develop psychiatric disorders, according to a 2005 study of the WHO of about 22 %. A more recent study (Cooper et al, 2007) reported an even higher point prevalence of 40.9 % using clinical diagnostic criteria.

Due to the atypical presentation of psychiatric disorders in people with ID, their limited abilities of expressing their selves and understanding speech and the impaired competency of introspection in these patients, psychiatrists are faced with a variety of diagnostic difficulties and challenges. Gaedt (1997) highlighted the following problem fields in the care of people with ID:

1. Diagnostic uncertainty increases the risk of false diagnosis.
2. Diffuse or extended indication bears the risk of pharmacological off-label-use.
3. Developmental deficits are misinterpreted as psychiatric symptoms.
4. There is a high co-morbidity with epilepsy.
5. These patients show an increased vulnerability to psychoactive agents.
6. Therapy with psychoactive drugs leads to gain of weight.
7. Challenging behavior is a burden for carers.
8. Expectations of carers concerning the effect of psychoactive drugs may be irrational.

Despite the diagnostic uncertainty in mentally ill people with ID, physicians have to follow important rules of a reasonable pharmacotherapy, which found consensus in several international guidelines such as published by the German Society for Psychiatry, Psychotherapy and Nervous Diseases (DGPPN) in 2003:

1. Therapy with psychoactive drugs has to be carried out accordingly to a specific indication. A defined psychiatric disorder has to be diagnosed and categorized exactly.
2. Therapy of a psychiatric disorder has to be carried out with an approved drug.
3. Combination of two or more pharmacological agents increases the risk for interactions and adverse side effects and therefore should be avoided.

Nevertheless, polypharmacy has become a clinical reality for people with ID. Prescription of psychoactive drugs is often not based in science and not evaluated appropriately (Matson, 2000). Furthermore, the occurrence of desired and undesired pharmacological effects is not systematically observed or insufficiently recorded. (Meins et al, 1993; Deb and Fraser, 1994; Singh et al, 1997; Hässler, 1998; Matson et al, 2000; Hennicke, 2008).

This has been put in words as early as 1958, when Greiner stated in his thesis:

"In the years to come, the retarded may claim an all-time record of having the greatest variety and largest tonnage of chemical agents shovelled into them."

Since then only a few studies have been conducted to research and examine the prevalence of psychopharmacotherapy in people with ID (Hässler, 2007; Hennicke, 2008; Stolker et al, 2002; Spreat et.al, 2004; Singh, 1997; Matson, 2000; Robertson et al, 2000; Didden et al, 1997; Brylewski and Duggan, 2004).

All these papers refer to psychopharmacological treatment in residential settings for people with ID or long-term departments of psychiatric hospitals. However, to our knowledge there is no study that systematically analyzes prescription patterns of psychopharmacologic drugs to inpatients with ID and co-existing psychiatric disorders in a specialized tertiary care treatment center.

METHODOLOGY

Our specialized center for the treatment of adults with ID and psychiatric disorders is one of 30 providers of inpatient psychiatric care for people with ID in Germany and treats approximately 300 inpateints annually.

Due to the fact that pharmacotherapy of our patients is systematically monitored according to the European project of pharmacological vigilance (Arzneimittelsicherheit in der Psychiatrie, AMSP) since 1996, we intended to analyze clinical data obtained according to the standardized AMSP (Arzneimittelsicherheit in der Psychiatry) protocol (Grohmann et al. 2004) by clinically experienced and continually trained raters (medical doctors only) on regular observation dates from 319 patients over a period from 2003 and 2007 in the first place.

Table 1. Groups of Psychiatric Disorders

Category	Psychiatric Diagnosis (relating to ICD-10)
0	no psychiatric diagnosis
1	chapter F1, excl. withdrawal state with delirium, psychotic disorder and amnesic syndrome
2	Chapter F2, referred to as „psychosis", incl.: schizoaffective disorders, psychotic disorders due to substance use
3	Chapter F3: affective disorders with indication for antipsychotic treatment, incl.: mania, bipolar affective disorder, severe depressive episode with psychotic symptoms, recurrent depressive disorder, severe current episode with psychotic symptoms
4	Chapter F3: affective disorders without indication for antipsychotic treatment, incl.: unipolar and recurrent depressive episodes without psychotic symptoms, persistent affective disorders and Chapter F4
5	Chapter F6
6	Dementia
7	Chapter F84: Pervasive developmental disorders (referred to as "autism")
8	Chapter F9
9	Delirium

Table 2. Groups of Psychoactive Drugs

Group	Psychoactive drug
1 a	Atypical antipsychotics
1 b	Typical sedating antipsychotics
1 c	Typical high-potency antipsychotics
2	Antidepressants
3	Mood stabilizers excl. carbamazepine, valproic acid and lamotrigine when prescribed as anticonvulsants in co-morbidity with epilepsy
4	Benzodiazepines

In the second part of the study we modified the design and reviewed archived medical records, obtaining data of discharge summaries of all inpatients in the sample years 1997, 2002 and 2007 regarding age, sex, residence, length of stay, degree of ID, main psychiatric diagnosis and psychotropic medication at the date of dismissal.

The total size of the sample after data acquisition then was 491, including 23 inpatients in 1997, 182 in 2002 and 286 in 2007.

The psychiatric diagnoses were grouped into categories relating to the International Classification of Diseases ICD-10 (WHO, 1992) (see Table 1). All prescribed psychoactive drugs were categorized into groups (see Table 2).

RESULTS

Analysis of AMSP Data (2003 - 2007)

Overall frequency of prescribed psychoactive drugs: Besides risperidone (18.18%), our patients were treated most frequently with anxiolytic or sedating drugs such as diazepam (24.45%), melperone (17.55%) and pipamperone (15.36%). Regarding antipsychotics we prescribed typicals (84.99 %) more often than atypicals (67.77 %).

Concerning polypharmacy (Figure 1) almost half of our patients with ID and psychiatric disorders were treated with one drug only (48.35 %). In 51.65% polypharmacy was detected. However, the AMSP protocol doesn't distinguish between psychoactive and somatic medication as antihypertensive, antidiabetic agents or else.

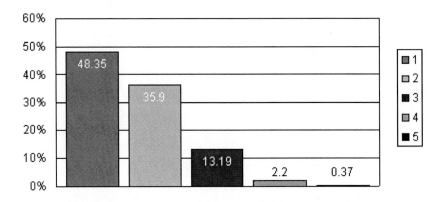

Figure 1. Number of drugs per patient (n=319).

Analysis of Data Obtained From Discharge Summaries (1997 - 2007)

There is a tendency that the average length of stay decreases in the course of the years from 56 days in 1997 to 28.3 days in 2007. Due to the small sample size in 1997 (N=23, versus N=286 in 2007) no significance could be calculated.

Figure 2 shows a significant increase in diagnosis of psychotic disorders in 2007 (44%) compared to 2002 (20.3%). This might be due to the establishment of a specialized outpatient clinic at our center with the opportunity to treat patients with mild or moderate degrees of problem behavior or psychiatric diseases and leaves inpatient treatment to the more severely ill patients. On the other hand overreporting in 2007 or underreporting in the years before has to be taken into consideration to explain this increase.

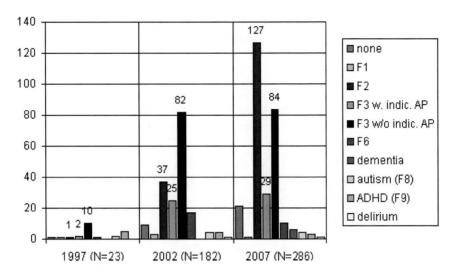

Figure 2. Diagnosis per year (count).

In 2007 personality disorders and affective disorders were diagnosed less than in 2002.

Regarding personality disorders, this might be due to a specific admission procedure to our psychotherapeutic program for inpatients with borderline personality disorder (Marsha Linehan`s dialectic behavioral therapy, adapted for patients with ID).

According to Tsiouris et al. (2003) challenging behaviors should not be considered as depressive equivalents in individuals with ID. This might be an explanation for the decreased diagnosing of affective disorders in 2007.

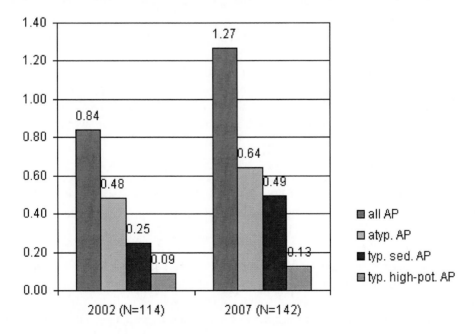

Figure 3. Antipsychotics per Patient.

In 2007 more atypical and sedating antipsychotics were prescribed (Figure 3). This results in an increased prescription of antipsychotics in general, whereas the use of typical high-potency antipsychotics doesn't differ between 2002 and 2007. This might be due to the increased number of psychotic disorders diagnosed in 2007.

In 1997 benzodiazepine medication was paramount (47.83%). The decrease of prescription of these drugs might be due to our efforts to avoid substance dependencies. This might also explain the increase in the prescription of sedating antipsychotics instead.

The re-increase in 2007 (10.84%) compared to 2002 (3.3%) could be a result of more frequent diagnosis of psychotic disorders, when anxiolytic therapy in acute psychotic episodes might be necessary.

Concerning the diagnostic group "affective disorders with indication for antipsychotic treatment" the same pattern of prescription as in the "psychosis" group was detected.

In the diagnostic group "affective disorders without indication for antipsychotic treatment" a greater amount of antipsychotic prescription, too, namely atypical antipsychotics as well as sedating antipsychotic agents was identified over the course of the years. Furthermore, patients in 2007 received less mood stabilizers.

DISCUSSION

This study reveals the fact that in a specialized tertiary care treatment center psychopharmacotherapy is still paramount. The hypotheses could not be proved that the number of prescribed psychoactive drugs decreases with the implementation and improvement of therapeutic strategies other than pharmacotherapy since 2002 (e.g. psychotherapy (including interpersonal psychotherapy), art, music, occupational and physical therapies) and with the systematic monitoring of severe adverse side effects (within the European project of pharmacovigilance, AMSP).

However, it is important to consider the establishment of the specialized outpatient clinic at our center in 2005 as a confounding variable.

We suggest that by this opportunity of an outpatient treatment for patients with mild and moderate degrees of problem behavior and mental disorder inpatient treatment is left to the more severely ill patients. Furthermore in this context it is necessary to emphasize that psychotic disorders have been diagnosed more often in 2007. In patients who are in an acute crisis or suffer from a severe mental illness psychopharmacological treatment often cannot be replaced.

Secondly, the possibility to continue treatment in the outpatient division of our center leads to a shorter length of stay and offers the possibility to dismiss patients with sedating antipsychotic medication, for example, which can be monitored, evaluated and reduced during continuing ambulant care. Thus, the average length of inpatient stay at our center could be reduced considerably from 56 days in 1997 to 28.3 days in 2007.

Although pharmacotherapy should be part of a multimodal approach to treatment (King, 2007) including psychotherapy comparatively few studies have been conducted to evaluate psychotherapeutic treatment options other than psychoeducation for patients with schizophrenia. Respectively, similar adaptations of existing psychotherapeutic strategies (as it has been achieved in the dialectical behavior therapy for borderline personality disorder) have to be implemented for these individuals, to meet the specific needs of people with ID and co-morbid psychosis.Eventually, a greater attention to diagnosis, outcome measures in clinical trials (King, 2007) and a constantly alert and critical attitude concerning prescription patterns of each physician worrying about people with ID has to be claimed.

REFERENCES

Brylewski J, Duggan L (2004): Antipsychotic medication for challenging behavior in people with learning disability. *Cochrane Database Syst Rev.* 3: CD000377

Cooper SA, Smiley E, Morrison J, Williamson A, Allan L (2007) Mental ill-health in adults with intellectual disabilities: prevalence and associated factors. *Br J Psychiatry,* 190: 27-35

Deutsche Gesellschaft für Psychiatrie, Psychotherapie und Nervenheilkunde (Ed., 2003): Praxisleitlinien in Psychiatrie und Psychotherapie; Band 6: Behandlungsleitlinie Psychopharmakotherapie. Darmstadt: Steinkopff.

Deb S, Fraser W (1994): The use of psychotropic medication in people with learning disability: towards rational prescribing. *Human Psychopharmacology*; 9: 259-272.

Didden R, Duker PC, Korzilius H (1997): Meta-analytic study on treatment effectiveness for problem behaviors with individuals who have mental retardation. *Am J Ment Retard.* 1997; 101(4): 387-99.

Gaedt C (1997): Psychopharmakotherapie bei Menschen mit geistiger Behinderung. In: Dosen A: Psychische Störungen bei geistig behinderten Menschen. Stuttgart, Jena, Lübeck, Ulm: G. Fischer; 287-333.

Greiner T (1958): Problems of methodology in research with drugs. *Am J Ment Deficiency*; 64: 346-352.

Grohmann R, Engel RR, Rüther E, Hippius H. (2004): The AMSP drug safety program: methods and global results. *Pharmacopsychiatry*; 37 Suppl 1: 4-11.

Hässler F (1998): Psychopharmakotherapie bei geistig Behinderten. *Psychopharmakotherapie,* 5: 76-80.

Hässler F, Fegert JM. (1999): [Psychopharmacological therapy of self-injurious behavior in mentally retarded individuals] *Nervenarzt.*; 70(11): 1025-8.

Hässler F (2007): [Diagnosis and treatment of localized developmental disturbances.] *MMW Fortschr Med.* 22; 149(47): 29-32.

Hennicke K (2008): Psychopharmaka in Wohnstätten der Behindertenhilfe. Vermutungen über eine zunehmend unerträgliche Situation. In: Hennicke K (Ed.) Psychopharmaka in der Behindertenhilfe – Fluch oder Segen? Dokumentation der Arbeitstagung der DGSGB, Kassel, 09. November 2007. Materialien der DGSGB, Band 17, Berlin 2008; 4-22

King B (2007): Psychopharmakology in intellectual disabilities. In: Bouras N, Holt G (eds., 2007): Psychiatric and Behavioral Disorders in Intellectual and Developmental Disabilities. Cambridge University Press. 17: 310-29.

Matson JL et al. (2000): Psychopharmacology and mental retardation: A 10 year review (1990-1999). *Research in Developmental Disabilities*; 21: 263-296.

Meins W, Auwetter J, Krausz M, Turnier Y (1993) Behandlung mit Psychopharmaka in unterschiedlichen Einrichtungen für geistig Behinderte. *Nervenarzt*; 64: 451-455.

Robertson J et al. (2000): Receipt of psychotropic medication by people with intellectual disability in residential settings. *J Intellect Disabil Res.*; 44(6): 666-76.

Singh NN, Ellis CR, Wechsler H (1997) Psychopharmacoepidemiology of Mental retardation: 1966 to 1995. *Journal of Child and adolescent psychopharmacology,* (Vol. 7); 4: 255-266.

Spreat S, Conroy JW, Fullerton A. (2004): Statewide longitudinal survey of psychotropic medication use for persons with mental retardation: 1994 to 2000. Am J Ment Retard.; 109(4): 322-31.

Stolker JJ et al. (2002): Psychotropic drug use in intellectually disabled group-home residents with behavioral problems. *Pharmacopsychiatry*; 35(1): 19-23.

Tsiouris JA, Mann R, Patti PJ, Sturmey P (2003): Challenging behaviors should not be considered as depressive equivalents in individuals with intellectual disability. *J Intellect Disabil Res.*; 47(1): 14-21.

World Health Organisation (1992). The ICD-10 Classification of Mental and Behavioral Disorders. *Clinical Descriptions and Diagnostic Guidelines*. Geneva: WHO.

Chapter 5

PREMENSTRUAL SYNDROME IN WOMEN WITH DOWN SYNDROME

L. Mason

Faculty of Health and Applied social Science,
Liverpool John Moores University, Liverpool, UK

INTRODUCTION

Premenstrual Syndrome (PMS) is defined as 'the cyclical occurrence or exacerbation of physical and / or behavioral symptoms that peak shortly before menses and then remit or lessen with the onset of menses (ACOG, 1995). Diagnosis is made on the degree of change in symptomatology between the luteal and follicular phase of the menstrual cycle. It also requires only a history of a single physical or mood symptom occurring cyclically. There are 150 symptoms described in the literature, classified under affective, cognitive, pain, neurovegetative, autonomic, CNS, electrolyte, dermatological and behavioral. The most commonly reported are fatigue, irritability, abdominal bloating, breast tenderness and labile mood.

Pre-menstrual syndrome has been reported to be associated with a number of interrelated factors. These include age, parity, biochemistry, psychopathology, lifestyle and menstrual characteristics. Women with Down syndrome (DS) differ from typical women in some of these factors and we hypothesised that they may therefore be at higher risk of PMS.

Firstly, obesity is associated with problems in the menstrual cycle (Masho et al, 2005) and is common in DS (Shepperdson, 1992; Rubin et al, 1998). Secondly, an uninterrupted natural cycle is suggested as a risk factor for PMS (Warner and Bancroft, 1990), and since few women with DS become pregnant, they may be at increased risk. Thirdly, typical women with PMS have been found to have lower levels of serotonin at certain times of their menstrual cycle (Rapkin et al, 1987) whilst low levels of serotonin are a characteristic of DS (Seidl et al, 1999).

It is recognised that people with intellectual disabilities (ID) generally have unmet health needs, which are partly determined by communication difficulties in describing symptoms generally (Lennox and Kerr, 1997), and in particular 'indicating the existence or location of the pain' (Lennox et al, 1997). Indeed recognition of PMS may be a major problem for women who are unable to understand and articulate their physical or emotional discomfort. Such symptoms are often internally experienced with no objective visible signs and so make recognition of PMS by carers an added complication. (Rubinow & Roy-Byrne, 1984). We therefore also speculated that recognition of PMS may be difficult for women with ID and their carers and that this condition may largely go unrecognised.

METHODOLOGY

A daily checklist used to diagnose PMS with typical women, the Calendar of Premenstrual Experience (COPE) (Mortola et al, 1990) was adapted for use with the DS population. The COPE is a 22 item 4 point rating scale. Construct validity has been measured using the Beck Depression Inventory (Beck et al, 1961) and the Profile of Mood State (McNair et al, 1971), whilst Feuerstein and Shaw (2002) reported high internal consistency on the behavior subscale and moderate correlation with the physical scale. Whilst adaptation incorporated the same items, a simple explanation and illustration for each symptom and the use of a colour graded tick box marked whether each symptom was present 'yes a lot', 'yes a little' or 'no' were added. A double page was dedicated to each day of the month. Following its' validation in a sample of typically developed women, the Diary was completed by 52 women with DS/carers over a two monthly cycles. These participants were also invited to take part in an interview to discuss completing the Diary, and around menstruation in general. Forty two of these agreed to be interviewed, whilst a further six carers, who were unable to complete the diary wanted to share their past experiences of their daughters' menstruation and were also interviewed. Twelve interviews were carried out face to face in participants homes, 47 were telephonic interviews. Interview topics included menarche, menstruation, self care and then focused on PMS.

FINDINGS

Results from the interviews showed that whilst most carers were unable to give the precise age, they were able to estimate their daughters age of menarche to within 2 or 3 months. The youngest age was 9 years, which occurred in two cases, and the oldest was nearly 19 years. The average age was between 12 and 13 years, and mode was 13 years. A significant proportion had not been provided with any information to prepare for menarche and thus described the first period as a 'shock'. This included five mothers who were not prepared for their daughters to start their periods and expressed their surprise when it happened, assuming that girls with DS matured later compared with the typical population. Comparison of the range and average age at menarche was similar to that reported in previous studies of women with DS and also women in general (Morabia & Costanza, 1998; Nakamoto, 2000).

Data from the Diary showed mean length of menses was 4.9 days, with a mode of 5 and mean cycle length of 27.7 days, which was consistent with the few studies undertaken in women with DS (Goldstein, 1988; Scola and Pueschel, 1992) and similar to the typical population. Taken together they provide evidence that women with DS might have a menstrual cycle of similar pattern to typically developed women (Fehring et al, 2006). Caution is needed however, as data were not collected in our study from women who were not menstruating or possibly not menstruating regularly. We suspect that some of the women may have had amenorrhoea, whilst others informed us that they were using Depo-Provera to reduce or halt their menstrual period and thus would not be suitable for inclusion in our study.

DISCUSSION

Speculation that women with DS might be at higher risk for PMS was not confirmed in our study, with PMS diagnosed, according to the Diary, in just 18-20% of our population. However, rather interestingly, 54% of mothers thought their daughter had or probably had PMS. The symptoms women and mothers usually identified as PMS were lethargy, tearfulness or mood swings, but also included spots, lack of concentration, incontinence, constipation or diarrhoea, breast swelling and tenderness, aggression, and food cravings.

In order to assess whether any specific symptoms were more prevalent in women with DS and whether the patterns over the cycle might vary when compared to typical women, a comparison of the patterns of the typical women (from the validation exercise) and those of women with DS was undertaken. However, symptom occurrence and symptom pattern were similar i.e. around half of each sample had few if any symptoms across the month, whilst the remainder had numerous symptoms throughout the month in no particular pattern. We also looked specifically at reporting frequency of "feeling bloated", which is one of the most common symptoms and one we felt might be difficult to articulate and thus could be under represented in the DS population. However the frequency was very similar for both the typical women with whom we validated our diary, and those with DS

Due to the high discrepancy between actual prevalence of PMS, according to the Diary and perceptions of its' occurrence we wondered whether any behaviors, especially emotional ones, that the carer cannot account for in any other way might have been labelled as a symptom of PMS. This is less likely to occur in the general population if the women themselves are able to tie in their symptoms with their approaching period. However, we found that most women with DS were, according to their mothers, unable to do this (Mason and Cunningham, 2007). Our data would support this hypothesis. One woman in our study had a very clear pattern whereby she developed acne pre-menstrually every month and which remitted with the onset of her period. Her mother did not consider that this might be PMS. In contrast, a woman with mood swings who was irritable and tearful was deemed as premenstrual even though her symptoms did not occur during the luteal phase. Indeed, a general pattern was observed by which symptoms such as irritability, mood swings and crying often led the mothers to label their daughters as premenstrual, irrespective of when they occurred in relation to the menstrual cycle. It is likely that may be partly due to lay perceptions of PMS, largely shaped by the media, that focus only on the emotional symptoms rather than the physical (Parsons, 2004).

Despite the high proportion of mothers believing that their daughters may have PMS, treatment was rarely sought for this condition. Indeed just 4 instances were described where advice had been sought, treatment had been given in 3 of these, and in two was deemed to be particularly successful. When asked why help had not been sought, it seemed that it just hadn't occurred to the mothers to do so. When prompted further there seemed to be 3 main reasons for inaction; the symptoms were not that bad, it was seen as being 'just one of those things', or it was something that the mothers themselves had had to put up with, the implication being that their daughters should do the same.

CONCLUSION

From the study findings demonstrate that many women with DS begin menstruating at a similar age to the typical population, and also have a similar menstrual cycle (although we acknowledge that our results must be treated with some caution). The hypotheses that PMS would be higher or go unrecognised in women with DS was not supported by our findings. The overestimation of PMS in our population may be due to lay perceptions of PMS, and compounded by the inability of women with DS to link any symptoms to the timing of their menstrual cycle. Whilst treatment was rarely sought for this condition, reasons for this were not compelling, yet it is possible that it could be effective in alleviating symptoms.

REFERENCES

ACOG. (1995) Premenstrual Syndrome (ACOG Committee Opinion). *International Journal of Gynecology and Obstetrics* 50, 80-84.

Beck AT., Ward CH., Mendelson M., Mock J. & Erbaugh J. (1961) An inventory for measuring depression. *Archives of General Psychiatry, 4*, 561-571.

Fehring RJ., Schneider M. & Raviele K. (2006) Variability in the phases of the menstrual cycle. *Journal of Obstetric Gynecologic and Neonatal Nursing, 35*, 376-384.

Feuerstein M. & Shaw WS. (2002) Measurement properties of the calendar of premenstrual experience in patients with premenstrual syndrome. *Journal of Reproductive Medicine, 47*, 279-289.

Goldstein H. (1988) Menarche, menstruation, sexual relations and contraception of adolescent females with Down syndrome. *European Journal of Obstetric, Gynecological and Reproductive Biology, 27*, 343-349.

Lennox NG., Cook A. & Diggerns JN (1997) Caring for adults with intellectual disabilities. *Modern Medicine of Australia, 3*, 79-87.

Lennox NG. & Kerr M P. (1997) Primary health care and people with an intellectual disability: the evidence base. *Journal of Intellectual Disability Research, 41*, 365-372.

Masho SW., Adera T. & South-Paul J. (2005) Obesity as a risk factor for premenstrual syndrome. *Journal of Psychosomatic Obstetrics and Gynaecology, 26*, 33-39.

Mason L. & Cunningham CC. (2007) *PMS in Women With Down Syndrome*. Final Report. Liverpool John Moores University, Liverpool.

McNair DM., Lorr M & Droppleman LF. (1971) *Profile of Mood States Manual*. Educational & Industrial Testing Service. San Diego, CA.

Morabia A. & Costanza MC. (1990) International variability in ages at menarche, first livebirth, and menopause. World Health Organization Collaborative Study of Neoplasia and Steroid Contraceptives. *American Journal of Epidemiology,* 148(12), 1195-1205.

Mortola JF., Girton L., Beck L. & Yen SSC. (1990) Diagnosis of premenstrual syndrome by a simple, prospective and reliable instrument: The calendar of premenstrual experiences. *Obstetrics and Gynecology,* 76, 302-307.

Nakamoto JM. (2000) Myths and variations in normal pubertal development. *Western Journal of Medicine,* 172(3), 182-185.

Parsons R. (2004) *The Portrayal of PMS on Television Sitcoms.* http://meowpower.org/archives/december04/ampioa3.html. Accessed 05/10/2005.

Rapkin AJ., Edelmuth E., Chang LC., Reading AE., McGuire MT. & Su TP. (1987) Whole-blood serotonin in premenstrual syndrome. *Obstetrics and Gynaecology,* 70, 533-537.

Rubin SS., Rimmer JH., Chicoine B., Braddock D & McGuire DE. (1998) Overweight prevalence in persons with Down syndrome. *Mental Retardation,* 36,1751-181.

Rubinow D. & Roy-Byrne P. (1984) Premenstrual syndromes: overview from methodological perspective. *American Journal of Psychiatry,* 141, 163-171.

Scola PS. & Pueschel SM. (1992) Menstrual cycles and basal body temperature curves in women with Down syndrome. *Obstetrics and Gynecology,* 78, 91-94.

Seidl R., Kaehler ST., Prast H., Singewald N., Cairns H., Gratzer M. & Lubec G. (1999) Serotonin in brains of adult patients with Down syndrome. *Journal of Neural Transmitters Suppl.* 57, 221-232.

Shepperdson B. (1992) *Growing Up With Down's Syndrome.* Cassell, London.

Warner P. & Bancroft J. (1990) Factors related to self-reporting of the pre-menstrual syndrome. *British Journal of Psychiatry,* 157, 249-260.

Chapter 6

WOMEN WITH AND WITHOUT INTELLECTUAL DISABILITIES AND PSYCHIATRIC DISORDERS: A COMPARISON OF THE LITERATURE

L. Taggart

Institute of Nursing Research, University of Ulster, N. Ireland

INTRODUCTION

This literature review compares and contrasts three key areas in women with and without intellectual disability (ID) focusing on: mental health conditions, the psych-social contextual background of how these conditions develop and the clinical presentation of these conditions. This chapter is based upon a more comprehensive review published previously (Taggart et al, 2008).

The World Health Organisation (WHO; 2000) has reported that mental ill health will double by the year 2020 and this will have important ramifications for women particularly, as they are more likely to develop mental health problems compared to men. Moreover, there is a strong body of evidence to show that people with ID are more likely to develop mental health problems compared to the non-ID population (Bouras & Holt, 2007). However, little is known about the mental health of women with ID.

WOMEN WITHOUT INTELLECTUAL DISABILITY AND PSYCHIATRIC DISORDERS

Women without ID have higher rates of depressive disorders, anxiety disorders, eating disorders, dementia, pre and peri-menstrual disorders, as well as borderline personality disorder (WHO, 2000). Although gender differences have not been reported for severe mental health illness (i.e. schizophrenia), disparities were found pertaining to clinical presentation. As women suffer from more mental ill-health compared to men, the WHO (2000) has argued that in addition to biological differences between the sexes, clinicians and researchers should also examine the woman's psycho-social/contextual world (i.e. poverty, juggling multiple roles, social isolation, restricted social support networks). It is the impact of these cumulative events that according to the WHO (2000) *'disempower'* and *'lower the self-esteem'* of these women thereby leading to mental health problems developing. In addition, women are also more likely to experience physical and sexual violence that also has been found to contribute to the development of mental ill health (Domestic Violence Data Source, 2005). Women present differently to men in accessing primary and mental healthcare settings, and they are more likely to be prescribed psychotropic medication, exhibit somatic symptoms, report suicidal behaviors and be hospitalised more compared to men.

Nevertheless, many women within mainstream psychiatry have reported being discriminated against as their specific gender needs have not been addressed (i.e. specific side-effects of psychotropic medication have not been examined during pregnancy, sexual victimisation within mixed hospital wards). As result, the WHO (2000) and the Dept of Health in England and Wales (Dept. of Health, 2002; 2003; 2006a,b) have highlighted the need for a gender-sensitive approach regarding the mental health care of women focusing upon risk factors, treatment/management and demonstrating examples of 'good practice'.

WOMEN WITH INTELLECTUAL DISABILITY AND PSYCHIATRIC DISORDERS

Little has been written regarding the mental health of women with ID, as historically women and also men with ID have been viewed as 'a *gendered, asexualised'* (Burns, 1993). Although there is growing evidence that people with ID are more likely to develop psychiatric disorders compared to the non-ID population (Bouras & Holt, 2007), prevalence rates between men and women with ID have rarely been explored.

Studies that have examined prevalence rates of depression, anxiety, dementia, severe mental illness (i.e. schizophrenia and bi-polar disorder), eating disorders and substance abuse among men and women with intellectual disabilities and these have been found to be contradictory. Disparities exists regarding staff reports versus self-reports, level of ID, sample, mental health inclusion/exclusion criterion and use of mainstream classification systems (i.e. DSM-4/ICD-10 versus DC-LD). Therefore, it is difficult to draw clear conclusions from these studies has to whether women with ID have higher rates of mental ill health compared to men with ID, and also with women without ID. More robust studies are required.

In attempting to understand the prevalence rates of these psychiatric disorders, the presentation also explored the psycho-social/ contextual background of how these women with ID developed these conditions. The authors purported that women with ID may be more likely to be disempowered and have lower levels of self-esteem compared to women without ID; factors that according to the WHO (2000) lead women to develop mental health problems. Women with ID not only experience the same psycho-social/contextual risk factors as women without ID (as above), but may also experience additional stressors as a result of having an ID (i.e. cognitive impairment, communication difficulties, limited coping strategies) (Lunsky, 2003l; James & Warner, 2005) (see Box 1). Alongside this, women with ID have also been reported to suffer from higher levels of physical and sexual violence compared to women without ID (Nosek et al., 1997, Sobsey, 2000, Sequeira et al., 2003) further affecting their self-esteem.

Box 1: Factors for women with Intellectual disability leading to 'disempowerment' and 'low self-esteem'

Physical conditions
Different genetic syndromes
Impairment of brain function
Severe and complex Epilepsy
Increased medical conditions (i.e. cardiovascular, cerebra-vascular and neurological problems)
Greater likelihood of being less active, having poorer nutrition and obese
Physical and sensory impairment
Increased use of antipsychotic medication

Intra Variables
Cognitive deficits
Poorer communication skills and comprehension
Limited social skills
Restricted coping styles
Poorer literacy and budgetary skills
Perceived lack of emotional support
Challenging Behaviors

Inter variables
Institutionalisation
Increased marginalisation
Stigma/labelling
Bullying
Being reinforced for passivity
Differing societal expectations
Lack of choice and meaning in one's life
No engagement in day to day activities
Less likely to be in a relationship/married/have children
More likely to live with their elderly parents
More likely to live in residential accommodation
Limited social support networks/friends
High levels of carer stress
More negative life events
Lack of talk therapies
Lack of accessible health information
Limited access to health screening
Not availing of healthcare services and exclusion from society

---

Adapted from Taggart, L., McMillan, R. & Lawson, R. (2008): Women with and without intellectual disability and psychiatric disorders: an examination of the literature. Journal of Intellectual Disabilities, 12(3), 191-211.

With regards to clinical presentation at primary, mental health and ID care settings little is known about how women differ from men with ID. More detailed research needs to be conducted into women and men with ID about their demographics, clinical presentation and treatment outcomes.

Few studies have examined the effects of gender in relation to ID services; in fact the authors have argued that ID services are gender-blind. The authors cite Clements et al. (2005) who indicated that this lack of gender awareness has even contributed to the development of challenging behaviors. One example that was highlighted involved women with ID residing in mixed residential units with men with ID, as well as male staff. As previously reported above a higher proportion of women with ID will have experienced physical and sexual violence, therefore some of these women may display challenging behavior as a means to escape from the emotional discomfort encountered by the distressed women. Despite the reports from the WHO (2000) and the Dept of Health (Dept. of Health, 2002, 2003, 2006a,b), they highlighted the need for gender sensitive psychiatric services: there is an absence within these mainstream reports and also the ID policies regarding the need for such services for women with ID. ('Valuing People' in (2001) England & Wales; 'The Same as You' (2001) in Scotland; 'Equal Lives' (2005) in Northern Ireland, and 'Vision for Change' (2006) in the Republic of Ireland).

CONCLUSION

The needs of women with ID have to be clearly visible at the center of each government's ID and also mainstream mental health strategies/policies. Likewise, appropriate funding and resources also need to be made available so services can be developed. A greater emphasis needs to be placed upon promoting the women's self-esteem and providing the opportunities for these women to be empowered.

Women with intellectual disabilities should be supported to use mainstream gender sensitive psychiatric service, this includes the development of single sex in-patient facilities as identified by the Dept. of Health (2002) for women without ID.

More evidence is required on the clinical conditions (i.e. prevalence/epidemiology, interplay of the biological, psychological and social causes), the contextual background (i.e. the factors that diminish, and also promote, self-esteem and empowerment) and clinical presentation (i.e how these women present themselves to primary healthcare, mainstream mental health and ID services). There is an also significant need for women with ID to be heard and that the meaning they ascribe to their lived experiences acted upon. Gender-sensitive psychiatric services are required for women with ID.

ACKNOWLEDGMENTS

We would like to acknowledge the commissioners of this review, Judith Trust, London.

REFERENCES

Bouras, N. & Holt, G. (Eds.) (2007). *Psychiatric and Behavioral disorders in development disabilities and mental retardation.* Cambridge: Cambridge University Press.

Burns, J. (1993) *Invisible women – women who have learning difficulties.* The Psychologist, 6th March, 102-105.

Clements, J., Clare I., & Ezelle, L. A. (2005) Real men, real women, real lives? Gender issues in learning disabilities and challenging behavior. *Disability & Society,* 10 (4), 425 – 435.

Department of Health (2002) Women's Mental Health: Into the Mainstream. *Dept of Health: HMSO, London.*

Department of Health (2003) Mainstreaming Gender and Women's Mental Health: Implementation Guidance. *HMSO, London.*

Department of Health (2006a) *Supporting women into the mainstream: Commissioning women-only community day services.* HMSO, London.

Department of Health (2006b) *The Mental Health of Women at Risk in the Criminal Care System.* HMSO, London.

Department of Health and Children (2006) Vision for Change. *Published by the Department of Health and Children, Dublin.*

Department of Health and Social Services & Public Safety (N. Ireland) (2005) Equal Lives: Review of policy and services for people with a learning disability in Northern Ireland. *Belfast: DHSSPS.*

Department of Health. (2001) *Valuing People: A new strategy for learning disability for the 21st century.* HMSO, London.

Domestic Violence Data Source (2005) *Family Violence Prevention Fund.* Department of Health: London.

James, M. & Warner, S. (2005) Coping with their lives - women, learning disabilities, self-harm and the secure unit: a Q-methodological study. *British Journal of Learning Disabilities,* 33, 120 – 127.

Lunsky, Y. (2003) Depressive symptoms in intellectual disability: does gender play a role? *Journal of Intellectual disability Research,* 47, (6), 417 – 427.

Nosek, M. A., Howland, & Young, M. E. (1997) Abuse of women with disabilities. *Policy implications. Journal of Disability Policy Studies,* 8, 157-175.

Scottish Executive (2001) *The same as you? A review of services for people with learning disabilities.* http://www.scotland.gov.uk

Sequeira, H., Howlin, P. & Hollins, S. (2003) Psychological disturbances associated with sexual abuse in people with learning disabilities. *British Journal of Psychiatry,* 183, 451-456.

Sobsey, D. (2000) Faces of violence against women with developmental disabilities. *Impact,* 13 (3), 2-3.

Taggart, L., McMillan, R. & Lawson, R. (2008): Women with and without intellectual disability and psychiatric disorders: an examination of the literature. *Journal of Intellectual Disabilities,* 12(3), 191-211.

World Health Organisation (2000) *Women's Mental Health: Evidence Based Review.* WHO: Geneva.

Chapter 7

STAFFS' KNOWLEDGE AND PERCEPTIONS OF WORKING WITH WOMEN WITH INTELLECTUAL DISABILITIES AND MENTAL HEALTH PROBLEMS

L. Taggart
Institute of Nursing Research, University of Ulster, N. Ireland

INTRODUCTION

There is strong empirical evidence to show that women without intellectual disabilities (ID) are more likely to develop mental health problems compared to men (WHO, 2000, 2007). These higher prevalence figures result not only from biological differences among the sexes, but also from a range of psycho-social experiences. These include: poverty, inequality, social isolation, restricted social support networks, juggling multiple roles, and physical and sexual violence. As an indirect consequence of these experiences, the WHO (2000, 2007) has argued that these events have lead women to be 'disempowered' and have 'low self-esteem', thereby leading to higher mental health rates.

People with ID are also more likely to develop mental health problems compared to the non-ID population (Bouras & Holt, 2007). However, little is known about the prevalence rates of mental health problems among men and women with ID, as those prevalence studies published contradict each other. Taggart et al (2008) argues that mental health prevalence rates among women with ID may be higher as not only these women will experience the same psycho-social events as women without ID, but also encounter greater levels of discrimination as a result of having an ID. Likewise, little is known about the cause of mental health problems in women with ID. The aim of this study was therefore to explore the possible risk factors that may lead, and resilient/protective factors that may protect, women with ID from developing a psychiatric disorder. This chapter is based upon a more comprehensive review published earlier (Taggart et al, 2008).

METHOD

A qualitative focus group methodology was used. Eight focus groups were conducted with a range of ID personnel (i.e. nurses, social workers, psychiatrists, psychologists, residential staff) across community, residential facilities and hospital settings throughout Northern Ireland. In total 32 professionals took part in the eight focus groups. The focus groups lasted approximately 60 minutes and were audiotaped. The focus groups were audiotaped and the transcriptions were subjected to a thematic content analysis using Newell & Burnard's (2006) framework.

The interview format was based upon a detailed literature review and followed a flexible structure. Questions were developed that focused upon the staffs' knowledge around the risk factors that may lead women with ID to develop mental health problems, and the resilient/protective factors that may protect women with ID from developing mental health problems. Ethical approval was obtained, written informed consent was sought and assurance of confidentiality was given.

FINDINGS

The findings are presented under the two main questions that were asked. Six risk factors were identified across the focus groups, it was observed that cumulatively these risk factors diminished the women's 'self-esteem' and 'disempowered' these women; these are.

Challenges of having both an ID and being female: Many of the staff reported that the women on their caseload knew they were different, being female and having an ID, leading to double disadvantage. The staff spoke of many of these women with ID being 'exploited', 'abused', 'stigmatised', made to feel 'different' and not 'fitting in' compared with their sisters, mothers, female staff and other women without an ID.

Unmet individual and societal expectations: Many of the staff across the focus groups highlighted that for many of the women with ID on their caseloads they felt they did not live up to 'individual and societal expectations' of what it means to be a woman. Not being married, not having a boyfriend / husband, not having children like their sisters, mothers and female staff, as result this comparison affected their self-esteem.

Dysfunctional family up-bringing: In all of the focus groups the staff reported stories of women with ID that grew up in 'dysfunctional families' and how this had affected the women's mental health later in adult life. This included parents who had mental health problems, parents with substance abuse problems, siblings and fathers who had physically assaulted and / or sexually abused these women as young girls.

Unstable relationships and loss of children: Some staff indicated that for those women with ID who were in a relationship / marriage and had children, if the relationship was unstable this could affect the women's mental health. Particularly if there were issues of domestic violence, substance abuse, and physical and sexual violence. In addition, some women with ID who had children had their children removed and caused further emotional distress and deterioration in the women's mental health.

Domestic violence: under-reported: A small number of the staff raised this issue and highlighted it was frequently 'under-reported'. Moreover, the staff highlighted the 'cyclical nature' of growing up within a culture of family violence and emotional mistreatment.

Negative life experiences: All the staff reiterated scenarios were many of these women with ID experienced an array of negative events, ranging from 'bereavement', 'lack of employment'/'structure', 'isolation'/'loneliness'/'lack of friends', 'substance abuse' and 'involvement with the courts'.

In terms of the protective/resilient factors, three main themes were identified by the staff, firstly being proactive in life by starting within 'families and school' thereby promoting emotional literacy skills, self-esteem and empowering these women to speak up for themselves. Secondly, many of the staff highlighted that women with ID should be supported to fully participate in their local communities in order to promote and maintain positive mental health, and improve their coping strategies and social skills. These included promoting broader friendship networks including personal relationships, and employment, educational and recreational opportunities. Thirdly, the majority of the staff identified the importance of 'early recognition of potential mental health problems/challenging behaviors'. This included employing screening tools and education of all staff regarding mental health promotion.

DISCUSSION

The findings of this study highlight that women with ID do experience the same psycho-social/contextual experiences as women without ID. Moreover, the staff across the focus groups have also highlighted the affect that these experiences have upon the women's self-esteem and subsequently their mental health. However, more detailed research is required to examine the relationship between self-esteem, and also disempowerment, in women with ID and how these intra variables mediate mental health.

Staff can be more proactive in the early recognition, assessment, treatment and long-term management of these risk factors (i.e. family/relationship/children issues, domestic violence, abuse, life events, structured environments, loneliness, and expectations). Likewise, staff can be involved in promoting opportunities for the women with ID to improve their self-esteem and empowerment (including choice, autonomy, friendships / relationships). There is also the potential for ID staff to develop inter-agency collaboration with mainstream women specific gender services (i.e. women only day centers/groups/therapy, women only wards, Nexus, Well Women Clinics, Women's AID).

Specific training is required for all front-line staff on women with ID and psychiatric disorders, knowing the risk as well as the protective factors. Training and education should also be offered to women with intellectual disability about these risk factors and support these women to develop health promoting behaviors/healthier lifestyles (i.e. weight management, physical health (pre-menstrual tension and menstruation), social support networks; develop relationships, being involved in education, employment and leisure opportunities). Women with intellectual disabilities should also be supported to use mainstream gender sensitive psychiatric services.

ACKNOWLEDGMENTS

We would like to acknowledge the commissioners of this review, Judith Trust, London.

REFERENCES

Bouras, N. & Holt, G. (Eds.) (2007). *Psychiatric and Behavioral disorders in development disabilities and mental retardation.* Cambridge: Cambridge University Press.

Newell R & Burnard P (2006) *Research for evidence-based practice.* Oxford: Blackwell.

Taggart. L, McMillan, R. & Lawson, A. (2008) Women with and without intellectual disability and psychiatric disorders: an examination of the literature. *Journal of Intellectual Disabilities,* 12 (3), 191-211.

World Health Organisation (2000) *Women's Mental Health: Evidence Based Review.* WHO: Geneva.

World Health Organisation (2007) Integrating Gender Analysis and Actions into the Work of the WHO. Geneva: World Health Organisation.

Chapter 8

FORENSIC PSYCHOTHERAPY AND PAEDOPHILIA IN INTELLECTUAL DISABILITIES

R. Curen

Respond, Stephenson Way, London. UK

FORENSIC PSYCHOTHERAPY AND LINKS WITH INTELLECTUAL DISABILITIES

Forensic psychotherapy can be broadly described as the psychodynamic treatment of violent offender patients. Forensic psychotherapy is conducted by psychologists, psychiatrists, psychotherapists and psychiatric nurses, in both the community and a range of secure settings. It is understood to be a treatment that uses the therapeutic relationship to consider offending behavior and then to modify that behavior. Attention to the transference and counter transference experienced in the consulting room is central to the treatment. A sound understanding of developmental theory and attachment theories are also essential when considering the aetiology of offending behaviors. Forensic psychotherapy is essentially an attempt to grapple with the core issues of aggression, perversion and hostility and their manifestation in behaviors inside and outside ofthe consulting room.

In the field of intellectual disabilities (ID) it is necessary to provide services for men and women who may have engaged in behaviors which put themselves and others at risk. These services have a broad spectrum ranging from what one might describe as 'sexually inappropriate' behavior - for example, masturbating in public - to rape. Paedphilia and those that rely on fetishistic enactments that might put themselves or others at risk, for instance auto-asphyxiation or frottage.

There are many psychoanalytic ideas that I have found helpful in developing our understanding of therapy and assessment with people with ID. Most notable are the theories of perversion developed first by Sigmund Freud (1905), then Edward Glover (1944) and elaborated on by Melvin Glasser (1996) and Estella Welldon (1988, 1996) and theories of delinquency developed by Donald Winnicott (1956) and David Campbell (1989).

Glasser's (1996) Core Complex has been an incredibly useful tool in advancing our understanding of patients with ID and paedophilic ideation. As I have said previously (2009)

Glasser indicates that the offender patient has two contradictory affects: one is aggression in response to a perceived threat and is concerned with survival. The other is an intense longing for complete merging or confluence with the object (object meaning a person or symbol of a person). However, since the object is invariably regarded as potentially engulfing, the patient fears that the loss of separate identity will inevitably follow. One possible reaction to this percieved threat is self-preservative aggression directed against the very object that is desired for intimacy and the gratification of their needs, security and containment. This poses diametrically opposed conflicts. The patient's solution to this is the use of sexualisation which converts aggression into sadism. The intention to destroy is then converted into a wish to injure and control. In this way the object is preserved and the possibiliity of the relationship is ensured, albeit in sado-masochistic terms.

Campbell (1989) has related Glasser's theory to adolescents and suggests that for them these double annihilation anxieties of engulfment and abandonment activate a self-preservative aggression - an aggression that attempts to destroy threats to physical or psychological survival. For the adolescent the threat to its survival and its mother are indistinguishable, hence the adolescent is in a bind as it cannot afford to destroy the object (mother) that threatens its survival as this is the same object on which it depends for survival.Glasser and Campbell agree that a way out of this bind exists in changing the aim of the aggression away from eliminating the mother and towards controlling her by sexualised aggression (sadism).

With these conpcepts in mind I'd like to discuss some of my work with a patient, whom I shall call Paul, who I have been seeing for 3 years:-

REFERRAL

In July 2003 Paul, who was 47 years old at the time, was initially referred by his Social Worker for a forensic risk assessment. The risk assessment report was completed and the following year Paul was referred for individual psychotherapy. Funding was agreed for 1 year with possible future funding available dependent on progress and funding being available.

PATIENT HISTORY

Paul is the youngest of 5 children. He has 3 sisters and 1 half sister. His mother was White British and his father of Afro-Carribean decent. He was placed in care at the age of 2 months. He has had no continuous contact with his family since childhood, although some occasional contact may have been preserved with family members during the early years of his time in care. The circumstances that originally brought Paul into care are uncertain. His mother is thought to have also had ID. His mother is now deceased and Paul has only recently been informed of this, although staff supporting him have known for many years. Paul has had no contact with his father. Recently Paul has been in contact with some of his sisters. His half sister is understood to have ID and Paul has no contact with her.

At the age of 2 months Paul was taken into a Nursery. He was soon transferred to Hospital because of 'frequent screaming bouts and lack of progress and developmental delays'. At 20 months he was transferred to another Nursery where a diagnosis of mental retardation was made and he was soon transferred to a hospital. He was often seen 'screaming and banging his head'. At 5 he attended an Educationally Sub Normal (ESN) school. He is said to have made good progress but 'unfortunately started to deteriorate when the house mother left. He started dropping things, was dribbling and chewed whatever he had in his hand.' At 13 he was sent to a secondary school but was found to be 'unsuitable'. He was also seen masturbating in public.

During his childhood Paul presented a number of disturbing behaviors with the diagnosis of 'Moderate ID with Behavior Impairment.' It appears that at reaching adolescence a number of previously reported behaviors had receded, but some sexually inappropriate behaviors were regularly reported.

Since school Paul has lived in large long-stay hospitals and later in smaller residential care homes.

LEVEL OF INTELLECTUAL DISABILITY

Paul has a 'moderate ID,' his full scale IQ having been assessed at 52. His social, educational and occupational histories are consistent with this level of intellectual disability. He is very knowledgeable about football, especially his favourite team, to which he seems positively attached.

FORENSIC HISTORY

Paul has no reported criminal convictions. Reports describe a history of allegations although it is unclear if there had been police involvement on all occasions.

Aged 28 approached two young boys. Held one in his arms and made 'homosexual movements' behind the other boy.

Aged 32 the priest from the local church wrote saying that some parents had complained about Paul touching the boys during a church service.

Aged 33 he was taken by a fellow resident to a friend's house where it was reported that the man paid £3 for sex.

Aged 39 had sex with a 16 year old boy who also had ID. Sexual activities took place after local scout group meetings.

Aged 40 he was suspended from the local scout group.

Aged 45 a sexual incident took place in the toilets where Paul attended his weekly therapy group sessions. Unsure if Paul or the other man initiated sexual contact.

Also aged 45 Paul assaulted a fellow worker by grabbing his bottom. Paul was asked to leave his work placement.

Aged 46 sexually assaulted a 16-year-old man with Down syndrome in the men's toilet of the college they both attended.

Also aged 46 Mr was seen staring at a young boy on a train. The boy challenged Paul who started retreating into his usual behaviors of mumbling and poking his eye. Staff travelling with Paul managed to diffuse the situation.

Aged 47 Paul was referred to Respond for a forensic risk assessment. The reason for the assessment as expressed in the referral form stated: '(Paul)…has homosexual urges and has spent a number of years coming to terms with this. He has minimal interaction with people outside of his home and attempts made by Paul to find a male partner (or simply fulfil his sexual urges) have resulted in Paul being involved in incidents of abuse…involving mainly young men in various situations.' This reason for referral was expanded upon in meetings where Paul was viewed as representing a risk to children and vulnerable persons and that risk management had become necessary. The referrers were concerned that Paul may still represent a risk to others and that Paul himself may be at risk of becoming a victim of sexual or physical abuse.

Paul said himself when asked why he thought he had been referred for a risk assessment stated that it was so that he could talk about his 'touching of children'. He indicated that he was a risk to children and that he could not be relied upon not to 'touch children on their bottoms'. He explained that he was trying not to touch children when he went shopping.

The risk assessment proceeded without interruption and Paul engaged in the process. The report described Paul as presenting with 'a confusing and diverse range of inappropriate behaviors that are of a sexualised quality, some of which should be described as predatory.' The assessor went on to note that Paul had 'no established internal inhibitors' and could offer 'no insight into his offending behaviors.' He harbours 'paedophilic thoughts' and is at 'high risk of enacting these without regard for consequence.' He has described himself as not like 'other child sex offenders because he has a learning disability'.

For me Paul's early abandonment and his history of sexualised behavior point to significant developmental deficiencies that are apparent in the consulting room via our developing therapeutic relationship. His ID is also a factor in the treatment to date due to the level of his arrested mental functioning. I believe that his state of mind is such that the use of interpretation and *thinking with* the patient is simply not possible. My understanding of the way his mind works makes me believe that a more direct and simplified way of working is most likely to facilitate the development of the work.

I have chosen material from a number of different sessions in order to demonstrate my clinical thinking and to discuss the presentation of Paul's paedophilic perversion in the transference and countertransference considerations. Paul's ID are also significant in trying to gain an understanding of his psychopathology. I have therefore, where appropriate, discussed the possible significance of these in terms of how they can affect the development of an individual's sexuality and sense of self.

DISCUSSION

Since starting work with Paul much of the clinical material has focused on his paedophilic thinking. As I shall demonstrate it is clear that Paul is aware of these thoughts, but is unable or unwilling to think about the consequences of his actions outside of what other people might think about them. For instance he is able to say that what he did was wrong, but he only seems to know about it through the eyes of other people who, for him, act as external measurements of how he is supposed to behave. He appears to be unaware of the reality of his acting out. For example the following dialogue comes from one of our sessions:

> Paul: There was a man called X, this young boy I'm not sure how old he is and he's moved in and I 'm trying to avoid him and I try not to touch him.
> Me: Are you attracted to him?
> Paul: Sometimes, but I try not to touch him up and I haven't touched him yet.
> Me: But maybe you feel like you would like to touch him.
> Paul: No I wouldn't do that, because he might make allegations to the staff, so I can be friends but mustn't touch him. I've been very careful.
> Me: You feel you need to be very careful.
> Paul: I do need to be careful. There is this other guy called Y and I have to be careful with him as well I cannot touch him. He touches me and I touch him, but it's not allowed as I'd be the one to get in trouble. He could get us in trouble. He touched me and then we could get in trouble and then get kicked out of the home, so I've stopped now.

Paul relies totally upon his fear of what might happen to him if he is discovered. The staff act as the external inhibitors to his acting out and this reality is what keeps him within reasonable boundaries of what is considered acceptable. The alternative is that he is at the mercy of impulses and stimulus driven behavior.

Stanley Ruszczynski (2006) highlights the number of writers who have paid attention to the understanding of perversion as the 'product of distortion and misrepresentation of reality' (p. 106). They stress the disowning of the reality of the difference of the generations and of the sexes. Ruszczynski continues by stating:

> Misrepresentation of reality is central to an understanding of the perversions and arises from a specific mechanism in which contradictory versions of reality are allowed to coexist simultaneously (p. 107).

I have been struck at times by Paul's apparent omnipotence and narcissism. For example in one session he described how another resident was caught with his girlfriend in the house:

> Me: There was the girlfriend who shouldn't have been in the house.
> Paul: I said I didn't want to have to keep looking out for people who shouldn't be there, I am the Health and Safety Officer.
> Me: And that means…
> Paul: I do have to look out for what people shouldn't be doing.
> Me: Like sexual things?
> Paul: Well yes and other things.

For Paul omnipotence is one of the mechanisms that he employs in order to avoid the reality of the oedipal destiny that obliges one to give these up in favour of being able to tolerate loss and ones dependence on others. The above dialogue looks like a form of omnipotent thinking but it is also an impoverishment of thought and of appropriate connections to the outside world. In this example he takes on the role of police/safety officer in an enactment of the castrating father, with him as castrator. Paul was abandoned at such a young age and his ID make it doubly hard for him to tolerate the fundamental facts of life.

For him the combination of aggression and sex is recruited to deny the facts of life and to destroy the potential in being able to relate to people.

Paul's stream of words often seems to be about nothing, in the sense of being connected to any genuine thought or feeling. I find that this way of communicating with the world and me is a manoeuvre against the pain of being in touch with intolerable feelings of loss and fragmentation. When he mumbles to himself and says, 'what next' I experience a pseudo-thinking which is more an attempt to ensure that he does not really experience me as someone with a mind and therefore as someone who is different and separable from himself. However, I ask myself if he really thinks like that and part of my task is to think about *what* I am to him, rather that *who* I am to him. If I develop this further I wonder too about *what* Paul is to me. For example, in a recent session he changes the subject from talking about an incident in which he sexually assaulted a 16-year-old in a toilet:

> Paul: No I thought he was 25 or 26 or 23 or 22 or 21.
> Me: But he was younger.
> Paul: I think so, but it's not going to happen again as staff will be with me at all times in the toilet.
> Me: And that stops it from happening again.
> Paul: Yes. I went to cooking yesterday and we made a quiche.

This way of being with me reminds me of being with a young child and many times throughout our sessions I am reminded of Paul's childlike manner. I sometimes experience it as an attempt to seduce me or to get me to collude with him and to therefore be disarmed. It is also an example of his inability to concentrate and that he always heads towards the closest stimulus to hand. This is the level at which he functions. Changing the subject is a concentration of object constancy rather than a truly defensive manoeuvre. Changing the subject is a challenge for me as I find it difficult to work with. My countertransference reaction is to get frustrated and become more of an investigating policeman (trying to get at what he is avoiding) and importantly maybe this is *what* he experiences me as. A number of times Paul has referred to himself as his home's Health and Safety Officer and this is not dissimilar to the role I find myself in – the therapist as the one looking out for danger and raising the alarm if something is amiss.

Paul's reaction to interpretations remains fixed. He often talks incessantly, often speaking over anything I try to say. It is sometimes difficult to know how much of what I say is actually understood. I keep my language as basic as I can and am careful not to allow any interpretations to be too complex. Yet he still continues to bat away most of my interventions, trying instead to conduct a monologue and to fill each session with his words. He often confuses tenses and contradicts himself within the same sentence. For example:

> Paul: I put my hand there and touched myself. It's disgusting (staring at hands and then smelling his fingers). I don't care what other people say.
> Me: You say it's disgusting.
> Paul: That's what they say.
> Me: What do you say?
> Paul: I agree.
> Me: So you touch yourself and then…

Paul: Then I stop. I do it on purpose when I'm being rude. But I need to think hard about it.

I find this kind of dialogue maddening and at times I have felt overwhelmed and I have used my clinical supervision to look at this by focusing not so much on the content but on my confusion. My countertransference is an important way of understanding Paul's state of mind. In sessions I can feel confused and disabled. I sense aggression in what he says although it is disturbing because he also seems so vulnerable and inadequate. My countertransference is vital in helping me to understand but in all of Paul's attitudes and the way he makes me feel there is something missing in him: there is no emotional content. It is our emotions, as well as our thoughts and our ability to relate that hold us together; I often wonder what holds Paul together? The answer I find is a fragile sense of self that is lonely and cut-off.

In another early session we returned to the paedophilia issue and I attempted to help him by introducing the idea that part of him might want to do something while the other might not, i.e. he might know it is wrong but that he might still feel like doing it. This session also demonstrated the denial and defendedness of his thinking. He seems to lack internal inhibitors (Finkelhor 1986) that could stop him from acting out some of his paedophilic thoughts and he therefore relies upon the external vigilance and constraints of the staff that monitor and supervise him. This can be viewed in a number of different ways; firstly he is well aware of his impulses and hence his potential for causing harm and therefore uses those around him as his control mechanism; and secondly he keeps himself in an unthinking position that is a defence against 'knowing' and being responsible for his actions.

In one session Paul focused on the doll's house and enacted a very sexualised scenario:

Paul: Can anyone see in the door?
Me: I don't think so. What do you think they would see?
Paul: Me playing crazy with the doll's house.
Me: No one can see.
Paul: Don't tell anyone, keep that quiet. (He moves back to the doll's house) They are all lying down and he (a sheep) can see up her skirt. Oh god. (laughs). Naughty (Dribble comes out of his mouth and he is seemingly excited. He puts the head of the sheep right up the skirt of the doll and laughs and dribbles more – I feel disgusted.)

Paul starts by asking if anyone can see him/us, as if we might be engaged in something not right – sex, craziness. He tries to get me to collude with him in this scene of the sheep and the doll. I find it difficult to watch, but strangely engrossing. I wonder whether he is aware of what he is showing me about his thoughts and I think about how aggressive this scene is in terms of what he does to the doll and to me sadomasochistically.

I also find that Paul is uninterested in what I think; he doesn't want me to think because the nature of his behavior is omnipotent and this points to a psychopathic element to his personality and behavior. I left the session needing to test whether it is my hate in the countertransference (Winnicott, 1949) that leaves me feeling no compassion for him. He is constantly trying to assert his power as if no one matters to him and he seems to work on a binary level. My mission at this point in the therapy is not to care for him but to try and create or achieve an experience in which Paul might learn to get to know something. The important function of the work is to help him to develop a capacity to think relatively, that is so obviously missing from the sessions.

CRITICAL REVIEW

This paper has brought to my attention the high and sometimes unrealistic expectations I unconsciously had before starting this work with Paul. I am also aware of the difference in my earliest formulation to my current one. I think I entered into this work in a rather naïve way, thinking that what was probably needed was for me, as therapist, to be aware of the patients projections and to quickly get to grips with his psychopathology and to then offer insightful and enlightening interpretations that would lead the patient to a better understanding of himself and the reasons behind his behavior. I also fell into a habit of acting like a policeman trying to get at the truth and to somehow extract a confession. I can now see, thanks to my supervision, that I was defended against the awfulness of Paul's history and of his existence. My countertransference reactions led me to act as policeman and inquisitor, desperately digging for the illusive truth. I now think that this is a familiar pattern for Paul as a way of galvanising interest (positive and negative) from those around him. Firstly, in order to make him safe and to contain him; and secondly, and maybe more importantly, to guard against knowing the reality of his life, by always externalising any responsibility for himself onto others.

I am also aware of the fact that it is my defence against contamination that leads me into the role of the policeman. It's much safer to stick to the facts than to delve further into the messiness and uncharted waters of Paul's psychopathology.

In terms of technique I often try to slow things down significantly in order to allow myself to fully take on board the sometimes obscured trajectory of Paul's thinking. The learning edge for me in this treatment is to be able to slow down and not act as the policeman in the room. I focus on discovering and understanding the symbolic meanings of his thinking, even if this is only a part-object experience of his life. Progress with Paul can only really be measured in terms of what I'm learning about my own working practice as well as my witnessing of him slowly coming to life in front of me (Alvarez 1992).

FORMULATION

Paul is a complex individual who needs to spend more time in treatment so that any reparative work can take place. His ID limits his ability to make sense of some of his experiences, specifically his early abandonment, and this will always be a permanent feature of his psychopathology. I see Paul's treatment as part of larger package of care that is necessary for him to feel contained enough not to act out sexually. His treatment is therefore unlike some other disturbed patients, in that he has little insight into his reasons for acting out. I mentioned earlier his lack of internal inhibitors and this leads to the current situation of needing constant monitoring and vigilance on the part of his carers. It is worth considering that Paul has in fact partly created this 'family' of watchful people as an effort to maintain his own safety as well as that of others.

Daniel Juda (2004) writes that:

...homosexual paedophilia may be a behavioral manifestation of self-structural deficiencies that are the result of subjectively experienced inadequate mirroring and poorly idealisable early parental objects. (p. 153)

Borrowing from Kohut, Juda encourages the analyst to become 'an adequate mirroring and later omnipotent object, to utilise whatever adequate capacities have survived or are strong enough to develop rapidly'. (p. 154) He sees homosexual paedophilia as a disorder that frequently requires a serious deficit in the person's self-formulation which prevents him or her from being able to empathise with the victim/self-object – just as an infant has not developed the capacity to experience reality from the mother's point of view (ibid).

This relates to Paul in terms of never really having had a mother (figure) who was there for him and who could help him to experience the others reality. What we are therefore left with is a problem of trying to locate Paul's capacity to form a positive attachment to me. The other problem for the future is whether I have the capacity to provide the adequate mirroring Paul would require.

CONCLUSION

I have said before (2009) that a central aim of psychotherapeutic treatment is to lessen the negative or unsupportive defences against internal conflict by supporting the patient to identify, address and attempt to integrate their internal dynamics. Hodges (2003) writes, 'this aim is hopefully achieved by making internal objects, inner worlds and their workings more available or accessible to the patient.' She continues by stating that a careful exploration of the meaning in the patient's behaviors can lead to a more useful expression of feelings.

More research needs to be undertaken, but experience suggests that interventions such as those described above can provide a thoughtful and containing space, for both the patient and also for those who work with them, supporting and supervising them in the community. Sex offenders with ID, and specifically those with paedophilic tendencies may sometimes find themselves beyond the reach of the criminal justice system and attendant treatment programmes. They are therefore highly dependent on care providers to offer imaginative and thoughtful interventions which respect their human rights and also recognise the impact of early trauma and of the experience of growing up and living with ID in a society that is at best often disinterested and that at worst openly hostile towards them. These interventions and treatments must ensure the safety of others whilst nurturing personal growth, developing personal responsibility, thereby increasing the possibility of change in his or her dangerous behavior.

REFERENCES

Alvarez, A (1992) Live Company: Psychotherapy with Autistic, Borderline, deprived and Abused Children. London: Routledge.

Campbell, D. (1989) From Practice to Psychodynamic Theories of Delinquency in Adolescence, in Cordess, C. and Cox, M. (eds.) Forensic Psychotherapy: Crime, psychodynamics and the Offender Patient, London: Jessica Kingsley.

Curen, R. (2009) 'Can they see in the door?':Issues in the Assessment and Treatment of Learning Disabled Sex Offenders, In Cottis, T. (ed) Intellectual Disability, Trauma and Psychotherapy. London. Routledge.

Finkelhor, D. (1986) A Sourcebook on Child Sexual Abuse, California: Sage.

Freud, S. (1905) 'Three Essays on the theory of sexuality'. In Strachey, J. (ed) The Standard Edition of the Complete Psychological Works of Sigmond Freud, Vol 7. London: Hogarth Press.

Glasser, M. (1996) Aggression and Sadism in the Perversions, in Sexual Deviation 3rd Edition,Rosen, I. (ed), Oxford: Oxford University Press.

Glover, E. (1944) Mental Abnormality and Crime, London. Macmillan.

Hodges, S. (2003) Counselling Adults with Learning Disabilities. Basingstoke: Palgrave.

Juda, D. (2004)The Usefulness of Self Psychology. In The Mind of the Paedophile; Psychoanalytic Perspectives, Socarides, C. with Loeb, L.R. (ed), London: Karnac.

Ruszczynski, S. (2006). The problem of certain psychic realities: aggression and violence as perverse solutions', in Aggression and Destructiveness: Psychoanalytic Perspectives, Harding, C.(ed). Hove: Routledge

Welldon, E., V. (1988) Mother, Madonna, Whore: the idealisation and denigration of motherhood. London: Guildford Press.

Welldon, E. V. (1996) Contrasts in Male and Female Sexual Perversions' in Cordess, C. and Cox, M. (eds.) *Forensic Psychotherapy: Crime, psychodynamics and the Offender Patient*, London: Jessica Kingsley.

Winnicott, D.W. (1949)Hate in the countertransference. *Inernational Journal of Psycho-Analysis*, 30: 69-75

Winnicott, D. W. (1956). The Antisocial tendency. In D. W. Winnicott *Collected Paper: through Paediatrics to Psycho-Analysis*. London: Karnac Books.

PART II. AGING AND LIFESPAN

As per the general population individuals with intellectual disabilities (ID) are living longer than previously. As a consequence there is an increase in age-related mental health disorders, particularly of dementia in Alzheimer's disease. The role of life events and their impact on the older population is highlighted by *Patti*. Such life events include moving residents, illness, loss of a close friend, and injury to oneself. The psychological and physical consequences of persons with ID surviving into middle-age and beyond is independently reported on by *Carr* and *Coppus and colleagues*. *Carr's* outstanding research of the follow-up of a cohort of children with Down syndrome for 40 years highlights the relative stability in neuropsychological scores over this time period. In contrast, *Sone and colleagues* and *Coppus and colleagues* demonstrate a number of health disorders and risk factors for mortality. Associated risk factors for mortality being older, physically handicapped, severity of ID, and presence of at least one ApoE allele. The emotions associated with imminent death remain under-researched in the field of ID. *Maaskant and colleagues* highlight the issues of understanding death and how best persons can be supported.

A significant proportion of the elderly ID population do not suffer any mental ill-health. However, they too may have un-met needs. *Brehmer* discusses the concept of 'frailty' in older persons with ID whilst *Hole and colleagues* emphasize the need for clear and explicit policies to maximise service delivery. *Willis and colleagues* discuss the issue of breast cancer screening, an issue with aptly highlights the need for the delivery of a well developed community service for all individuals.

Chapter 9

PSYCHOSOCIAL ASPECTS OF AGING IN DOWN SYNDROME: THE IMPACT OF LIFE EVENTS

P.J. Patti

George A. Jervis Clinic,New York State Institute for Basic Research in Developmental Disabilities, New York, USA

INTRODUCTION

Exposure to life events can have a direct as well as an indirect influence on physical and mental health. In the general population, negative life situations have been associated with the onset of depression in both young and older adults (Brilman & Ormel, 2001; Kraaji et al, 2002; Muscatell et al, 2009). For people with dementia, changes in routine or living situations can increase the risk of deterioration and have a negative effect on physical health and mortality (Mirotznik & Kamp, 2000; Butler et al, 2004; Waite et al, 2004).

People with intellectual disabilities (ID) were reported to respond to life events in a similar way as people in the general population. Experiencing one or more life events in the previous 12 months was associated with increased risk of mental health problems (Cooper et al, 2007). A growing number of studies have reported a significant relationship between life events exposure and psychiatric problems in adults with ID (Hastings et al, 2004, Owen et al, 2004; Hamilton et al, 2005; Esbensen & Benson, 2006). Personal loss, moving to a new residence and changing jobs have been implicated as risk factors for mental and physical ill health. Adults with ID who experienced more negative life events were also reported to exhibit more behavior problems and depressive symptoms Esbensen & Benson, 2006). A study of referrals to a mental health service revealed that depression, personality disorder and adjustment reaction were reliably associated with multiple exposure to life events (Tsakanikos et al, 2007). In a review, Hulbert-Williams and Hastings concluded that there is reasonable evidence based on studies conducted thus far that life events are associated with psychological problems in people with ID (Patti et al, 2005).

The most frequent life events experienced by adults with ID residing in an institutional setting included staffing and residence changes, conflicts with staff and others, death of relative or close friend, and personal injury or physical illness (Owen et al, 2004). Life events exposure was associated with an increased frequency of aggressive/destructive behavior and the presence of affective disorder. In a population-based sample of adults with ID receiving community and residential services (n=1155), the most frequent life events in the previous 12 months were moving residence (15.5%), illness of close relative or friend (9%), conflict with friend, neighbor or relative (8.8%), illness or injury to self (8.5%), and death of close friend/relative (8.3%) (Hastings et al, 2004).

LIFE EVENTS EXPOSURE IN ADULTS WITH DOWN SYNDROME

Few studies investigated life events in adults with Down syndrome (DS). Hamilton et al (2005) included 129 DS adults in a sample of 624 ID adults (mean age 34.2 years). A strong relationship between life events frequency and emotional/behavioral problems was found in DS adults who were functioning in the mild range but not for those in the moderate to severe range of ID. Owen et al (2004) included only 6 DS adults in their residential sample of 93 adults with ID. Only one published study to date compared the frequency and types of life events in older adults with and without DS. Patti et al (2005) analyzed life events experienced by 211 adults living in community group homes over a 5 year period. The types of life events are listed in Table 1.

Table 1. Common life events in older adults with and without DS[1]

Relocations
Change in residence
Nursing home placement
Environmental/Social Changes
Change in day treatment program
Change in living conditions
Other: change in peer group, social relationships
Losses/Separations
Death of parent
Death of family member
Other: death of a peer, change/loss of a roommate or friend
Medical Events/Changes
Hospitalization(s)
Seizure-onset
Fracture
Pneumonia
Other: cataract removal, other surgeries, new medical conditions.

[1](Patti et al, 2005)

Relocations and medical events were significantly greater in the DS group, whereas a significantly lower number of occurrences in all life events categories were found in the non-

DS group. These findings suggest that adults with DS in the sixth decade of life experience a greater number of life events than their non-DS counterparts of similar or older ages.

A follow-up study explored the number of relocations over a 5 and 10 year period, and current or final placement in a cohort of 140 adults with and without DS (Patti et al, 2009). Data on 61 DS adults (mean age 61.8 years) was compared with 79 non-DS adults (mean age 70.7 years). The DS group encountered significantly more relocations (i.e. changing group homes, nursing home placement) over time due to functional decline associated with dementia than the non-DS group. A mean of 1.07 and 1.26 relocations respectively occurred during a 5 and 10 year period for the DS group compared to a mean of 0.59 and 1.00 in the non-DS group. Placement in a nursing home for end of life care was significantly higher in the DS group (39% versus 9%) whereas the majority (91%) in the non-DS group remained in a group home setting. Mortality data also revealed significant differences between the two groups. Of the 44 who died in the DS group the locations of death were nursing home 46%; hospital 39% and group home 16%; for the 25 who died in the non-DS group it was group home 52%, hospital 28% and nursing home 20%.

THE EFFECTS OF MULTIPLE LIFE EVENTS OVER TIME

It is likely that in different situations people with ID will experience one or more life events as they age through the lifespan. When and where they occur can have a bearing on health status and placement. Most studies looked at life events exposure over 12 months. Hastings et al (2004) reported 46.3% in a population sample to encounter at least one life event in 12 months and 17.4% to encounter two or more. Those living in an institution were more likely to have been exposed to at least one recent event than those residing in a community setting. Owen et al (2004) reported long-stay hospital residents to encounter an average of 3.50 negative events in 12 months. An average of 4.68 life events for the previous 2 years was reported in 624 adults with ID living in family/foster care or a staffed accommodation (Hamilton et al, 2005) and an average of 1.17 life events was reported in 281 adults with ID seen in a mental health clinic (Tsakanikos et al, 2007).

From the above studies, life events exposure can vary based on where a person resides. The number of life events exposure, however, may be less important than the types of events experienced. The effects of specific life events (e.g. death of parent, physical illness, relocation) may be difficult to fully assess within a 12 month period as their consequences can take longer to affect a person. The cumulative exposure of life events with the additional onset of medical frailties associated with aging can combine to create a stressful period for people with DS and can often result in relocation (Patti et al, 2005; 2009).

As seen in Figure 1, multiple life events can lead to a change in behavior and, if accompanied by a medical illness or condition, affect quality of life. For DS adults, age and functional decline are important factors in life events exposure since they can have consequences on the provision of care and placement. Functional decline was found to be greater in older DS adults in comparison to age-specific controls with ID but without DS (Prasher, 1996; Prasher & Chung, 1996). The principal factor causing decline in DS adults is the increased incidence of dementia (Prasher, 1999). However, a loss in functioning in DS adults before age 50 may be due to depression rather than dementia and can be effectively treated with positive results (Tsiouris & Patti, 1997). Regardless of the causative factors, functional decline is a distinguishing feature in the behavioral phenotype of adults with DS. It is imperative to formulate a differential diagnosis whenever functional decline occurs in an adult with DS so proper treatment strategies can be implemented (Patti, 2005).

Possible Interactions of Different Life Events on Behavior

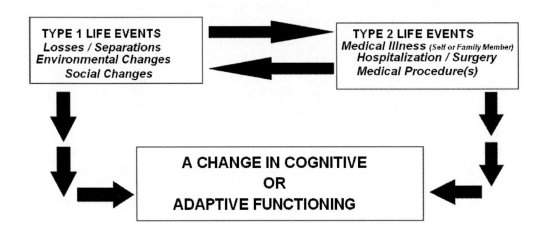

Figure 1. Possible Interactions of Different Life Events on Behavior.

AGE AND THE EFFECTS OF SOCIAL AND ENVIRONMENTAL EVENTS

Adults with DS are often the youngest offspring in the family, with elderly parents, and siblings who are generally older than themselves (Seltzer et al, 1993). For those living at home, the death of a parent can lead to a change in location (e.g. moving in with a relative, moving to a group home). This constitutes two life events occurring in a limited time period. The transition to a new or unfamiliar setting may pose challenges for the individual and possibly lead to behavioral and adjustment difficulties. An early study suggested that people with DS display more psychological problems in adapting to minor changes in daily routine starting at age 40 years (Haveman et al, 1994). This is often around the same time when families may seek placement for DS adults, typically after the death of a parent or when they can no longer be cared for by other family members. In a recent report, placement out of the home and parental death were predictors of change in health, functional abilities and behavior problems (Esbensen et al, 2008). For older adults with and without DS living in group homes, the death of a parent or family member, changing day programs, and loss/separation of a friend or roommate were more frequent occurrences in the lives of adults with DS (Patti et al, 2009).

Changes in group home placement or other relocations regardless of the underlying reasons can have a negative effect. Separation from familiar staff and peers can cause behavioral and adjustment problems especially for those DS adults who may also be experiencing early signs of dementia. The impact of relocation was found to have a negative effect on mortality and physical health status for some elderly patients (Butler & Orrell, 2004; Meehan et al, 2004). Patti and colleagues suggested that the increased number of relocations and placements encountered by older DS adults may even contribute to their accelerated rate of decline even when dementia is taken into account (Patti et al, 2009)

THE EFFECTS OF MEDICAL EVENTS IN OLDER PEOPLE WITH DS

Age 40 years appears to be a turning point for DS adults since they were found to have a higher risk of health, functional and cognitive problems as they age. Prior to age 40, DS adults are at lower risk for dementia and functional decline (Esbensen et al, 2008) although they remain predisposed to mood and anxiety disorders (Patti & Tsiouris, 2006). Other reports indicated that until the age of 40 years the rates of mortality were similar for adults with DS and other types of ID (Strauss & Eyman, 1996; Esbensen et al, 2007). Dementia was reported to occur in more than half the DS population between age 50 and 60 years with Alzheimer disease being the predominant form (Patti, 2005). The average age of onset was found to be between 50 and 55 years, with a range from 38 to 70 years (Coppus et al, 2006). For adults with DS surviving to middle age, the development of dementia is frequent but not inevitable, and some will reach old age without clinical features of dementia (Margallo-Lana et al, 2007).

The general consensus is that adults with DS tend to experience more medical changes after age 50 years than those without DS. This coincides with the increased incidence of dementia in DS adults (Patti, 2005; Meehan et al, 2004; Coppus et al, 2006). The onset of age-related medical problems can result in a loss of previously attained skills and reduce independence. Medical events such as late-onset seizures, pneumonia, fractures, and new medical conditions occur more often in older DS adults than non-DS adults. Often a person displaying age-related decline needs to be moved to an alternative setting for increased care or for safety management issues (Patti et al, 2005).

CONCLUSION

Professionals working with the elderly ID population need to monitor older adults who have experienced one or more life events because they are at risk for consequential change in their behavior or functioning. Indications are that life events exposure can have a cumulative effect over time which can impact behavior, health and stability. Relocations and medical life events appear to occur more often in older adults, and their effects may not be immediately recognized by family members or group home staff. Further studies investigating life events and changes in older adults with ID are necessary to identify and evaluate their effects on physical or mental health.

REFERENCES

Brilman EI, Ormel J. Life events, difficulties and onset of depressive episodes in later life. *Psychol Med.* 2001 Jul;31(5):859-869.

Butler R, Orrell M, Ukoumunne OC et al. Life events and survival in dementia: a 5-year follow-up study. *Aust N Z J Psychiatry,* 2004 Sep;38(9):702-705.

Cooper SA, Smiley E, Morrison J et al. Mental ill-health in adults with intellectual disabilities: prevalence and associated factors. *Br J Psychiatry,* 2007 Jan;190:27-35.

Coppus A, Evenhuis H, Verberne GJ et al. Dementia and mortality in persons with Down's syndrome. *J Intellect Disabil Res.* 2006;50:768-77.

Esbensen AJ, Benson BA. A prospective analysis of life events, problem behaviors and depression in adults with intellectual disability. *J Intellect Disabil Res.* 2006 Apr;50(Pt 4):248-258.

Esbensen AJ, Seltzer MM, Greenberg JS. Factors predicting mortality in midlife adults with and without Down syndrome living with family. *J Intellect Disabil Res.* 2007;51:1039-50.

Esbensen AJ, Seltzer MM, Krauss MW. Stability and change in health, functional abilities, and behavior problems among adults with and without Down syndrome. *Am J Ment Retard.* 2008 Jul;113(4):263-277.

Hamilton D, Sutherland G, Iacono T. Further examination of relationships between life events and psychiatric symptoms in adults with intellectual disability. *J Intellect Disabil Res.* 2005 Nov;49(Pt 11):839-844.

Hastings RP, Hatton C, Taylor JL et al. Life events and psychiatric symptoms in adults with intellectual disabilities. *J Intellect Disabil Res.* 2004 Jan;48(1):42-46.

Haveman MJ, Maaskant MA, van Schrojenstein Lantman HM et al. Mental health problems in elderly people with and without Down's syndrome. *J Intellect Disabil Res.* 1994 Jun;38 (Pt 3):341-355.

Hulbert-Williams L, Hastings RP. Life events as a risk factor for psychological problems in individuals with intellectual disabilities: a critical review. *J Intellect Disabil Res.* 2008 Nov;52(11):883-95

Kraaij V, Arensman E, Spinhoven P. Negative life events and depression in elderly persons: a meta-analysis. *J Gerontol B Psychol Sci Soc Sci.* 2002 Jan;57(1):87-94.

Margallo-Lana ML, Moore PB, Kay DW et al. Fifteen-year follow-up of 92 hospitalized adults with Down's syndrome: incidence of cognitive decline, its relationship to age and neuropathology. *J Intellect Disabil Res.* 2007;51:463-477

Meehan T, Robertson S, Stedman T et al. Outcomes for elderly patients with mental illness following relocation from a stand-alone psychiatric hospital to community based extended care units. *Aust N Z J Psychiatry,* 2004;38:948–952

Mirotznik J, Kamp LL.Cognitive status and relocation stress: a test of the vulnerability hypothesis. *Gerontologist,* 2000 Oct;40(5):531-9.

Muscatell KA, Slavich GM, Monroe SM et al. Stressful life events, chronic difficulties, and the symptoms of clinical depression. *J Nerv Ment Dis.* 2009 Mar;197(3):154-160.

Owen DM, Hastings RP, Noone SJ et al. Life events as correlates of problem behavior and mental health in a residential population of adults with developmental disabilities. *Res Dev Disabil.* 2004 Jul-Aug;25(4):309-320

Patti PJ, Amble KB, Flory MJ. Life events in older adults with intellectual disabilities: Differences between adults with and without Down syndrome. *J Policy Pract Intellect Disabil.* 2005; 2:149-155.

Patti P.J., Amble K. & Flory M. Placement, relocation and end of life issues in aging adults with and without Down syndrome: A retrospective study. 2009, Manuscript under review.

Patti PJ, Tsiouris JA. Psychopathology in adults with Down syndrome: Clinical findings from an outpatient clinic. *Int J Disabil Human Dev.* 2006;5(4):357-64.

Patti PJ. Depression, dementia and Down syndrome. In Sturmey P, ed. Mood disorders in people with mental retardation. Kingston, NY: NADD Press, 2005:131-155

Prasher VP. Age-associated functional decline in adults with Down's syndrome. *Eur J Psychiatry,* 1996;10:129-135.

Prasher VP, Chung MC. Causes of age-related decline in adaptive behavior in adults with Down syndrome: Differential diagnosis of dementia. *Am J Ment Retard.* 1996;10:1175-1183.

Prasher VP. Adaptive behavior. In: Janicki MP, Dalton AJ, eds. Dementia, aging, and intellectual disabilities: A handbook. Philadelphia: Taylor & Francis, 1999:157-178

Seltzer MM, Krauss MW, Tsunematsu N. Adults with Down syndrome and their aging mothers: diagnostic group differences. *Am J Ment Retard.* 1993;97(5):496-508

Strauss D, Eyman R K. Mortality of people with mental retardation in California with and without Down syndrome, 1986–1991. *Am J Ment Retard.* 1996;100:643-653

Tsakanikos E, Bouras N, Costello H et al. Multiple exposure to life events and clinical psychopathology in adults with intellectual disability. *Soc Psychiatry Psychiatr Epidemiol.* 2007 Jan;42(1):24-28.

Tsiouris JA, Patti PJ. Drug treatment of depression associated with dementia or presented as "pseudodementia" in older adults with Down syndrome. *J Appl Res Intellect Disabil.* 1997;10:312-322.

Waite A, Bebbington P, Skelton-Robinson M et al. Life events, depression and social support in dementia. *Br J Clin Psychol.* 2004 Sep;43(Pt 3):313-324.

Chapter 10

FOUR TO FORTY YEARS: THE PATTERN OF DEVELOPMENT OF A COHORT WITH DOWN SYNDROME

J. Carr
Formerly of St George's Hospital, London, UK

INTRODUCTION

The study described here, set up by the UK Medical Research Council's Psychiatric Genetics Research Unit, concerned all the infants born with Down syndrome (DS), in part of South East England in the year December 1963-November 1964. The psychological part of the study ran from six weeks to 4 years, then continued to, so far, 11, 21, 30, 35 and 40 years. Here the focus is on the findings from 4- 40 years.

BACKGROUND TO THE STUDY

Fifty-four babies were referred to the study. Forty-five remained in the family home, nine went out of home soon after birth. Over the years there were losses to the study, all but three through deaths, so that by age 40 years 34 remained in the study, men and women being equally represented.

The test instruments used changed over time. These were: up to four years, the Bayley Scales of Mental and Motor Development (Bayley 1964, 1969); at 11 years the Merrill-Palmer Scale (Merrill-Palmer 1948) and the Reynell Language Scales (Reynell 1969); from age 21 onwards the Leiter International Performance Scale (Leiter 1980), British Picture Vocabulary Scale (Dunn et al 1982), the vocabulary sub-test from the Pre-School and Primary Scale of Intelligence (Wechsler 1967), the Analysis of Reading Tests (Neale 1958) and Arithmetic-Mathematics Test (Vernon 1960).

RESULTS

In this paper mean scores are given for those 34 people present throughout the study. Data on all present at each single stage can be found in Carr (submitted).

From six weeks to four years mean IQs declined from 73 at six weeks to 44 at four years (Carr 1975). From four to 11 years mean IQ declined by less than one point, then increased to 21 years by just over five points (probably because verbal items, included in the Merrill-Palmer test at 11 were absent from the Leiter Scale at 21 and thereafter). From 21 to 40 years mean IQ declined by just over three points. (Table 1). So the rapid decline seen in early childhood, widely documented in other reports (eg, Ludlow & Allen 1979, Morgan 1979) was not continued into adulthood.

Table 1. Means and standard deviations of test scores/ages from 4-40 years

Years, chronological age	4	11	21	30	35	40
IQ (n=34)	40.8	39.6	44.9	43.4	43	41.5
sd	11.1	10.8	14	14.5	13.5	12.9

Language - age in months						
Expression(n=18)		52.2	66.8	72.5	68.9	65.6
sd		15.4	18.5	18.4	15.6	20.1
Comprehension (n=30)		45.3	57.3	61.83	60.2	59.1
sd		10.9	19.6	28.1	28.1	27.8

Reading – age in months						
Accuracy (n=14)			94.6	96.5	97.1	99.5
sd			18.8	18.3	18.1	19.8
Comprehension n=11)			82.6	86.2	86	84.4
sd			11	15.3	16	16.9

Arithmetic – age in months (n=26)						
			63	63.5	62.5	62.3
sd			7.2	8.9	8.2	8.3

Language

At four years three-quarters of the cohort used two words, just over half of these using them to make their wants known (Carr, 1975). At age 11 years the mean language ages were around 4 years (Table 1). At 21 years and again at 30 years both means rose, then declined slightly. These figures are derived from all those able to score on each test – just over half the cohort in the case of expression and nearly 90% in the case of comprehension. When mean comprehension was calculated for only those able to score also on the test of expression the two means are much closer, within a maximum of 4 months of each other, with no consistent advantage to either score.

Reading and Arithmetic

Only two-fifths of the cohort scored on the reading tests. At age 21 years the mean age for accuracy was 7 years 10 months and mean comprehension 6 years 9 months. Figures for comprehension then remained stable, but those for accuracy continued to rise, reaching 8 years 3 months at age 40. Mean arithmetic age at age 21 was 5 years 3 months, and this remained almost unchanged over the years. While the highest reading age achieved was 12 years three months the highest arithmetic age gained was seven years. For those who at age 40 years scored on both tests mean reading accuracy age was 8 years 3 months, and mean arithmetic age nearly three years lower, at 5 years 6 months.

Self-Help

In this paper the focus is on four basic skills, assessed from age 11 years onwards using the Health Behavior and Skills schedule (Wing 1980).

**Table 2. Means and standard deviations of self-help scores,
11-40 years (n=34)**

Years, chronological age	11	21	30	35	40
Total s/h (max=58)	39	49.3	48.5	46.4	46.5
sd	9.6	11.1	12.6	13.5	13.8
Feeding (max=11)	9.2	10.3	10.3	9.8	9.6
sd	2.1	1.5	1.7	2.4	2.2
Washing (max=17)	7.4	12.2	11.8	10.8	10.9
sd	2.8	4.3	5.8	5.5	5.6
Dressing (max=17)	11.2	14.6	14.6	14.1	14.7
sd	2.8	3.8	3.7	4.4	4.6
Toilet (max=13)	11.1	11.9	11.8	11.8	11.5
sd	3.1	2.1	2.5	2.6	3.2

Mean total self-help rose from 11 to 21 years, then declined slightly. Mean scores for washing and dressing followed a similar track, but feeding and toiletting appeared fairly well established by age 11 years and changed little after that. Both individual and total self-help scores were strongly related to IQ, at p=<.01 or better.

DIFFERENCES BY GENDER, PLACE OF REARING AND SOCIAL CLASS

Mean IQs of females have been consistently higher than those of males, the difference being significant at age 21 years; means of those brought up at home have been higher, though not significantly so, than those of the six brought up out of home; means of those from manual working class families have been higher, again non-significantly, than those from non-manual working class families.

Females had higher scores on all tests throughout the study. After controlling for IQ the difference was significant for expression and comprehension of language at age 35 years and for expression at age 40 years. Mean IQs of those brought up in their own homes have been somewhat higher than were those of the six brought up out of home, but the differences were small and diminished over time. Those from manual working class families had higher mean scores on IQ and self-help; those from non- manual working class families had higher mean scores on language (significant for comprehension at age 21 years and for expression at age 30years and for both at age 40 years); and for reading accuracy and comprehension at age 21 years and for reading comprehension at age 30 years; and for arithmetic at age 21 years.

CONCLUSION

Three findings from this study, although not peculiar to it, stand out for the writer. First, the wide variability - in abilities, personalities, interests - in people with DS; second, the overall superiority of females; and third, the close association of IQ with all the skills measured. This is particularly significant in view of the fact that the rapid decline in IQ in early childhood, seen in this and other studies, was halted after four years old, contrasting with results from some earlier studies (Cornwell & Birch 1969, Morgan 1979) which showed mean IQs declining by 12 and 25 points between the ages of 4 and 17 years. Language scores too increased to adulthood, declining slightly thereafter. Of the basic academic skills, reading is a relative strength for people with DS and was the only one of the skills assessed to increase throughout the study. Nevertheless, only two-fifths of the cohort gained a score on the test, and over half could not read any word, while arithmetical skills were very limited and hardly changed over 20 years. It seems that numeracy and literacy played only a small part in the regimes of the cohort's day placements, including in further education, and a strong case could be made out, in the interest of promoting the people's ability to live independently, for more emphasis on these topics in adult life.

REFERENCES

Bayley, N. (1964). *Manual of Directions for Infant Scales of Development.* National Institute of Mental Health.

Carr, J. (1975). Young Children with Down's Syndrome. London. Butterworths.

Carr, J. Forty years of life with Down's Syndrome. Submitted.

Cornwell, A.C. & Birch, H.G. (1969). Psychological and social development in home-reared children with Down's Syndrome (Mongolism). *American Journal of Mental Deficiency*, 74, 341-350.

Dunn, L.M., Dunn, L.M., Whetton, C. & Pintilie, D. (1982). The British Picture Vocabulary Scales. *Windsor: NFER-Nelson*.

Leiter, R.G. (1980). *Leiter International Performance Scale: instruction manual.* Chicago: Stoelting & Co.

Ludlow, J.R. & Allen, L.M. (1979). The effect of early intervention and pre-school stimulus on the development of the Down's syndrome child. *Journal of Mental Deficiency Research*, 23, 29-44.

Merrill-Palmer Scale of Mental Tests (1948). New York: Harcourt Brace & World.

Morgan, S.B. (1979). Adaptive skills in Down's Syndrome children. Mental Retardation, 17, 247-249.

Neale, M.D. (1958). *Neale Analysis of Reading Ability manual.* London: Macmillan.

Reynell, J. (1969). *Reynell Developmental Language Scale.* Slough, Bucks: National Foundation for Educational Research.

Vernon, P. (1960) *Intelligence and attainment tests.* London. University of London Press.

Wechsler, D. (1967). *The Wechsler Pre-School and Primary Scale of Intelligence.* New York: Psychological Corporation.

Wing, L. (1980).MRC handicaps, behavior and skills schedule in epidemiological research. *Acta Psychiatrica Scandinavcia,* Supplement 285, 62,241-247.

Chapter 11

SURVIVAL IN ELDERLY PERSONS
WITH DOWN SYNDROME

A.M.W. Coppus[1], H.M. Evenhuis[2], G.J. Verberne[3], F.E. Visser[4],
B.A. Oostra[5], P. Eikelenboom[6], W.A. van Gool[6], J.C. Janssens[7], and
C.M. van Duijn[8]

[1]Department of Epidemiology & Biostatistics, Erasmus MC,
Rotterdam, The Netherlands
[2]Department of General Practice, Intellectual Disability Medicine, Erasmus MC,
Rotterdam, The Netherlands
[3]Dichterbij, Center for the Intellectually Disabled, Gennep,
The Netherlands
[4]s'-HeerenLoo-Midden Nederland, Center for the Intellectually Disabled, Ermelo, The
Netherlands
[5]Department of Clinical Genetics, Erasmus MC, Rotterdam,
The Netherlands
[6]Department of Neurology, Academic Medical Center, Amsterdam,
The Netherlands
[7]Department of Public Health, Erasmus MC, Rotterdam, The Netherlands
[8]Department of Epidemiology & Biostatistics, Erasmus MC, Rotterdam, The Netherlands

INTRODUCTION

In recent decades there has been a distinct trend toward longer survival in persons with Down syndrome (DS) (Baird & Sadovnick, 1988), increasing from 9 years in 1929 to 12 in 1949 and 49 years in 1997 (Yang et al, 2002). In developed countries recent estimates indicate a mean age of death of older than 50 (Bittles et al, 2007, Glasson et al, 2003; Glasson et al, 2002; Janicki et al, 1999; Bittles et al, 2002). Despite major progress, persons with DS still show greater mortality rates early in life, as well as in later stages of life (Yang et al, 2002), suggesting that there still may be differences from the general population. In this chapter we further explore survival in older persons with DS. A expansion of this work is published elsewhere (Coppus et al, 2008).

METHODOLOGY

In a prospective longitudinal cohort study of dementia and mortality, 506 persons with DS aged 45 and older were followed for a mean of 4.5 years (range 0.0-7.6 years). All participants were monitored annually until they died (n = 109) or their representatives withdrew them from the study (n = 7), up to the reference date of January 1, 2007. At the time of study entry, each person received a complete assessment including interviews with relatives, caregivers, and their general practitioner. The medical records were reviewed to examine past or present disorders (e.g., cardiovascular risk factors, epilepsy and depression), mobility, and the possible use of drugs. All persons obtained a general physical and neurological examination and, if compliant, a venapuncture. The same questionnaires and interviews were used annually from 1999-2007.

Pre-morbid severity of intellectual disability was classified using the International Classification of Diseases, Tenth Revision (ICD-10) (WHO, 1992). The diagnosis of dementia was based on the ICD-10 Symptom Checklist for Mental Disorders (WHO, 1993), in particular, dementia and Alzheimer's disease, and according to the guidelines produced by an international consensus panel established under the auspices of the Aging Special Interest Group of the International Association for the Scientific Study of Intellectual Disabilities (IASSID) (Aylward et al, 1997). The diagnosis of dementia was supported using two observer-rated questionnaires, the Dementia Questionnaire for persons with an Intellectual Disability (DMR) (Evenhuis, 1992; 1996) and the Social Competence Rating Scale for persons with an Intellectual Disability (SRZ) (Krayer & Bildt, 2004).

Vital status was obtained using follow-up interviews and written correspondence. Information on causes of death was obtained from relatives or the primary caregivers of the deceased and was augmented with information from medical reports or autopsy records.

The risk of mortality according to participant characteristics and clinical diagnoses was investigated using Cox proportional hazards models, adjusting for age at baseline as a covariate. Follow-up time was defined according to date at entry and date at death or January 1, 2007. The risks of mortality between groups were compared by estimating hazard ratios in the Cox models. Survival analyses were performed in persons for whom complete data were available (75.8%).

The relationship between rate of decline in DMR and SRZ and risk of mortality was investigated in persons without dementia using a mixed-model repeated-measures procedure (Wothke, 2000). Decline in functioning was investigated in patients with at least 5 years of follow-up (n = 483), totaling five measurements of cognitive, functional and social ability. Mean DMR and SRZ scores were compared between survivors and decedents.

RESULTS

A total of 506 persons with DS were studied, of whom 304 were men (60.1%). At baseline the mean age was 51.9 for men (range 45-70) and 52.0 for women (range 45-77). The risk of mortality according to patient characteristics and different health conditions are described in Tables 1 and 2. Older persons at baseline, those with physical handicaps, those living in institutions, and those with a severe to profound level of intellectual disability were more likely to have died during follow-up (Table 1). The presence of at least one APOEε4 allele was associated with greater mortality risk.

Table 1. Mortality risk by baseline characteristics

Characteristics	HR (95%CI)*	p-value
-Age	1.15 (1.12-1.19)	p<0.001
-Sex	1.10 (0.75-1.63)	p=0.62
-Severity of Intellectual Disability	1.84 (1.22-2.77)	p=0.003
-Institutionalised	1.67 (1.08-2.57)	p=0.02
-APOEε4 present	1.58 (1.00-2.50)	p=0.05

*HR = Hazard Rate ,CI = confidence Interval.

Mortality risk was significantly related to morbidity (Table 2). We found a significant increase in mortality risk in those with dementia. In contrast to the general population, impaired mobility, severity of intellectual disability, the presence of epilepsy and visual impairment, not cardiovascular risk factors or sex, predicted survival. Finally, the Cox analysis was repeated including all covariates found to be related to mortality in a multivariate survival analysis. Only dementia (HR: 4.03, 95%CI = 2.16-7.49; p <0.001), age at baseline (HR: 1.11, 95%CI = 1.05-1.16; p <0.001) and a restricted mobility (HR: 1.92, 95%CI = 1.06-3.46; p = 0.03) remained significantly associated with mortality risk.

Table 2. Mortality risk by morbidity at baseline

Characteristic	HR (95%CI)*	p-value
Prevalent demented	2.91 (1.94-4.36)	p<0.001
Incident demented	1.97 (1.32-2.94)	p<0.001
Epilepsy	2.29 (1.50-3.48)	p<0.001
Depression	1.41 (0.91-2.19)	p=0.12
Cardio vascular risk factors	0.96 (0.59-1.57)	p=0.88
Visual impairment	2.33 (1.54-3.55)	p<0.001
Hearing impairment	1.55 (0.94-2.56)	p=0.08
Mobility with restriction	2.76 (1.85-4.14)	p<0.001

*HR = Hazard Rate,CI = Confidence Interval.

A decrease in function over the annual assessment periods was observed in the DMR and SRZ scores in all patients without dementia. Participants who had died after 5 years of follow-up showed significantly greater decline in functioning, than those who survived at all levels of performance (p < 0.001). Although it is difficult to detect a decline in those with the lowest level of performance, this decline, monitored by screening tests even in this group, is related to mortality. A relative preservation of cognitive and functional ability was associated with better survival.

CONCLUSION

Age and dementia have long been recognized as major predictors of mortality. This study demonstrates that other factors, such as severity of Intellectual Disability, mobility, morbidity, and social and functional skills also significantly contribute to survival.

REFERENCES

Aylward EH, Burt DB, Thorpe LU, Lai F, Dalton A. Diagnosis of dementia in individuals with intellectual disability. *J Intellect Disabil Res*.1997;41 (Pt 2):152-164.

Baird PA, Sadovnick AD. Life expectancy in Down syndrome adults. *Lancet,* 1988;2:1354-1356.

Bittles AH, Bower C, Hussain R, Glasson EJ. The four ages of Down syndrome. *Eur J Public Health.* 2007;17:221-225.

Bittles AH, Petterson BA, Sullivan SG, Hussain R, Glasson EJ, Montgomery PD. The influence of intellectual disability on life expectancy. *J Gerontol A Biol Sci Med Sci.* 2002;57:M470-472.

Coppus AM, Evenhuis HM, Verberne GJ, Visser FE, Oostra BA, Eikelenboom P, van Gool WA, Janssens AC, van Duijn CM. Survival in elderly *J Am Geriatr Soc.* 2008 ;56:2311-6.

Evenhuis HM. Evaluation of a screening instrument for dementia in ageing mentally retarded persons. *J Intellect Disabil Res.* 1992;36 (Pt 4):337-347.

Evenhuis HM. Further evaluation of the Dementia Questionnaire for Persons with MentalRetardation (DMR). *J Intellect Disabil Res.* 1996;40 (Pt 4):369-373.

Glasson EJ, Sullivan SG, Hussain R, Petterson BA, Montgomery PD, Bittles AH. Comparative survival advantage of males with Down syndrome. *Am J Hum Biol.* 2003;15:192-195.

Glasson EJ, Sullivan SG, Hussain R, Petterson BA, Montgomery PD, Bittles AH. The changing survival profile of people with Down's syndrome: implications for genetic counselling. *Clin Genet.* 2002;62:390-393.

Janicki MP, Dalton AJ, Henderson CM, Davidson PW. Mortality and morbidity among older adults with intellectual disability: health services considerations. *Disabil Rehabil.* 1999;21:284-294.

Krayer DWK, G.N. Bildt,AA.de. SRZ/SRZ1, Sociale Redzaamheidsschalen, Handleiding; 2004.

World Health Organization, ICD-10: International Statistical Classification of Diseases and related Health Problems, 10th revision. 1992.

World Health Organisation (1993). The ICD-10 Classification of Mental and Behavioral Disorders. Diagnostic Criteria for Research. Geneva: WHO.

Wothke. Longitudinal and multi-group modeling with missing data. Modeling longitudinal and multilevel data: practical issues, applied approaches and specific examples: Mahwah,NJ: Lawrence Erlbaum Associates; 2000.

Yang Q, Rasmussen SA, Friedman JM. Mortality associated with Down's syndrome in the USA from 1983 to 1997: a population-based study. *Lancet,*2002;359:1019-1025.

Chapter 12

HOW DO PERSONS WITH SEVERE AND PROFOUND INTELLECTUAL DISABILITIES EXPERIENCE THEIR APPROACHING DEATH AND HOW CAN THEY BE SUPPORTED

M. Maaskant[1], R.M. van de Kerkhof[2], H. van Bomme[3], and W. van de Wouw[4]

[1]Governor Kremers Center of the University of Maastricht (Dpt. Health Care and Nursing Science), the Netherlands
[2]Lunetzorg, Eindhoven, the Netherlands
[3]Severinus, Veldhoven, the Netherlands
[4]Máxima Medisch Centrum, Eindhoven, the Netherlands

INTRODUCTION

A person's life is finite. When confronted with their approaching death, people will react in their own ways. This is true for persons with intellectual disabilities (ID), as it is for others. During the last decade, there has been an increase in publications on death and dying of persons with ID (Table 1). Publications on this topic tend to focus on persons with mild and moderate ID. In this text, we focus on persons with severe and profound ID. We explain how these persons experience their approaching death and how their mourning can take place. We suggest methods to recognise behavioral signs and we give suggestions for supporting these persons.

We base our text and suggestions on several publications on development, death and dying in persons with ID, and on our own experiences with this topic. Current knowledge is still scarce, and a lot of the required knowledge is still lacking. We see this text as a beginning and hope that others will follow.

Table 1. Recent publications on death and dying of persons with ID

Blackman 2002; 2003; 2008
Brickell & Munir, 2008
Dodd et al, 2005; 2008
Dowling et al, 2006
Gault 2003
Gilrane et al, 2007
Hollins et al, 2003
Mappin & Hanlon, 2005
McEvoy et al 2002
McEvoy & Smith, 2005
Meeusen et al, 2006
Read 2007
Read & Elliott, 2007
Tuffrey-Wijne 2007

UNDERSTANDING DEATH

It is not plausible that persons with profound ID have a clear understanding of the concept of death. Persons with profound ID experience the world from a concrete level: the only things that exist are those that can be seen, felt, heard, smelled or touched. They are not able to make a distinction between their own body and its surroundings (Meeusen et al, 2006). Their communication is limited and usually non-verbal. They do not recognize their own emotions or of others; consequently it is not possible to talk about emotions with them. There is no conscious understanding of life and thus not of death either. Or, one might say, caregivers (family, other close relatives, professional staff) are not really able to know if they feel or know those things.

A message about their nearing death will not be meaningful to them in ways we assume for others. Accordingly, persons with profound ID will not pass the stages of grief, i.e., denial, anger, bargaining, depression, acceptance (Embregts, 2002). At least, it is not noticeable for caregivers that persons with profound ID pass through these stages.

However, persons with profound ID will notice their decreasing abilities and physical infirmities, and may react to that with anger or irritation. The loss of abilities and functions usually impacts on established structures and patterns as well. Caregivers' behaviors or mood (either consciously or unconsciously) will change as well, because they react on the sad message by being upset, sad, angry or resigned. Persons with profound ID will feel that something is going on and react on these changes as well.

Persons with severe ID have a better understanding of emotions, life and death than persons with profound ID. Nevertheless, they do not fully understand the concept of death. Persons with severe ID watch the world around them from their own perspectives. They are capable of distinguishing between their own personalities and those of others, but hardly can put themselves in somebody else's position (egocentric thinking) (Meeusen & Van Bommel, 2006). They more or less are able to connect illness and death of others and themselves. They even may conclude that before the message has been told. With these persons, consciousness is in its formative stages, as are certain values and norms. They cling to established structures and patterns, because in this way the world is reliable and manageable. Basic emotions as 'sadness' and 'joy' are recognized. It is possible to talk about these emotions with them. Imagination and reality tend to be mixed up. In this phase of magic thinking, involving the creation of imaginary pictures help them to come to terms with death.

Apparently, persons with severe ID do not pass the stages of grief, because they lack the real understanding of the concept of death. They may name death, but hardly realize what death really means. For example, they may think that death is reversible or temporary. When they heard about their own nearing death, they may react soberly or deny it later on or regard it as an exciting event. Their magic thinking may not only result in unreal ideas, but also in fearful perceptions of death, often linked with concrete impressions (their soul really will leave the body when dying, thereby making a hole in the body).

The increasing loss of functions and abilities may result in feelings of sadness and anger
These feelings are being taken out on one and all, alternating with needs for closeness.

Expressions of anger and jealousy towards those who are healthy may be present. They may ask for a lot of (negative) attention in order to cope with the changing situations they notice but in fact do not really understand.

UNDERSTANDING SIGNALS

Persons with profound and severe ID usually have limited communication skills and must rely on caregivers who try to understand their signals and behavior. In dying processes, it is essential that caregivers are able to see and understand behavior and body language.

Instruments for detecting distress (e.g., DISDAT (Regnard et al, 2007) and pain in nonverbal clients (e.g., KIDPAINS (Van Hastenberg & van Dongen, 2007), video analyses (Embregts, 2002; Heijoop, 1982), life stories and empathic stories (Hewitt, 1998; Meininger, 2006) are useful for this.

In addition, carers should know about experiencing pain (e.g., high pain thresholds in Prader Willi syndrome), aberrant reactions to medication, misdiagnosing symptoms (e.g., challenging behavior attributed to the aetiology of ID instead of physical discomfort or illness).

SUPPORT

It is not useful to try to make persons with profound ID who are terminally ill understand what death really is. It is essential to offer closeness by offering physical contact in a warm, familiar and safe atmosphere. Soft voices, respectful touching, soft favourite music and favourite cuddly toys or other materials are therefore useful.

It is valuable for daily life that established structures and patterns are being continued as much as possible when abilities and functions decrease, unless good alternatives are available. It also is important to recognize concrete experience and changes (in both persons and circumstances) and to offer room for reactions on these changes.

Caregivers must be aware of the ways their attitudes may have changed because of their knowledge about the illness and it prospects. It is logical that their attitudes change (consciously or unconsciously), but they have to be aware of its impact for the ill persons.

For persons with severe ID, it is also not useful to try to elucidate the concept of death. For them, it is important just to be there (especially non-verbally) and to offer trust and safety. This can be reached by making daily life clear and familiar with as much established structures and patterns as possible, since the world becomes fearful and unreliable when these structures and patterns disappear.

Play and drawings are useful instruments to express emotions and experiences. Questions by persons with severe ID have to be answered as concretely and literally as possible. However, imaginations of death (magic thinking) have to be cleared up in order to prevent fear about sickness and death. In the meantime, attention has to be paid to their imaginations that may appear rather childish. Such childish imaginations belong to the social-emotional stage of persons with severe ID (Meeusen et al, 2006).

Caregivers must not feel undaunted when an ill person with severe ID is not willing to talk about illness and death or is not willing to include the exact topic in play. It is not useful to try to break the defence mechanisms or to disagree. It is important to respect the feelings. The topic can possibly be talked about via less emotionally charged themes or via indirect play.

As the developmental level is higher, persons with severe ID will ask more questions. From a developmental age of approximately 4 years, more 'why-questions' will be asked, both verbally and non-verbally. It is essential to answer these questions, but in small, manageable doses at appropriate moments and in suitable situations.

Whenever possible, persons involved must maintain their autonomy, even when it only regards rather small things. As with persons with profound ID, caregivers have to be aware of their own attitudes and the way they express their (logical) emotions. Their behavior and emotions must not result in additional fear, sadness and unsteadiness related to the persons they take care of.

CONCLUSION

This text deals with experiencing approaching death of persons with profound and severe ID and how they can be supported. It is very important that persons with ID are being supported when they are confronted with loss and/or when they are terminally ill or dying.

Naturally, everyone reacts in his own way to sad messages. For persons with ID, the level of ID and social-emotional development impact their reactions in rather substantial ways. But level of ID is not the only impact; earlier experiences, parenting, education, religion, and culture impact the reactions as well.

The descriptions we gave, are given as guidelines, not as set facts. We strongly recommend and hope to develop the topic further and that others will do the same. Evaluating methods to support terminally ill persons with (profound and severe) ID is essential, not only for them but for caregivers as well.

REFERENCES

Blackman, N. (2003). Loss, Attachment and Learning Disability. London: Woth Publishing.

Blackman, N. (2008) The Development of an Assessment Tool for the Bereavement Needs of People with Learning Disabilities. *British Journal of Learning Disabilities*, 36, 3, 165-170.

Blackman, N.J. (2002) Grief and Intellectual Disability: A Systemic Approach. *Journal of Gerontological Social Work*, 38, 1-2, 253-263.

Brickell, C., Munir, K. (2008) Grief and its complications in individuals with intellectual disability. *Harvard* Review of *Psychiatry*, 16, 1, 1-12.

Dodd, P., Dowling, S., Hollins, S. (2005) A Review of the Emotional, Psychiatric and Behavioral Responses to Bereavement in People with Intellectual Disabilities. *Journal of Intellectual Disability Research*, 49, 7, 537-543.

Dodd, P., Guerin, S., McEvoy, J., Buckley, S., Tyrrell, J., Hillery, J. (2008) A Study of Complicated Grief Symptoms in People with Intellectual Disabilities. *Journal of Intellectual Disability Research*, 52, 5, 415-425.

Dowling, S., Hubert, J., White, S; Hollins, S. (2006) Bereaved Adults with Intellectual Disabilities: A Combined Randomized Controlled Trial and Qualitative Study of Two Community Based Interventions. *Journal of Intellectual Disability Research*, 50, 4, 277-287.

Embregts, P.J.C.M. (2002) Effects of video feedback on social behavior of young people with mild intellectual disability and staff responses. *International Journal of Disability, Development and Education*, 49, 1, 105-116.

Gault, J. (2003) Bereavement: helping a patient with a learning disability to cope. *Nursing Times*, 99, 1, 26-27

Gilrane McGarry, U., Taggart, L (2007) An exploration of the support received by people with intellectual disabilities who have been bereaved. *Journal of Research in Nursing*, 12, 2, 129-144.

Heijkoop, J. (1982) Videobandanalyse, unieke informatiebron bij mediatietherapie (Videotape analysis: A unique information source in mediation therapy.) *Gedragstherapie*, 15, 1, 58-64.

Hewitt, H. (1998) Life-story books for people with learning disabilities. *Nursing Times*, 94, 33, 61-63.

Hollins S., Blackman N, Dowling S., Brighton, C. (2003) When somebody dies. London: The Royal College of Psychiatrists.

Mappin, R., Hanlon, D. (2005) Description And Evaluation Of A Bereavement Group For People With Learning Disabilities. *British Journal of Learning Disabilities*, 33, 3, 106-112.

McEvoy, J., Reid, Y., Guerin, S. (2002) Emotion recognition and concept of death in people with learning disabilities. *British Journal of Developmental Disabilities*, 48, 95, 2, 83-89.

McEvoy, J., Smith, E. (2005) Families Perceptions of the Grieving Process and Concept of Death in Individuals with Intellectual Disabilities. *British Journal of Developmental Disabilities*, 51, 100, 1, 17-25.

Meininger, H.P. (2006) Narrating, Writing, Reading: Life Story Work as an Aid to (Self) Advocacy. *British Journal of Learning Disabilities*, 34, 3, 181-188.

Meeusen R, Van Bommel H, Van de Wouw W, Maaskant M. Perceptions of death and management of grief in people with intellectual disability. *Journal of Policy and Practice in Intellectual Disabilities*, 2006, 3, 2, 95-104.

Read, S. (2007) An exploration of the supports received by people with learning disabilities who have been bereaved. *Journal of Research in Nursing*, 12, 2, 145-146.

Read, S., Elliott, D. (2007) Exploring a continuum of support for bereaved people with intellectual disabilities: a strategic approach. *Journal of Intellectual Disability Research*, 11, 2, 167-181.

Regnard C, Reynolds J, Watson B, Matthews D, Gibson L, Clarke C. Understanding distress in people with severe communication difficulties: developing and assessing the Disability Distress Assessment Tool (DisDAT). *Journal of Intellectual Disability Research*, 2007, 51, 4, 277-92.

Tuffrey-Wijne IMM. Palliative care for people with intellectual disabilities. Maastricht: PhD-Thesis Maastricht University, 2007.

Van Hastenberg-van Dongen KAJ. Translating Pain; assessing expressive pain behavior of children with severe to profound intellectual disabilities. Maastricht: PhD-Thesis Maastricht University, 2004.

Chapter 13

THE FRAILTY SYNDROME IN OLDER PERSONS WITH INTELLECTUAL DISABILITIES

B. Brehmer

University of Vienna, Faculty of Psychology, Liebigg. 5.Vienna Austria

INTRODUCTION

Whereas frailty publications involving the general population substantially increased during the last two decades, research on frailty related issues in people with intellectual disabilities (ID) does not exist. Nevertheless, the word "frailty" has been used in ID literature more often recently, with its use mostly limited to aging issues of family carers (e.g. Barton, 1998). But still, in the field of ID the concept of frailty has no empirical foundation. Currently, frailty researchers discuss frailty and disability as different but overlapping concepts.

This study referred to the **theoretical work by Rockwood** (1994). He suggested a dynamic frailty model: Frailty is like a balance beam, in which the balance between assets and deficits determines whether a person can maintain good health and independence. Clearly, his perception of frailty does not solely focus on physiological symptoms but defines frailty as a dynamic, complex interaction of biological, psychological, cognitive and social factors. Further, Rockwood (2000) postulates five criteria for defining frailty:

- multisystemic instability,
- allowance for heterogeneity within a population,
- change over time,
- association with an increased risk of adverse outcomes,
- association with aging.

The **development of the frailty measurement** for this study was based on in-depth analysis of about 200 articles on frailty. The analysis suggested the development of a new assessment tool, because no instrument fulfilled the criteria by Rockwood or assessed "multisystemic impairments". Most instruments included only physical symptoms, rarely cognitive or psychological health outcomes and only one measurement (Schuurmanns et al., 2004) considered social factors.

First, all previous frailty variables were sorted in four domains (physical, psychological, cognitive and social) to fulfil the criterion "multisystemic instability" by Rockwood. Like in previous research publications the instrumental activities of daily living (IADL) were grouped into the cognitive domain, although for some of those items a good physical health is also necessary (e.g. washing clothes). These four lists were presented to 42 multi-professional experts (general physicians, geriatricians, clinical psychologists and educational scientists with experience in ID), who were instructed to rank the items within these lists according to what they thought were the most important factors for the development of frailty. For example, according to their expertise the activities of daily living (ADL) items, falls, a worsened mobility and balance and also incontinence are the most important variables of the physical domain. The experts were also asked to rank the four domains and they perceived the physical domain to be of highest importance for the development of frailty, with the psychological coming second and the cognitive third. The social domain was deemed least important.

Two other Rockwood criteria are central for the **design of a frailty questionnaire**: "change over time" and "association with an increased risk of adverse outcomes". The criterion "change over time" affects the wording of the items. Typical items would be "Has your vision <u>changed</u>?", "Did it get <u>worse</u>?" and "<u>Since when</u> did it get worse?" This response format considers the fact that people with severe or profound disabilities might have always suffered from restrictions in one or more area(s), which would be no indicator for frailty.

Concluding, the present study used a **two-fold frailty criterion**:

[1]   Negative health outcomes in three or four domains according to the criterion "multisystemic impairment".

[2]   A minimum of six negative health outcomes: Steverink's "Groningen Frailty Indicator" (2001) used a cut off of five and above for frailty with a maximum score of 15. Therefore, the present study used a cut off of six and above for defining a person as frail (maximum score of 33).

Frailty data was collected by trained interviewers through self-report and third party interviews. They were conducted within the Austrian part of the POMONA II EU-project "Health Indicators for People with Intellectual Disabilities", in a representative sample of 190 people with ID, aged between 18 and 76 years (Brehmer, 2008). Data was gathered between November 2006 and November 2007. The frailty questionnaire was included in the POMONA protocol.

RESULTS

First, psychometric properties of the frailty instrument will be presented, the frail sample will be characterised, and the course of frailty will be discussed.

In a first step Cronbach's Alpha was calculated for the 33 frailty variables. Cronbach's Alpha was satisfying with a value of .803. After exclusion of 14 inappropriate items (low adjusted item–scale correlations), Cronbach's Alpha rose to a value of 0.854 and Guttman's split half reliability was of similar satisfaction with a value of 0.72. An exploratory factor analysis explained a total variance of 59.81% with three resulting factors. The first factor represented the physical domain, including all ADL items. The second component contained all IADL items. Those variables were positively related to the first factor. The third factor included all mental health/psychological items. The social items were excluded before calculation, because of their low reliability.

Characteristics of the Frail Sample

Altogether, 17 subjects (9%) of the sample (age 18 to 73 years) fulfilled both frailty criteria. For the general population Ostir (2004) estimated that 10-25% of the population older than 65 years are frail. Considering that life expectancy is approximately 10 to 15 years lower for people with ID, the prevalence for people with ID over 50 years was 27% and therefore quite similar to the general population.

The median age in the frail sample was 61. Non-frail persons seemed to be significantly younger with a median age of 39 (p= .000). So Rockwood's criterion "association with aging" was verified for people with ID.

The level of disability was determined through appraisal by third parties (front line staff and the interviewer). The frail population included more persons with mild or moderate disability (82%; n= 14) and only three people with severe disability. This result supports the hypothesis that disability and frailty are different constructs.

No differences could be observed between the frail and non-frail subgroups concerning gender and living situation. Frail people with ID were located more often in institutional settings (65%) and more often in urban regions (53%). Although some researchers (e.g. Fried, 2001) reported higher frailty prevalence in the general population for women, only a trend could be detected in the ID population: Women with ID (frail 53% vs. non-frail 48%) are more frequently frail than men (frail 47% vs. non-frail 52%).

Frailty Developmental Course

To date some researchers have suggested theoretical etiology models of frailty, but none have been statistically verified (e.g. Morley, 2002, Mühlberg and Sieber, 2004). In the present study the frailty development can be described in a retrospective way. The following is one example:

> Jennifer is a 45-year-old woman with Down-Syndrome, who still lives with her family. Jennifer relies on assistance during the interview. Her medical history shows high blood pressure. She is obese (BMI 33).

> **Jennifer's Frailty Course:**
> Seven years ago, Jennifer's social life changed – two of her friends moved away and one family member died. She described this event as traumatic. More than five years ago her vision and hearing ability and two years ago her physical strength began to decline. Since then she has become more anxious to fall and hurt herself. Her carer mentioned that she generally

became more nervous and anxious. Both Jennifer and her carer name a general health decline, problems with her memory skills and grip strength. They cannot provide an exact date to the three negative changes. Therefore she had to stop working in the last months.

For the whole frailty subgroup it can be noticed that the frailty process started around the age of 50 years and was continuing since eight years. Typically frailty started with negative changes in the social or psychological domain. The most frequently mentioned changes in the last stage were: an awareness of a general health decline, increased medication and psychological changes like memory difficulties.

CONCLUSION

Based on the knowledge of frailty in the general population, this concept was successfully introduced to the ID population and this type of research seems to be very helpful to trace health changes. Although the specially constructed questionnaire had satisfying psychometric properties, the wording, the item content (e.g. the social domain) and the interview technique should be revised with the participation of self-advocates.

Also, findings reveal a similar prevalence rate to the general population. Frailty and disability are two different challenges: People with ID can additionally develop the frailty syndrome, which typically has its onset after the age of 50. However, the impact of the disability level and/or the disability aetiology on the frailty condition in later life needs clarification. It remains unclear whether the frailty syndrome of persons with a severe or profound ID progresses faster and thus in a different way compared to persons with a mild or moderate ID. For better understanding of the interaction between intellectual disability and frailty and for the development of prevention strategies, longitudinal research is recommended.

REFERENCES

Barton, R. (1998). Family involvement in the pre-discharge assessment of long-stay patients with learning disabilities: a *qualitative study*. *Journal of Intellectual Disabilities*, 2, 79-88.

Brehmer, B., Zeilinger, E. & Weber, G. (2008). Gesundheit von erwachsenen Menschen mit intellektueller Behinderung. Bericht zum POMONA Projekt. Psychologie in Österreich, 5.

Fried, L.P., Tangen, C.M. & Walston, J. (2001) Frailty in older adults: Evidence for a phenotype. *Journal of Gerontology: Medical Science*, 56A, M146-M156.

Morley, J.E., Perry, H.M. III, Miller, D.K. (2002) Editorial: Something about frailty. Journal of Gerontology: *Medical Science*, 57A, M698-M704.

Mühlberg, W., Sieber C. (2004) Sarcopenia and frailty in geriatrics patients: implications for training and prevention. *Zeitschrift für Gerontologie und Geriatrie*, 37, 2-8.

Ostir, G.V, Ottenbacher, K.J, Markides, K.S. (2004) Onset of frailty in older adults and the protective role of positive affect. *Psychology and Aging*, 19, 402–408.

Rockwood, K., Fax, R.A., et al. (1994) Frailty in elderly people: an evolving concept. *Canadian Medical Association Journal*, 150, 489-495.

Rockwood, K., Hogan, D.B., Mac Knight, C. (2000) Conceptualization and measurement of frailty in elderly people. *Drugs Aging*, 17, 295-302.

Schuurmans, H., Steverink, N. und Lindenberg, S. (2004) Old or frail: What tells us more? Journal of Gerontology: *Medical Science*, 59A, 962-965.

Steverink, N., Slaets, J.P.J, Schuumans, H. und Van Lis, M. (2001) Measuring frailty: developing and testing the GFI. *Gerontologist*, 41.

Chapter 14

SUPPORTING AGING ADULTS WITH INTELLECTUAL DISABILITIES

R. Hole[1], T. Stainton[1]. and L. Willson[1]

[1]School of Social Work, University of British Columbria
Okanagan, Canada

INTRODUCTION

Dramatic changes in life expectancy for individuals with intellectual disabilities (ID) have occurred in the last 50 years (Bigby, 2002); and, research on adults with ID consistently demonstrates that the life expectancy of individuals with a disability continues to rise as health and social conditions continue to improve (Delorme, 1999; Heller, 2000; Lawrence & Roush, 2008). These trends in the population of adults with ID reflects the changing demographics in Canada; in 2006[1], there were approximately 47, 290 adults between the ages of 45-64 and 7,260 adults over the age of 65 years living with ID[2] (Participation and Activity Limitation Study, 2006). As a result, supports and services for seniors with developmental disabilities and their families are an increasingly urgent issue. As one focus of a 3-year research project in British Columbia [B.C.], Canada, this paper outlines findings of a descriptive qualitative study that explored the views of adults with ID and their family members concerning services and supports for aging adults with ID.

METHODOLOGY

Focus groups and individual interviews were conducted with 35 self-advocates and 70 family members throughout the province of B.C. Interviews centered on four broad topic

---

[1] According to the 2006 census the population of Canada was 31,612,897.

[2] These rates are an underestimation of this population. According to Boyd (1997), prevalence rates of 1-3% have been used to estimate the number of aging adults with developmental disabilities. However, it is difficult to accurately identify precise figures because there are a large number of individuals still unknown to formal service providers.

areas: transition services for young adults; residential services; non-residential services; and, services for seniors. In total, 11 self-advocates and 11 family members participated in the interviews focusing on services to seniors. The interviews were digitally recorded and, subsequently, transcribed verbatim. Thematic analysis (Braun & Clarke, 2006) was used to compare, contrast, and categorize the data into themes (both within and across transcripts). For this paper, findings related to the topic "services for seniors" are presented.

FINDINGS

Voices of Self-Advocates

The findings of this study reflect a diversity of views with respect to aging adults' plans and hopes for the future. When asked about their future hopes and wishes, many participants expressed their desire to continue participating in the activities they currently enjoy. Participants also talked about their desire to retire and to be a "senior" while emphasizing particular leisure activities that they would enjoy: e.g., music, photography, and arts and crafts. Thus, for many participants, retirement was associated with opportunity to pursue other activities such as travel and participate in leisure activities. Interestingly, when talking about retirement, many participants expressed the desire to keep working. The diversity of views with respect to future plans and desires points to the importance of assessing the individual needs and wishes of each person when planning with them for their future.

When asking participants about their future concerns several themes emerged. Crawford (2004) found that self-advocates expressed concern about issues of isolation; loneliness; no one being there to listen; no one with authority to speak on their behalf; and, lack of relationships, generally. Similarly, the participants in the present study expressed concerns relating to issues of relationships and security; particularly about aging parents, living arrangements, and loneliness. For example, one participant expressed, "...if my dad dies, what will the future be for me?" Another participant was dissatisfied that he had to move to a different neighbourhood than the one where he and his mother had lived. He shared, "and one thing is my mom died of a heart attack...it was hard for me to take...I didn't have any choice [where to live]...so I found it was too far for me." Finally, loneliness was an issue that participants spoke to with respect to aging and not being able to get out as often. For example, one participants shared, "I wish I could do more like I want to be doing more so I wouldn't feel so like I'm not all alone I feel sometimes like during the day when everybody is working I feel I should be doing something but I'm not."

Voices of Family Members

The findings from the interviews with family members of aging adults with ID reflect the current Canadian landscape where the increasing lifespan of aging adults and their unique needs are emerging in a context where the social care architecture – programs, services, systems, and policies – are fragmented and lagging in response to the growing demographic changes (Stainton, Hole, Charles, Yodanis, Powell, & Crawford, 2006). Thus, prominent findings centerd on the identification of barriers to supports and gaps in services as well as the importance of "proactive planning" as opposed to "crisis planning".

Repeatedly, family members expressed concerns about barriers to and gaps in supports and services. For example, with respect to formal services family members stressed concerns pertaining to funding and the implications that scarce resources have for individual choice. In particular, family members stressed the importance of choice with respect to aging in place. Family members wanted to ensure that their loved one will live in a home where she/he was content, comfortable, and safe: family members wanted to know that their loved one would be okay and happy. With respect to informal supports and services, many family members shared that their experiences of support networks dissolving/changing over time led to uncertainty and concerns with respect to future supports for their aging adult child. For example, one parent stated, "…as you get older a lot of these people will pass and a lot of them move away and your support system kind of does almost eradicate and there's not much you can do about it, it's all very…Life goes on and you just seem to be stuck here and life goes on for the people who are leaving ___ life takes them elsewhere… [who will be around when I'm no longer here?]" The uncertainty relating to possible supports and services and concerns for the future led to many family members stressing the importance of planning for the future. In particular, participants distinguished between "crisis planning" and "proactive planning".

Repeatedly family members of aging adults with ID expressed the importance of pro-active planning for the future rather than waiting for a crisis to happen. For these family members, there was recognition of the need to create some kind of plan to provide stability in the face of future changes. In fact, the need for proactive planning was articulated as a response to concerns about the future. For example, one parent expressed, "…everybody is concerned what's going to happen when we're not longer around right and our group, the parents who have kept their kids at home and I mean they're in their sixties, seventies and eighties and they're still, their children are still at home with them." And, another aging parent shared, "I'm really concerned. I'm sixty-three and she's eighteen so there's a huge difference and I will be gone for many years of her life and I'm the only one left. So it is a real source of concern for me, for somebody to watch out for her when I'm gone." Thus, there was a strong argument articulated by these participants that planning for the future was paramount and urgent, and the participants emphasized that such planning should be pro-active. Finally, in exploring what pro-active planning might look like, participants emphasized the following key points: the importance of living arrangements, the importance of choice, the value of social networks, and, the need for attending to legal issues – particularly ensuring that aging adults with an intellectual disability had an advocate.

CONCLUSION

Adults with ID are living longer and more independently than ever before. Given the primacy that families in this study placed on proactive planning and the underlying concerns about their loved one's future, a number of recommendations become paramount. Currently, the services and systems in place to support aging adults with ID and their families are fragmented leaving family members uncertain as to the various options available. Clear and explicit policy to guide action and practice is needed. Families and individuals need support to plan for the future that places primacy on choice and self-determination; such an emphasis implicates the value and importance of transparency with respect to different options. Such options might explore concepts such as aging in place, residential options as one ages, non-residential supports, retirement plans, and, ongoing work and leisure activities. Finally, as aging brings to the fore issues of transition and uncertainty, options for legal and financial planning need to be unequivocally addressed in the planning process.

REFERENCES

Bigby, C. (2002). Aging people with a lifelong disability: challenges for the aged care and disability sectors. *Journal of Intellectual & Developmental Disability*, 27(4), 231-241.

Braun V & Clarke V. (2006)Using thematic analysis in psychology. *Qualitative Research in Psychology*, 3, 77-101.

Crawford, C. (2004). Coming of Age: Securing Positive Futures for Seniors with Intellectual Disabilities. L'Institut Roeher Institute. June, 2004, 54 pages.

Delorme, M. (1999). Aging and people with developmental disabilities. In I. Brown, & M. Percy (Eds.), Developmental disabilities in Ontario (First Edition ed., pp. 189-195). Toronto, Ontario: Front Porch Publishing, Toronto.

Heller, T., Miller, A. B., Hsieh, K. & Sterns, H. (2000). Later life planning: Promoting knowledge of options and choice making, *Mental Retardation*, 38, 5, 395-406.

Lawrence, S. & Roush, S. E. (2008). Examining pre-retirement and related services offered to service-users with an intellectual disability in Ireland. *Journal of Intellectual Disabilities*, 12, 3, 239-252.

Participation and Activity Limitation Survey. (2001). Statistics Canada.

Stainton, T., Hole, R., Charles, G., Yodanis, C., Powell, S., & Crawford, C. Residential Options for Adults with Developmental Disabilities: Quality and Cost Outcomes. The Ministry of Children and Family Development, Province of British Columbia. Oct, 2006. 60 pages.

Chapter 15

TALKING TO OLDER WOMEN WITH INTELLECTUAL DISABILITIES ABOUT PARTICIPATING IN BREASTCANCER SCREENING

D.S. Willis[1], C.K. Kennedy[1] and L. Kilbride[1]

[1]School of Nursing, Midwifery & Social Care, Edinburgh Napier University, Edinburgh, Scotland

INTRODUCTION

The greater longevity in people with intellectual disabilities (ID) means that they will also experience the same age related illnesses as those in the general population (Tuffrey-Wijne et al, 2007). One of the most common age related illnesses is cancer (McPherson et al, 2006). Cancer Research UK (2009) report that in 2006, there were 154,162 deaths from cancer, accounting for 27% of all deaths in the UK. Forty seven percent of all cancer deaths occur from cancers of the lung, bowel, breast and prostate (Cancer Research UK, 2009). Relatively little, however, is known about cancer with respect to incidence, morbidity and mortality in people with ID; as research on morbidity and mortality generally relates to respiratory and cardiovascular conditions rather than cancer (Hogg et al. 2001).

The prevailing health message from the Scottish and other Governments across the developed world, places responsibility fro health with the individual (Scottish Executive, 2005). Cancer prevention therefore tends to focus on early detection, by raising public awareness to the early warning signs so that early treatment is obtained through mass population screening programmes. There are currently 3 national cancer screening programmes in operation in the UK, breast, cervical and bowel cancer. The focus of this summary is breast screening as breast cancer is the most common cancer in women with over 45,000 cases diagnosed in 2005 and accounts for approximately 31% (nearly 1 in 3) of all female cancers (Cancer Research UK, 2009).

All women aged between 50 and 70 years of age in the UK are eligible to attend the free National Health Service Breast Screening Programme (NHSBCSP) as long as they are registered with a general practitioner. Women are invited to attend every 3 years and invitations are centrally organised and automatically sent to eligible women from local screening units. Greater longevity means more women with ID will become eligible to participate in the NHSBCSP, but low up-take of the service amongst women with ID is reported (NHS Health Scotland 2004).

It is estimated that between 5–10% of breast cancers are inherited with the genes BRCA1 and BRCA2 being identified as responsible (McPherson et al. 2006). After hereditary factors, sex and increasing age amplify the risk of getting breast cancer. Risk factors associated with development of the disease include: excessive alcohol intake (Tjonneland et al, 2007), high fat diets (Blackburn et al, 2003), low physical exercise, obesity (Key et al, 2003) and being nulliparous (McPherson et al, 2006). For women with ID, these risks pose serious problems as people with ID generally have higher incidences of obesity, lower levels of exercise, a poorer diet and high level of nulliparity compared to the general population (Bell & Bhate, 1992; Carlson & Wilson, 1996; Rimmer, 1994; Melville et al, 2005). In their favour, they are considered low consumers of alcohol and have protective factors such as low oestrogen levels (Carlson & Wilson, 1996) and earlier menopause (Carr & Hollins, 1995; Cosgrove et al, 1999; Schupf et al, 1997, 2003; Seltzer et al, 2001).

The incidence of breast cancer in women with ID is disputed and little epidemiological evidence has been undertaken. UK evidence suggests a lower incidence of breast cancer than the general population (Jancar & Jancar, 1977; Carter & Jancar, 1983; Jancar, 1990; Cooke, 1997) and is supported by epidemiological work conducted in Australia (Sullivan et al, 2003, 2004c; Sullivan and Hussain, 2004b). In contrast, population data in Finland suggested a comparable incidence to the general population (Patja et al, 2001). There is a suggestion that breast cancer may be even lower in women with Down syndrome (DS). Genetic work conducted on the genes on chromosome 21 (the chromosome abnormality responsible for DS) suggest chromosome 21 may have a negative effect on tumour onset and progression (Zorick et al, 2001; Benard et al, 2005). Cellular work conducted on well differentiated stroma (a connective tissue cell in organs found in the loose connective tissue) is thought to explain the absence of breast cancer in DS (Satge´ et al, 1998; Hasle et al, 2000; Satge´ & Sasco, 2002a,b; Sullivan & Hussain, 2004b). A review of the epidemiological evidence about DS and breast cancer can be found in Willis et al (2008a).

Low up-take in women with ID is well documented (Piachaud et al, 1998; Piachaud & Rohde,1998; Djuretic et al., 1999; Sullivan et al, 2003, 2004a,b; Pehl & Hunt, 2004) although 3 studies note higher up-take (Davies & Duff, 2001; Biswas et al, 2005; Gesualdi, 2006). Low up-take in women with ID has been seen associated with a number of potential barriers to breast screening. These barriers are wide ranging and include not being registered with a doctor, poor literacy skills, physical and intellectual ability level, ill health, moving home/area, transport, fear of the procedure, radiographer's, GP and carers attitudes (Stein, 2000; Davies & Duff, 2001, Sullivan et al. 2003, 2004b,c; Biswas et al, 2005; Isaacs, 2006; NHS Cancer Screening Programme, 2006). A number of strategies have been employed to improve breast screening up-take (usually educational interventions to the women and their carers)(Pehl & Hunt, 2004; Symonds & Howsam, 2004; Isaacs, 2006). A critical review of this literature can be found in Willis et al (2008b).

Whether women with ID should attend breast screening has been debated especially those with severe/profound, mental, or physical disabilities and women with DS (Satge´ & Sasco, 2002a,b; Sullivan and Hussain, 2004). Stronger evidence is available for women with DS due to the reported lower incidence of breast cancer and because they may be more vulnerable to ionising radiations, particularly X-rays (Satge´ & Sasco, 2002a,b). There are alternatives to breast screening such as breast examination and awareness however not all women with ID have the motor or cognitive skills to perform or understand breast checks. Carers could perform the breast checks but feel untrained to provide such support, or suggest it is the remit of the health professionals (Davies & Duff 2001; Poynor, 2003; Sullivan et al, 2004c). Failure of carers to address health needs can be seen as failing in the duty to care (Nursing and Midwifery Council, 2004), although, The Royal College of Nursing (1999) state that only trained specialists should perform breast checks. Given the numbers of carers that would need to be involved, the possibility of training carers to undertake breast checks seems uneconomical (Gillings-Taylor, 2004).

Participatory research approaches are used and recommended in health care, it is disappointing that to date women with ID have been asked on a limited basis about why they do not participate in breast screening. Two unpublished studies (Pehl,1999; cited in Pehl & Hunt, 2004; Proulx, 2008) have asked women with ID about participating in breast screening. Although Sullivan et al (2004c) planned to conduct interviews with women with ID, they were prevented from doing so by clinicians working on the study who felt interviews could only be conducted with women with mild ability. It was surmised that interviews with women with moderate/severe ability, would be unduly influenced by the necessary assistance needed from their carer to undertake the interview.

This study however gained ethical and management approval and one-to-one semi-structured interviews with 14 women with ID, 13 allied professionals, 12 support workers/paid carers and 3 family carers have been carried out. These were supported by periods of focused observation of health related activity, such as going to hospital or doctors appointments.

Detailed analysis is ongoing but preliminary examination of the data suggests that breast cancer screening is not well understood by women with ID, unless they have experienced breast cancer. The pain of the procedure was also identified a barrier. Data also suggests that carers have big role to play in monitoring health. Whilst undertaking the work, a number of difficulties such as accessing the women were addressed. People with ID are often seen as voiceless but those deemed to have capacity should be empowered to present their views about the care they receive as in this study. Without expressing their views, any health inequalities experienced by people with ID will be perpetuated and remain unchallenged and their experiences will not be acknowledged.

ACKNOWLEDGMENTS

Beth Alder, Edinburgh Napier University.

REFERENCES

Bell A. & Bhate M. (1992) Prevalence of overweight and obesity in Down's syndrome and other mentally handicapped adults living in the community. *J Intellect Disabil Res.* 36: 359–64.

Benard J., Beron-Gaillard N. & Satge´ D.C.L. (2005) Down's syndrome protects against breast cancer: is a constitutional cell microenvironment the key? *Int J Canc.* 113: 168–70.

Biswas M., Whalley H., Foster J.& Friedman E. (2005) Women with learning disability and uptake of screening: audit of screening uptake before and after one to one counselling. *J Public Health*, 27: 344–7.

Blackburn G.L., Copeland T., Khaodhiar L. & Buckley R.B. (2003) Diet and breast cancer. *J Women's Health*, 12: 183–92.

CancerResearch UK (2009) http://info.cancerresearchuk.org/cancerstats/mortality/ cancerdeaths/ (accessed March 24th 2009).

Carlson G. & Wilson J. (1996) Menstrual management and women who have learning disability: service providers and decision making. *J Intellect Disabil Res.* 2: 39–57.

Carr J. & Hollins S. (1995) Menopause in women with learning disabilities. *J Intellect Disabil Res.* 39: 137–139.

Carter G. & Jancar J. (1983) Mortality in the mentally handicapped: a fifty year survey at the Stoke Park Group of Hospitals (1930–1980). *J Ment Defic Res.* 41: 312–6.

Cooke L.B. (1997) Cancer and learning disability. *J Intellect Disabil Res.* 41: 312–6.

Cosgrove M.P., Tyrrell M., McCarron M., Gill M. & Lawlor B.A. (1999) Age at on set of dementia and age of menopause in women with Down's Syndrome. *J Intellect Disabil Res.* 43: 461–6.

Davies N. & Duff M. (2001) Breast cancer screening for older women with intellectual disability living in community group homes. *J Intellect Disabil Res.* 45: 253–7.

Djuretic T., Laing-Morton T., Guy M. & Gill M. (1999) Concerted effort is needed to ensure these women use preventative services. *Brit Med J.* 318: 537–8.

Gesualdi G. (2006) Screening for cancer in women with developmental disabilities: are they receiving the appropriate standard of care? *Excpt Par Mag.* 4: 61–5.

Gillings-Taylor S. (2004) Why the difference? Advice on breast examination given to carers of women who have learning disability and women who do not. *J of Learn Disabil.* 8: 175–89.

Hasle H., Haunstrup Clemmensen I. & Mikklesen M. (2000) Risks of leukaemia and solid tumours in individuals with Down's syndrome. *Lancet*, 355: 165–9.

Hogg J., Northfield J. & Turnbull J. (2001) Cancer and people with learning disabilities. Kidderminster, BILD Publications.

Isaacs R. (2006) Breast screening for women with learning disabilities. *Synergy*, 3: 15–8.

Jancar J. (1990) Cancer and mental handicap: a further study (1976–1985). *Brit J Psychiatry*, 156: 531–3.

Jancar M.P. & Jancar J. (1977) Cancer and mental retardation (a forty year review). *Bristol Med Chir J.* 92: 3–7.

Key T.J., Appleby P.N., Reeves G.K., Roddam A., Dorgan J.F. et al. (2003) Body mass index, serum sex hormones, and breast cancer risk in postmenopausal women. *J Natl Canc Inst.* 95: 1218–26.

McPherson K., Steel C.M. & Dixon J.M. (2006) Breast cancer – epidemiology, risk factors and genetics. In: Dixon J.M., editor. ABC of breast disease. 3rd ed. Oxford, Blackwell Publishing.

Melville C.A., Cooper S.-A., McGrother C.W., Thorp C.F. & Collacott R. (2005) Obesity in adults with Down syndrome: a case–control study. *J Intellect Disabil Res.* 49: 125–33.

NHS Cancer Screening Programme (2006) Equal access to breast and cervical screening for disabled women. Sheffield, NHS Cancer Screening Programmes.

NHS Health Scotland (2004) Health needs assessment people with learning disabilities. Glasgow, NHS Scotland.

Nursing and Midwifery Council (2004) Code of professional conduct. London, Nursing and Midwifery Council.

Patja K., Pukkala E. & Iivanainen M. (2001) Cancer incidence among people with intellectual disability. *J Intellect Disabil Res*. 45: 300–7.

Pehl J. & Hunt A. (2004) Improving access to breast screening. *Pract Res*. 7: 32–4.

Pehl J. (1999). Accessibility of breast screening services for women with learning disabilities in South Derbyshire. Practice and Research.

Piachaud J. & Rohde J. (1998) Screening for breast cancer is necessary inpatients with learning disability. *Brit Med J*. 316: 1979–80.

Piachaud J., Rohde J. & Pasupathy A. (1998) Health screening for people with Down's syndrome. *J Intellect Disabil Res*. 42: 341–5.

Poynor L. (2003) Being 'breast aware'. Pract Res, 6: 11–4.

Proulx, R., Mercier, C., Jutras, S., & Major, D. (August, 2008). Challenges in access to breast cancer screening for women with intellectual disability. 13th IASSID World Congress, Cape Town.

Rimmer J. (1994) Cardiovascular risk factors levels in adults with mental retardation. *Am J Ment Retard*. 98: 510–8.

Royal College of Nursing (1999) Developing roles: nurses working in breast care. London, RCN.

Satge' D.C.L. & Sasco A.J. (2002a) A reduced breast cancer incidence in Down syndrome. *Brit Med J*. 324: 1155.

Satge' D.C.L. & Sasco A.J. (2002b) Breast screening should be adapted in Down's syndrome. *Brit Med J*. 324: 1155–6.

Satge' D.C., Sommelet D., Geneix A., Nishi M., Malet P. et al. (1998) A tumour profile in Down syndrome. *Am J Med Genet*. 78: 207–16.

Schupf N., Zigman W., Kepell D., Lee J.H., Kline J. et al. (1997) Early menopause in women with Down Syndrome. *J Intellect Disabil Res*. 41: 264–7.

Schupf N., Pang D., Patel B.N., Silverman W., Schubert R., et al. (2003) Onset of dementia is associated with age at menopause in women with Down's syndrome. *Ann Neurol*. 54: 433–8.

Scottish Executive (2005) Delivering for health. Edinburgh, Scottish Executive.

Seltzer G.B., Schupf N. & Wu H.S. (2001) A prospective study of menopause in women with Down's Syndrome. *J Intellect Disabil Res*. 45: 1–7.

Stein K. (2000) Caring for people with learning disability: a survey of general practitioners' attitudes in Southampton and Southwest Hampshire. *Br J Learn Disabil*. 28: 9–15.

Sullivan S., Hussain R., Slack-Smith L.M. & Bittles A.H. (2003) Breast cancer uptake of mammography screening services by women with intellectual disabilities. *Prev Med*. 37: 507–12.

Sullivan S.G., Hussain R., Threlfall T. & Bittles A.H. (2004a) The incidence of cancer in people with intellectual disabilities. *Canc Caus Cont*. 15: 1021–5.

Sullivan S.G. & Hussain R. (2004b) Appropriate breast cancer screening for women with intellectual disability. *Brit Med J*. 328: 1979.

Sullivan S.G., Slack-Smith L.M. & Hussain R. (2004c) Understanding the use of breast cancer screening by women with intellectual disabilities. *Soc Prev med*. 49: 398–405.

Symonds D. & Howsam K. (2004) Breast awareness in learning disabilities. *Can Nurs Pract*. 3: 8–10.

Tjonneland A., Christensen J., Olsen A., Stripp C., Thomsen B.L. et al. (2007) Alcohol intake and breast cancer risk: the European Prospective Investigation into Cancer and Nutrition (EPIC). *Cancer Causes Control*, 18: 361–73.

Tuffrey-Wijne I., Hogg J. & Curfs L. (2007) End-of-life and palliative care for people with intellectual disabilities who have cancer or other life-limiting illness: a review of the literature and available resources. *JARID*, 20: 331–44.

Willis, D. S., Satge, D. & Sullivan, S. G. (2008a). Breast cancer surveillance in women with intellectual disabilities. *Internat J of Human Dev*. 7, 407-413.

Willis, D. S., Kennedy, C.M. & Kilbride, L. (2008b). Breast cancer screening in women with learning disabilities: current knowledge and considerations. *Brit J Learn Dis*. 36, 171–184.

Zorick T.S., Mustacchi Z., Bando S.Y., Zatz M., Moreira-Filho C.A. et al. (2001) High serum endostatin levels in Down syndrome: implications for improved treatment and prevention of solid tumours. *Eur J Hum Gen*. 9: 811–4.

Chapter 16

LIFESPAN RELATED DISEASES IN THE ADULTS WITH PROFOUND AND MULTIPLE INTELLECTUAL DISABILITIES

S. Sone[1]; K. Araki[1], T. Ezoe[1], H. Saijo[1], H. Hamaguchi[1], Y. Takeda[1], H. Nakayama[1], K. Motohashi[1], H. Inada[1], T. Hirayama[1], H. Suzuki[1] ,Y. Hirayama[1], K. Kurata[1], and M. Arima[1]

[1]Tokyo Metropolitan Higashiyamato Medical Center for Developmental and/or Multiple Disabilities, Higashiyamato, Tokyo

INTRODUCTION

In Japan many pediatric neurologists have undertaken clincal duties at facilities for persons with profound intellectual and multiple disabilities (PIMD). Health problems are managed in conjunction families and caregivers. Such interventions haves lead to marked increase in the life expectancy of persons with PIMD. Nowadays more than 80% of the residents of the facilities for the persons with PIMD are over 20 years old, and more than 10% are over 50 years.

As in other countries, in Japan also, it is necessary to assemble knowledge about diseases related to the increase in lifespan of persons with intellectual disabilities (ID). Epidemiological concerns regarding the diagnostic and therapeutic guidelines of co-existing diseases are of ongoing concern when applied to persons with PMID.

AIM

The aim of this initial research study was to determine the prevalence rate, diagnostic methods and treatment of lifespan related diseases in PMID, with a view to developing a more reliable and valid evidence based study.

METHOD

The period of this research was April 2005 to March 2006. Participants were randomly chosen adults with PIMD who lived in the facilities. Thirteen facilities participated in this study with 50 adults recruited from each facility.

Fifteen diseases were specifically chosen as lifespan related diseases: Type 2 diabetes mellitus, obesity, ischemic heart disease, cerebral infarction, cancer, periodontitis, hypertension, osteoporosis and hyperuricemia were chosen from the diseases common in Japanese adults. Then pneumonia, bone fracture, scoliosis, constipation, abnormal urinatkon and urinary stones were chosen from the diseases common in persons with PIMD.

The diagnosis of type 2 diabetes mellitus, obesity, hypertension and hyperuricemia were made using the same criteria as used in the general population. For example, cancer was expected to have been diagnosed pathologically, and periodontitis diagnosed by dentists. However, patients who were diagnosed with a cerebral infarction seldom received computed tomography for diagnosis. Patients who were diagnosed with ischemic heart disease seldom received electrocardiograms. Osteoporosis was diagnosed mostly by decrease of bone mineral density on bone X-ray films or by a past history of bone fracture. Bone fractures were diagnosed by an orthopeaditrician. Two thirds of scoliosis were diagnosed by X-ray (Cobb angle ranges from 15 to 147 degree), and the rest were diagnosed by physical sign. The most common diagnostic criteria of constipation was that the patient had no defecation for more than 3 days, and that the patient had received some laxative medication on the third day. Pneumonia was diagnosed by the combination of clinical signs, X-ray and blood examination. Diagnosis of gastroesophageal reflux was made from signs such as outflow of the food after the meal, or recurrent vomiting of black, bloody or coffee-ground vomit. Special examinations for diagnosis were performed in a half of the patients.

We asked the physicians working at the facilities to answer a questionnaire questioning whether they patients had the diseases or not and if so,, how they were diagnosed and treated. The answers were analyzed with F test or *kai-square test.*

RESULTS

Six hundred and sixteen questionnaires were sent back from the facilities. Sixty-eight were eliminated because of the lack of gender or age, or inadequate answers. The total number of participants were 548 (271 men and 277 women). The mean age was 38 years and 6 months.

Prevalence rates of diseases common amongst the general Japanese population found for persons with PMID were as follows; Type 2 diabetes mellitus 1.4%, obesity 0.2%, cerebral infarction 0.3%, periodontitis 63.8%, cancer 1.8%, osteoporosis 35.4% and hypertension 4.6%. Ischemic heart disease and hyperuricemia were not found. In more than 10% of cases, periodontitis, osteoporosis and hyperuricemia was undiagnosed. The prevalence rates of cancer, brain infarction and ischemic heart disease (which were the commonest causes of death in Japan), were markedly less than that for the general Japanese population. The prevalence rate of osteoporosis was higher for the PMID population as compared to the general Japanese population. The prevalence rates of hypertension, hyperuricemia and type 2 diabetes mellitus tended to increase with age and were markedly higher for persons over the age of 50 years. No age-related change in rates was found for the other health conditions.

The prevalence rates of diseases common among persons with PIMD was as follows; constipation 82%, scoliosis 57%, pneumonia 21%, gastroesophageal reflux 12%, bone fracture 7%, abnormal urination 10% and urinary stone 4%. These rates were much higher than reported for the general Japanese population. The age-related prevalence rates of bone fracture and urinary stone increased slightly as people got older.

DISCUSSION

The prevalence rates of periodontitis, osteoporosis, constipation, scoliosis, pneumonia gastroesophageal reflux and abnormal urination were found to occur in more than 10% of persons with PMID. These diseases are areas to focus resources on in terms of early detection and treatment.. Hypertension, cancer and type 2 diabetes mellitus, bone fracture and urinary stones, whose prevalence rates were less than 10% are diseases which professionals should have increased awareness off.

From this study, it can be seen that adults with PIMD can suffer a wide range of diseases. The involvement of several specialists will be necessary to provide good medical care to all adults with PIMD.

CONCLUSION

Adults with PIMD can suffer from diseases common to the general population. They may occur less often but can remain undetected and untreated for a significant length of time. Particular attention should be paid to those conditions associated with ID. Periodontitis, osteoporosis and constipation were conditions specifically highlighted in this study. Cancer and type 2 diabetes mellitus require detection as soon as possible.

PART III. BIOLOGICAL AND BIOBEHAVIORAL ISSUES

Molecular genetics and the biobehavioral aspects of intellectual disabilities (ID) are becoming areas of considerable interest, and undoubtedly will lead to a number of clinically significant breakthroughs over the next few decades. Particular syndromes receiving attention include Down syndrome, Fragile X, Prader-Willi and autism. *Hagerman* comprehensively reviews the bio-behavioral aspects of Fragile X and discusses future targeted treatments. A number of biological markers are now being investigated as factors in aggression and self abusive behavior. *Brown and colleagues* highlight areas of ongoing future research.

The Society for the Study of Behavioral Phenotypes as now been established for a number of years and investigates and highlights particular behavioral phenotypes associated with particular syndromes. Down syndrome is a good example of phenotypic behavior which is discussed further by *Cuskelly and colleagues*. Other specific phenotypic syndromes included Angelman's syndrome, CHARGE syndrome, Cornelia de Lange and Prader Willi syndrome. *Wulffaert and colleagues* report their findings regarding challenging behavior across these different groups and highlight the importance of genetic and environmental factors. Fetal alcohol and fetal tobacco syndromes are uncommon but are potentially of huge concern. *Tanaka* brings these two syndromes to our attention.

Chapter 17

FRAGILE X: A FAMILY OF DISORDERS AND ADVANCES IN TREATMENT

R. Hagerman

Department of Pediatrics, University of California at
Davis Medical Center USA

PHENOTYPIC OVERVIEW

The fragile X mutations including the premutation (55-200 CGG repeats) and the full mutation (>200 repeats) in the Fragile X Mental Retardation 1 gene (*FMR1*) lead to a broad spectrum of phenotypic involvement throughout the lifespan. The full mutation causes fragile X syndrome (FXS), the most common cause of inherited intellectual disabilities (ID) and the most common know cause of autism or autism spectrum (ASD) disorder (ASD). However individuals with FXS may not be intellectually impaired, particularly females, and they often present with learning disabilities or emotional difficulties. Autism occurs in approximately 30% of children with FXS and an additional 30% have an ASD (Harris, 2008). Hyperactivity, anxiety, mood instability, hand flapping and hand biting occur in the majority of children affected with FXS and these symptoms combined with language delays typically lead to diagnostic testing between 2 and 3 years of age (Bailey et al, 2003).

The full mutation leads to methylation of the gene and a subsequent block of transcription of *FMR1*. Consequently a deficit of *FMR1*-mRNA and *FMR1* protein (FMRP) occurs in males with a full mutation and a significant deficiency of FMRP occurs in females with a full mutation leading to the features of FXS. The level of FMRP is inversely correlated with the degree of clinical involvement including IQ and the severity of connective tissue involvement leading to the physical features of prominent ears, hyperextensible finger joints, and flat feet (Loesch et al, 2004). Macroorchidism and a long face are often seen during and after puberty.

The premutation can also lead to clinical involvement in a subgroup of children and in older carriers, although the mechanism of involvement is very different from the full mutation. Although the majority of premutation carriers have normal intellectual involvement, there is an enhanced level of *FMR1*-mRNA produced by the premutation (Tassone et al, 2000).The FMR1-mRNA levels are 2 to 8 times normal, leading to a gain of function effect or RNA toxicity which causes premutation specific disorders. These disorders include the fragile X-associated tremor/ataxia syndrome (FXTAS) and fragile X-associated primary ovarian insufficiency (FXPOI). In addition, psychiatric disorders including anxiety and depression are more common in premutation carriers than the general population (Hessl et al, 2005; Roberts et al, 2009). Boys with the premutation are also more likely to have ADHD and ASD compared to their brothers without the premutation, suggesting a neurodevelopmental effect of the premutation (Farzin et al, 2006).

FXTAS occurs in approximately 40% of older male carriers of the premutation and it includes an intention tremor, ataxia, neuropathy, autonomic dysfunction including hypertension and erectile dysfunction, and cognitive decline leading to dementia mainly in males. It is a progressive condition that typically begins in the 60s but the rate of progression is variable (Leehey et al, 2008). Brain atrophy and white matter disease are part of the diagnostic criteria for FXTAS (E. Berry-Kravis et al, 2007) and 60% of males and 13% of females with FXTAS have enhanced T2 signal intensity in the middle cerebellar peduncles (MCP sign) (Adams et al, 2007).

FXTAS is less common in women with less than 10% of female carriers experiencing tremor and ataxia with aging presumably because of the protective effects of the second X chromosome (Coffey et al, 2008). However, women with the premutation appear to experience autoimmune problems more commonly than age matched controls including hypothyroidism, and fibromyalgia (Coffey et al, 2008). Hypertension and neuropathy symptoms including numbness, tingling or pain in the lower extremities are also seen in the majority of older women with the premutation (Coffey et al, 2008).

Approximately 16 to 20% of women with the premutation also have FXPOI before the age of 40 (Sullivan et al, 2005; Wittenberger et al, 2007). Although FXPOI is also related to the RNA toxicity of the premutation, the occurrence of FXPOI is not associated with the subsequent development of FXTAS (Coffey et al, 2008).

The mechanism of RNA toxicity appears to be related to dysregulation of proteins in the neuron and perhaps to sequestration of proteins into eosinophilic intranuclear inclusions in neurons and astrocytes throughout the brain, in ganglia of the peripheral nervous system and in the Leydig cells of the testicles (Gokden et al, 2008; Greco et al, 2002; 2006; Tassone et al, 2007). The age of onset of FXTAS and the number of inclusions in the brain is correlated to the CGG repeat number. There is up-regulation of heat shock proteins, α B crystallin and lamin A/C leading to subsequent disruption of the lamin A/C structure on the inside of the nucleus (Arocena et al, 2005; Iwahashi et al, 2006).

The treatment of FXTAS includes the use of a variety of medications known to improve tremor including primidone or B blockers (Hagerman et al, 2008). Sometimes medications that improve the tremor of Parkinson's disease can be helpful in FXTAS and Botox has also been beneficial in cases. Treatment of hypertension, hypothyroidism and depression or anxiety when present is essential. If significant neuropathic pain is present then gabapentin or duloxetine can be helpful in our clinical experience (Hagerman et al, 2008). A controlled trial of memantine which can block glutamate toxicity is in progress for FXTAS but results are not available yet. Molecular techniques to lower levels of *FMR1*-mRNA may be a future treatment for FXTAS once the blood brain barrier problem for delivering medications to the CNS is solved.

Targeted Treatments in FXS

The advances in the neurobiology of fragile X have led to the development of new targeted treatments for FXS. FMRP is an RNA transport protein that also negatively regulates the translation of many messages in the neuron (Bassell & Warren, 2008). Therefore, when FMRP is absent, it leads to up-regulation of many proteins that are important for synaptic maturation and plasticity (Qin et al, 2005). FMRP is an inhibitor of protein translation that is required for long term depression (LTD) controlled by the metabotropic glutamate receptor 5 system (mGluR5)(Bear et al, 2004). Therefore in the absence FMRP there is downstream enhancement of protein production leading to enhanced LTD or weak synaptic connections throughout the brain in FXS and these changes are thought to be the main cause of the behavioral and cognitive problems of FXS (Bear et al, 2008). This concept has lead to the use of mGluR5 antagonists in FXS. In animal models of fragile X, the mGluR5 antagonists, such as fenobam, lithium and MPEP have rescued the fragile X phenotype including behavioral and cognitive deficits and seizures (de Vrij et al., 2008; McBride et al, 2005; Yan et al, 2005). A genetic rescue of the fragile X mouse through crossing it with an mGluR5 deficient mouse has lead to improvement of the dendritic spine phenotype in addition to behavioral and cognitive improvements (Dolen & Bear, 2008).

Recently mGluR5 antagonists have been utilized in adults with FXS, specifically fenobam in a single dose study to assess the pharmacokinetics and toxicity. There was a lack of toxicity seen with one dose and improvement in behavior and in the prepulse inhibition deficit in 50% of the patients with FXS (Berry-Kravis et al, 2009). This study documents the need of controlled trials of fenobam and other mGluR5 antagonists. An open trial of lithium, which has some activity in down regulating the mGluR5 system, demonstrated positive effects in behavior and a suggestion of cognitive improvements in individuals with FXS (Berry-Kravis et al, 2008).

There is also evidence that the GABA$_A$ system is down regulated in individuals with FXS (D'Hulst & Kooy, 2007) so agonists for this system have been proposed, but not yet tried (Hagerman et al, 2009). Currently a controlled trial of R-Baclofen, a GABA$_B$ agonist that has a more potent effect in down regulating the mGluR5 system than regular Baclofen is taking place but results are not yet available.

Recent evidence has demonstrated that the matrix metalloproteinase 9 (MMP9) protein is up-regulated in the absence of FMRP in the knock out mouse model of FXS (Bilousova et al, 2009). Newborn fragile X knockout mice were treated with minocycline, which is an antibiotic that down regulates the MMP9 system. After 1 month of treatment with minocycline at birth there was significant maturation of the dendritic spines so that they were comparable to normals. They subsequently documented improvement in an anxiety task and in a spacial task. This data suggests that minocycline would be beneficial in individuals with FXS and trials have been initiated in humans with FXS.

Currently a variety of approved medications can be helpful for children and adults with FXS. Medications commonly used include stimulants for the ADHD symptoms in children, selective serotonin reuptake inhibitors (SSRIs) for the anxiety, irritability and depression, although the latter is more common in carriers, and atypical antipsychotics or anticonvulsants, such as valproate, for mood stabilization and aggression (Hagerman et al, 2009). Aripiprazole (Abilify) is a remarkable new generation atypical antipsychotic that has usually a beneficial effect on hyperactivity, anxiety and mood instability in patients with FXS when used in low doses (Hagerman et al, 2009).

Both speech and language therapy and occupational therapy in addition to special education support are essential in the education of children with FXS (Braden, 2002; Scharfenaker et al, 2002). In addition, counseling to help with behavior management is often necessary (Hills-Epstein et al, 2002). The use of assistive technology, particularly computers can also facilitate educational supports for these children and they typically enjoy working on the computer (Greiss-Hess et al, 2009).

EPIDEMIOLOGY DIAGNOSTIC TESTING AND SCREENING

The full mutation occurs in 1 in 2500 alleles and the premutation occurs in 1 per 130 to 250 females and 1 per 250 to 810 males in the general population (Hagerman, 2008; Song et al, 2003). Because the premutation is relatively common, it is usually under diagnosed as is FXS. If you suspect the diagnosis fragile X DNA should be ordered and this can be carried out by almost all commercial laboratories and many hospitals and University molecular laboratories. Typically both PCR and Southern blot testing are carried out so that all full mutations and premutations are identified.

Once an individual is identified with an *FMR1* mutation in a family there are many individuals who are either carriers or significantly affected by FXS in the family. Therefore cascade testing is recommended in the family, such that all types of involvement can be identified and treated (McConkie-Rosell et al, 2007). Genetic counseling is recommended for all family members who are at risk for carrying a mutation. The family can also be referred to the National Fragile X Foundation (www.fragilex.org) for further information and contact information for the local parent support group.

Recently a new blood spot test for utilization in screening studies for fragile X mutations (Tassone et al, 2008). This test has facilitated trial programs of newborn screening in several locations in the country. Such studies will clarify the prevalence figures in all ethnic and racial groups in the US.

More intensive screening of high risk populations, such as those with autism or ID, those with POI, and those with tremor and/ or ataxia or cognitive decline are candidates for screening. With the advent of new targeted treatment for fragile X syndrome the need to identify patients with this disorder has intensified. The future looks bright for those with FXS because the combination of targeted treatments and intensive behavioral/educational programs should lead to a significantly improved outcome.

ACKNOWLEDGMENTS

This work was supported by grants from NICHD grant HD036071, NIA grant AG032115, NCRR grant DE019683 and the Health and Human Services Administration of Developmental Disabilities grant 90DD0596.

REFERENCES

Adams, J. S., Adams, P. E., Nguyen, D., Brunberg, J. A., Tassone, F., Zhang, W., et al. (2007). Volumetric brain changes in females with fragile X-associated tremor/ataxia syndrome (FXTAS). *Neurology, 69*(9), 851-859.

Arocena, D. G., Iwahashi, C. K., Won, N., Beilina, A., Ludwig, A. L., Tassone, F., et al. (2005). Induction of inclusion formation and disruption of lamin A/C structure by premutation CGG-repeat RNA in human cultured neural cells. *Hum Mol Genet, 14*(23), 3661-3671.

Bailey, D. B., Jr., Skinner, D., & Sparkman, K. L. (2003). Discovering fragile X syndrome: family experiences and perceptions. *Pediatrics, 111*(2), 407-416.

Bassell, G. J., & Warren, S. T. (2008). Fragile X syndrome: loss of local mRNA regulation alters synaptic development and function. *Neuron, 60*(2), 201-214.

Bear, M. F., Dolen, G., Osterweil, E., & Nagarajan, N. (2008). Fragile X: translation in action. *Neuropsychopharmacology, 33*(1), 84-87.

Bear, M. F., Huber, K. M., & Warren, S. T. (2004). The mGluR theory of fragile X mental retardation. *Trends Neurosci, 27*(7), 370-377.

Berry-Kravis, E., Abrams, L., Coffey, S. M., Hall, D. A., Greco, C., Gane, L. W., et al. (2007). Fragile X-associated tremor/ataxia syndrome: Clinical features, genetics, and testing guidelines. *Mov Disord, 22*(14), 2018-2030.

Berry-Kravis, E., Sumis, A., Hervey, C., Nelson, M., Porges, S. W., Weng, N., et al. (2008). Open-label treatment trial of lithium to target the underlying defect in fragile X syndrome. *J Dev Behav Pediatr, 29*(4), 293-302.

Berry-Kravis, E. M., Hessl, D., Coffey, S., Hervey, C., Schneider, A., Yuhas, J., et al. (2009). A pilot open-label single-dose trial of fenobam in adults with fragile X syndrome. *Journal of Medical Genetics*, jmg.2008.063701.

Bilousova, T. V., Dansie, L., Ngo, M., Aye, J., Charles, J. R., Ethell, D. W., et al. (2009). Minocycline promotes dendritic spine maturation and improves behavioral performance in the fragile X mouse model. *J Med Genet, 46*(2), 94-102.

Braden, M. (2002). Academic interventions in fragile X. In R. J. Hagerman & P. J. Hagerman (Eds.), *Fragile X Syndrome: Diagnosis, Treatment and Research, 3rd edition* (pp. 428-464). Baltimore: The Johns Hopkins University Press.

Coffey, S. M., Cook, K., Tartaglia, N., Tassone, F., Nguyen, D. V., Pan, R., et al. (2008). Expanded clinical phenotype of women with the FMR1 premutation. *Am J Med Genet A, 146A*(8), 1009-1016.

D'Hulst, C., & Kooy, R. F. (2007). The GABAA receptor: a novel target for treatment of fragile X? *Trends Neurosci, 30*(8), 425-431.

de Vrij, F. M., Levenga, J., van der Linde, H. C., Koekkoek, S. K., De Zeeuw, C. I., Nelson, D. L., et al. (2008). Rescue of behavioral phenotype and neuronal protrusion morphology in Fmr1 KO mice. *Neurobiol Dis, 31*(1), 127-132.

Dolen, G., & Bear, M. F. (2008). Role for metabotropic glutamate receptor 5 (mGluR5) in the pathogenesis of fragile X syndrome. *J Physiol, 586*(6), 1503-1508.

Farzin, F., Perry, H., Hessl, D., Loesch, D., Cohen, J., Bacalman, S., et al. (2006). Autism spectrum disorders and attention-deficit/hyperactivity disorder in boys with the fragile X premutation. *J Dev Behav Pediatr, 27*(2 Suppl), S137-144.

Gokden, M., Al-Hinti, J. T., & Harik, S. I. (2008). Peripheral nervous system pathology in fragile X tremor/ataxia syndrome (FXTAS). *Neuropathology*.

Greco, C. M., Berman, R. F., Martin, R. M., Tassone, F., Schwartz, P. H., Chang, A., et al. (2006). Neuropathology of fragile X-associated tremor/ataxia syndrome (FXTAS). *Brain, 129*(Pt 1), 243-255.

Greco, C. M., Hagerman, R. J., Tassone, F., Chudley, A., Del Bigio, M. R., Jacquemont, S., et al. (2002). Neuronal intranuclear inclusions in a new cerebellar tremor/ataxia syndrome among fragile X carriers. *Brain, 125*(8), 1760-1771.

Greiss-Hess, L., Lemons-Chitwood, K., Harris, S., Borodyanskaya, M., Hagerman, R. J., Bodine, C., et al. (2009). Assistive Technology Use by Persons With Fragile X Syndrome: Three Case Reports. *AOTA: Special Interest Section Quarterly: Technology, 19*(1), 1-4.

Hagerman, P. J. (2008). The fragile X prevalence paradox. *J Med Genet, 45*(8), 498-499.

Hagerman, R. J., Berry-Kravis, E., Kaufmann, W. E., Ono, M. Y., Tartaglia, N., Lachiewicz, A., et al. (2009). Advances in the treatment of fragile X syndrome. *Pediatrics, 123*(1), 378-390.

Hagerman, R. J., Hall, D. A., Coffey, S., Leehey, M., Bourgeois, J., Gould, J., et al. (2008). Treatment of fragile X-associated tremor ataxia syndrome (FXTAS) and related neurological problems. *Clin Interv Aging, 3*(2), 251-262.

Harris, S. W., Goodlin-Jones, B. et al. (2008). Autism Profiles of Young Males with Fragile X Syndrome. *Am J Mental Retardation*.

Hessl, D., Tassone, F., Loesch, D. Z., Berry-Kravis, E., Leehey, M. A., Gane, L. W., et al. (2005). Abnormal elevation of FMR1 mRNA is associated with psychological symptoms in individuals with the fragile X premutation. *Am J Med Genet B Neuropsychiatr Genet, 139*(1), 115-121.

Hills-Epstein, J., Riley, K., & Sobesky, W. (2002). The Treatment of Emotional and Behavioral Problems. In R. J. Hagerman & P. J. Hagerman (Eds.), *Fragile X Syndrome: Diagnosis, Treatment, and Research, 3rd Edition*. Baltimore: Johns Hopkins University Press:339-362.

Iwahashi, C. K., Yasui, D. H., An, H. J., Greco, C. M., Tassone, F., Nannen, K., et al. (2006). Protein composition of the intranuclear inclusions of FXTAS. *Brain, 129*(Pt 1), 256-271.

Leehey, M. A., Berry-Kravis, E., Goetz, C. G., Zhang, L., Hall, D. A., Li, L., et al. (2008). FMR1 CGG repeat length predicts motor dysfunction in premutation carriers. *Neurology, 70*(16 Pt 2), 1397-1402.

Loesch, D. Z., Huggins, R. M., & Hagerman, R. J. (2004). Phenotypic variation and FMRP levels in fragile X. *Ment Retard Dev Disabil Res Rev, 10*(1), 31-41.

McBride, S. M., Choi, C. H., Wang, Y., Liebelt, D., Braunstein, E., Ferreiro, D., et al. (2005). Pharmacological rescue of synaptic plasticity, courtship behavior, and mushroom body defects in a Drosophila model of fragile X syndrome. *Neuron, 45*(5), 753-764.

McConkie-Rosell, A., Abrams, L., Finucane, B., Cronister, A., Gane, L. W., Coffey, S. M., et al. (2007). Recommendations from multi-disciplinary focus groups on cascade testing and genetic counseling for fragile X-associated disorders. *J Genet Couns, 16*(5), 593-606.

Qin, M., Kang, J., Burlin, T. V., Jiang, C., & Smith, C. B. (2005). Postadolescent changes in regional cerebral protein synthesis: an in vivo study in the FMR1 null mouse. *J Neurosci, 25*(20), 5087-5095.

Roberts, J. E., Bailey, D. B., Jr., Mankowski, J., Ford, A., Sideris, J., Weisenfeld, L. A., et al. (2009). Mood and anxiety disorders in females with the FMR1 premutation. *Am J Med Genet B Neuropsychiatr Genet, 150B*(1), 130-139.

Scharfenaker, S., O'Connor, R., Stackhouse, T., & Noble, L. (2002). An integrated approach to intervention. In R. J. Hagerman & P. J. Hagerman (Eds.), *Fragile X Syndrome: Diagnosis, Treatment and Research, 3rd edition* (pp. 363-427). Baltimore: The Johns Hopkins University Press.

Song, F. J., Barton, P., Sleightholme, V., Yao, G. L., & Fry-Smith, A. (2003). Screening for fragile X syndrome: a literature review and modelling study. *Health Technol Assess, 7*(16), 1-106.

Sullivan, A. K., Marcus, M., Epstein, M. P., Allen, E. G., Anido, A. E., Paquin, J. J., et al. (2005). Association of FMR1 repeat size with ovarian dysfunction. *Hum Reprod, 20*(2), 402-412.

Tassone, F., Adams, J., Berry-Kravis, E. M., Cohen, S. S., Brusco, A., Leehey, M. A., et al. (2007). CGG repeat length correlates with age of onset of motor signs of the fragile X-associated tremor/ataxia syndrome (FXTAS). *Am J Med Genet B Neuropsychiatr Genet, 144*(4), 566-569.

Tassone, F., Hagerman, R. J., Taylor, A. K., Gane, L. W., Godfrey, T. E., & Hagerman, P. J. (2000). Elevated levels of FMR1 mRNA in carrier males: a new mechanism of involvement in the fragile-X syndrome. *Am J Hum Genet, 66*(1), 6-15.

Tassone, F., Pan, R., Amiri, K., Taylor, A. K., & Hagerman, P. J. (2008). A rapid polymerase chain reaction-based screening method for identification of all expanded alleles of the fragile X (FMR1) gene in newborn and high-risk populations. *J Mol Diagn, 10*(1), 43-49.

Wittenberger, M. D., Hagerman, R. J., Sherman, S. L., McConkie-Rosell, A., Welt, C. K., Rebar, R. W., et al. (2007). The FMR1 premutation and reproduction. *Fertil Steril, 87*(3), 456-465.

Yan, Q. J., Rammal, M., Tranfaglia, M., & Bauchwitz, R. P. (2005). Suppression of two major fragile X syndrome mouse model phenotypes by the mGluR5 antagonist MPEP. *Neuropharmacology, 49*(7), 1053-1066.

Chapter 18

BIOMARKERS OF AGGRESSIVE AND SELF-ABUSIVE BEHAVIOR

W.T. Brown[1], I.L. Cohen[1], R. Freedland[1], M. Flory[1], J.H. Yoo[1], J. Pettinger[1], and J.A. Tsiouris[1]

[1]NYS Institute for Basic Research in Developmental Disabilities, Staten Island, New York USA

INTRODUCTION

As part of a large survey of the incidence of aggressive and self-abusive behaviors among >4,500 New York State residents with intellectual deficiency (MRDD), we are interested in determining whether biomarkers can be identified that correlate with such behaviors. Serotonin and testosterone have been implicated in past studies among general populations. George and colleagues (2001) compared the cerebral spinal fluid concentrations of 5-hydroxyindoleacetic acid (5-HIAA a marker of serotonin) and testosterone obtained from perpetrators of domestic violence and a group of healthy comparison subjects. They found that CSF serotonin is lower in non-alcoholic individuals with domestic violence histories, while CSF testoterone is higher in alcoholic individuals with domestic diolence histories. Among genetic factors, functional polymorphisms of MAO-A have been linked to antisocial behavior. Caspi and colleagues (2002) found that maltreated children with a genotype conferring high levels of MAOA expression were less likely to develop aggressive and antisocial problems as adults.

Cohen and colleagues (2003) found the MAO-A low expresion genotype was associated with greater severity of autism. Their results showed the low expression allele was significantly correlated with a lower IQ by a mean of 22 points, and the differences became more marked over time. Meyer-Lindenberg and colleagues (2006) studied the impact of the MAO-A genotype on brain structure and function assessed with MRI in a large sample of healthy human volunteers finding that the low expression variant, associated with increased risk of violent behavior, predicted pronounced limbic volume reductions and hyperresponsive amygdala during emotional arousal, with diminished reactivity of regulatory prefrontal regions, compared with the high expression allele. Mice studies have shown that heterozygous deficiency for an enzyme involved with the metabolic degradation of catecholamines in the brain (COMT) is associated with increased aggressive behavior (Gogos et al, 1998). Among subjects with diagnosed genetic syndromes, including Fragile X, Prader-Willi, and Williams, aggressive profiles are more common.

In our survey, we have collected data using a modified Modified Overt Aggression Scale with 100 questions relating to the aggressive behaviors of the subjects in our study (Tsiouris & Cohen Scale, modified from Yadofsky). Factor analysis revealed four factors: "aggressive displays" which include mild to moderate aggression and destructive behaviors, verbal aggression, self-injurious behavior, and severe aggressive behaviors which are being analysed. Approximately 5% of our population exhibited such behaviors on a daily basis. The next phase of our project is to analyze potential genetic factors (MAOA, 5HTT, HTR1B, PH2, DRD2, DAT, DARPP-32, and CREB1) and other biomarkers among selected subsets of our subjects with either severe aggressive or self-abusive behaviors to search for such correlations that point to etiological contributions. Our hypothesis is that functional polymorphisms in genes related in the serotonin and dopamine pathways may modulate the severity of aggressive features. The findings of this study we anticipate may help lead to the targeted development of effective treatments.

REFERENCES

Caspi A, McClay J, Moffitt TE et al., Role of Genotype in the Cycle of Violence in Maltreated Children. *Science,* 297: 851 -854, 2002.

Cohen IL, Liu X, Schutz C et al., Association of Autism Severity with an MAOA Functional Polymorphism. *Clinical Genetics,* 64:190-197, 2003.

George DT, Umhau JC, Phillips MJ et al., Serotonin, testosterone and alcohol in the etiology of domestic violence. *Psychiatry Research,* 104: 27-37, 2001.

Gogos JA, Morgan M, Luine V et al., Catechol-O-Methyltransferase-deficient mice exhibit sexually dimorphic changes in catecholamine levels and behavior. *PNAS,* 95; 9991-6, 1998.

Meyer-Lindenberg A, et al. Neural mechanisms of genetic risk for impulsivity and violence in humans. *PNAS,* 103: 6269–74, 2006.

Chapter 19

Do Behavioral Problems in Children with Down Syndrome Suggest a Phenotypic Pattern?

Cuskelly M[1], Chant D[2], Hayes A[3], and Jobling A[1]

[1]The University of Queensland, Center of Excellence for Behavior Support and School of Education, Brisbane, Australia,

[2]The University of Queensland, Department of Psychiatry, Brisbane, Australia

[3]Australian Institute of Family Studies. Melbourne, Australia

Introduction

There is increasing interest in identifying phenotypic patterns in the behaviors of groups of individuals with the same syndrome (Hodapp & DesJardines, 2002). Behavioral phenotypes exist when certain behaviors occur more frequently in individuals with the same syndrome in comparison to those without the syndrome, or if particular patterns typically occur in one group more predictably than in others (Dykens, 1995).

One of the areas in which behavioral phenotypes may manifest is in the area of behavioral problems. While there has been some work on this issue with individuals with Down syndrome (DS) it is inconclusive, partly because approaches to the question have differed. The most pragmatic approach is to determine if there are behavior problems that occur in the majority of children with DS and then to ascertain if these differ from the problems seen in other children with and without an intellectual disability.

Dykens and Kasari (1997) identified behavior problems listed on the Child Behavior Checklist (CBCL; Achenbach 1991) which were reported by parents to occur in 50 percent or more of children with DS. They found six items met this criterion (stubborn; disobeys; speech problems; can't concentrate, argues a lot, and prefers being alone). Parents indicate if a behavior is very or often true of their child (2), somewhat or sometimes true (1), or not true (0). Unfortunately, it is not clear from Dykens and Kasari's report whether the behaviors identified were only those that received a score of 2 or if they also included those that received a score of 1.

In an earlier study, Pueschel et al (1991) compared children with DS and their nearest same-sex sibling using the CBCL. Significant differences between groups were found by Pueschel et al. (1991) on only 12 of the 118 items of the CBCL. Four of these were related to immaturity in comparison to peers, three to difficult behavior, two to sleeping difficulties, two to problems with attention, and one to speech problems. There was no indication that these behaviors occurred in the majority of children with DS, so while they indicated an increased propensity to engage in these behaviors they are not evidence of a behavioral phenotype as defined earlier.

METHODOLOGY

Participants

Sixty-nine families (95% of those invited) agreed to take part in an interview study about a range of family experiences. All had a child with DS between the ages of 4 years 6 months and 15 years 6 months. Complete data were available for the analyses reported here on only 62 families. The children with DS had a mean chronological age of 9.9 years (SD = 3.7) and a mean IQ of 43.4 (SD = 8.3) as assessed on the Stanford-Binet Intelligence Scale: Fourth Edition (SB:IV; Thorndike et al, 1986).

Instruments

The Child Behavior Checklist/4-18 (CBCL; Achenbach, 1991) is an 118 item checklist that gathers information about problem behaviors in children between the ages of 4 and 18 years and is completed by the child's parents. Individual items were used in the analysis reported here. This is the same version used by Dykens and Kasari (1997).

Part Two of the AAMR Adaptive Behavior Scale (ABS: Part Two) (Nihira et al, 1993) was used in the study as it was developed for use with individuals with an intellectual disability, unlike the CBCL. This instrument was included to ensure that there was an opportunity to discover whether there were any behaviors, additional to those on the CBCL, that were common in the children with DS.

Procedure

The data presented here are part of a larger study examining life in families with a child with DS. For the data collection associated with the broader study both parents were interviewed in their home on two occasions. At the end of the first interview both parents were given sufficient copies of the CBCL to enable them to complete one for each child between the ages of 4 and 18 years who lived in the family home. They were asked to complete these forms before the second interview and not to discuss their responses with each other until all forms had been completed. At the beginning of the second interview, the CBCLs were inspected to ensure they were complete and to discuss any difficulties parents had found in completing them. These were resolved and the forms completed before the second interview commenced. The SB:IV and ABS data were collected by a psychologist after the interviews had been completed. Only mothers responded to the ABS.

RESULTS

High Frequency Problem Behaviors

Table 1. Items from the CBCL reported to be 'somewhat or sometimes true' or 'very or often true' of their child with DS by 50 percent or more of parents

	Mother		Father	
Item	Somewhat or sometimes true	Very or often true	Somewhat or sometimes true	Very or often true
1. Acts too young for age	33.4[a]	57.1	33.3	55.6
3. Argues a lot	33.3	17.5	0	0
8. Can't concentrate, can't pay attention for long	50.7	30.2	36.5	49.2
11. Clings to adults or too dependent	0	0	44.4	12.7
19. Demands a lot of attention	31.7	27	44.4	28.6
22. Disobedient at home	57.1	15.9	59	8.2
23. Disobedient at school	53.9	6.4	46.1	4.7
29. Fears certain animals, situations, places	40.3	14.5	46	14.3
38. Gets teased a lot	46	4.8	0	0
41. Impulsive or acts without thinking	36.5	20.6	44.4	12.7
61. Poor school work	37.7	18	34.9	17.5
62. Poorly coordinated or clumsy	55.5	11.1	55.7	11.5
63. Prefers being with older kids	45.3	6.3	0	0
64. Prefers being with younger kids	48.4	9.4	42.9	7.9
74. Shows off/clowns	53.1	9.4	54	6.3
79. Speech problems	19.6	68.9	26.2	65.6
86. Stubborn, sullen or irritable	51.5	17.3	59.1	9.8

[a]Percentage of parents to indicate the behavior occurred at this level.

Those behaviors that were reported to be "somewhat or sometimes true" and "very or often true" for 50% or more of the children with DS were collated separately for mothers and fathers and are presented in Table 1. Two items were reported to be "very or often true" for 50% or more of the children on mothers' report: *Acts too young for age* and *Speech problem*. The same items met this criterion on the fathers' reports. *Can't concentrate, can't pay attention for long* was endorsed as occurring frequently in their child by 49.4% of fathers. No behaviors were reported to be "very or often true" for 50% or more of the siblings of a child with DS on either mothers' or fathers' reports.

The same analysis was conducted with the items of Part Two of the ABS and the results are presented in Table 2. These data were collected from mothers only. No item was found to be reported to occur frequently for 50% or more of the group.

Table 2 Items from Part Two of the ABS reported to occur occasionally or frequently in their children by mothers of children with DS

Item	Occurs occasionally	Occurs frequently
1.4. Pushes, scratches, or pinches others	46.6[a]	6.7
1.7. Throws objects at others	44.3	6.7
3.3. Teases others	40.0	13.3
4.1. Tries to tell others what to do	41.7	20.0
4.2. Demands services from others	45.3	18.3
6.2. Withdraws or pouts when thwarted	56.7	5.0
6.3. Becomes upset when thwarted	68.3	15.0
9.2. Pretends not to hear and does not follow instructions	48.3	16.7
9.3. Does not pay attention to instructions	60.0	16.7
9.4. Refuses to work on assigned subject	53.3	10.0
9.5. Hesitates for long periods before doing assigned tasks	45.0	20.0
13.1. Interrupts group discussion by talking about unrelated topics	48.3	5.0
14.2. Uses other's property without permission	50.0	18.3
37.2. Withdraws or pouts when criticized	53.4	3.3
37.3. Becomes upset when criticized	51.7	13.3
38.4. Acts silly to gain attention	46.7	13.3

[a]Percentage of parents to indicate the behavior occurred at this level.

DISCUSSION

In the sample included in this study, only two behaviors, acting younger than chronological age and having a problem with speech received a score of 2 for 50% or more of the children from both mothers and fathers. One behavior indicating difficulty with attention was reported to occur frequently by fathers only. No item on the ABS Problem Behavior Scale was reported to occur frequently for the majority of the group of children with DS. No parent listed any additional problem behaviors after completing the CBCL, although they were invited to do so.

The lack of agreement with the results of Dykens and Kasari (1997) maybe a product of methodological differences (they may have included items that were reported to occur occasionally) or to sample differences. There is insufficient information to rule out the first possibility.

Certainly, for a behavior to be considered to be a part of a behavioral phenotype it should occur predictably in the majority of the individuals within a diagnostic group. Acting younger than chronological age is common in children with an intellectual disability, irrespective of etiology so does not meet the criterion for a phenotypic characteristic (Dekker et al, 2002; Keogh et al, 1989). Speech difficulties may be considered to be characteristic of children with DS but can hardly be considered to be a behavior problem. This study, therefore, suggests that there is no phenotype for behavior problems for children with DS.

Some caution needs to be taken when considering these results. The CBCL was not developed for use with children with intellectual disability and there may be problems specific to this group that will not be picked up by that instrument. The inclusion of the problem behavior checklist from the ABS goes some way to addressing this issue.

ACKNOWLEDGMENT

This research was supported by a grant from the Australian Research Council. We are grateful to all the families who assisted with this research.

REFERENCES

Achenbach, T.M. (1991). *Manual for the Child Behavior Checklist/4-18 and 1991* Profile. Burlington, VT: Department of Psychiatry, University of Vermont.

Dekker, M.C., Koot, H.M., van der Ende, J., & Verhulst, F.C. (2002). Emotional and behavioral problems in children and adolescents with and without intellectual disability. Journal of Child Psychology and Psychiatry, 43, 1087-1098.

Dykens, E.M. (1995). Measuring Behavioral phenotypes: Provocations from the "new genetics". *American Journal on Mental Retardation*, 99, 522-532.

Dykens, E.M., & Kasari, C. (1997). Maladaptive behavior in children with Prader-Willi syndrome, Down syndrome, and nonspecific mental retardation. *American Journal on Mental Retardation*, 102, 228-137.

Hodapp, R.M. & DesJardins, J.L. (2002). Genetic etiologies of mental retardation: Issues for interventions and interventionists. *Journal of Developmental and Physical Disabilities*, 14, 323-338.

Keogh, B.K., Bernheimer, L.P., Haney, M., & Daley, S. (1989). Behavior and adjustment problems of young developmentally delayed children. *European Journal of Special Needs Education*, 4, 79-89.

Nihira, K., Leland, H., & Lambert, N. (1993). AAMR Adaptive Behavior Scale - Residential and Community (2nd Ed.), Examiner's manual. Austin, TX: PRO-ED.

Pueschel, S.M., Bernier, J.C., & Pezzullo, J.C. (1991). Behavioral observations in children with Down's syndrome. *Journal of Mental Deficiency Research*, 35, 502-511.

Thorndike, R.L., Hagan, E.P., & Sattler, J.M. (1986). Stanford-Binet Intelligence Scale: *Fourth Edition*. Chicago, IL: The Riverside Publishing Company.

Chapter 20

CHALLENGING BEHAVIOR IN ANGELMAN SYNDROME, CHARGE SYNDROME, CORNELIA DE LANGE SYNDROME, AND PRADER-WILLI SYNDROME

J. Wulffaert[1], Y.M. Dijkxhoorn[1] and I.A. van Berckelaer-Onnes[1]
[1]Department of Clinical Child and Adolescent Studies, Leiden University, the Netherlands

INTRODUCTION

The research group *Severe Developmental Disorders* of the department of Clinical Child and Adolescent Studies of Leiden University, the Netherlands, started a study on the behavioral phenotype in Cornelia de Lange syndrome in 2004.

A fruitful cooperation with the Dutch Cornelia de Lange Parent Support Group resulted in comparable studies in different genetic syndromes. In this paper we will report preliminary results on challenging behavior in Angelman, CHARGE, Cornelia de Lange, and Prader-Willi syndrome. We will compare the differences within, but also between different groups, hence gathering insight into the syndrome-specificity of the behavior.

METHODOLOGY

Participants and Procedure

All parents of the Dutch Parent Support Groups of Angelman syndrome ($N = 142$), CHARGE syndrome ($N = 55$), Cornelia de Lange syndrome ($N = 71$), and Prader-Willi syndrome ($N = 223$) were requested by letter to participate. For CHARGE syndrome additional participants were gathered through a Dutch outpatient clinic at the University Medical Center Groningen. The Dutch version of the Developmental Behavior Checklist – Primary Carer (DBC-P; Einfeld & Tonge, 2002) was used to collect data on challenging behavior. Parents received the questionnaire by post and were asked to return it through an included pre-paid envelope. See Table 1 for the final number of participants after removing questionnaires with too many missing values according to the questionnaire manual.

Table 1 Participants of the study that filled out the DBC-P

Syndrome	N	Age range in years	M age	SD age
Angelman	74	2 – 42	17.3	10.38
CHARGE	24	1 – 23	11.9	6.36
Cornelia de Lange	34	1 – 46	17.6	13.24
Prader-Willi	60	0 – 48	17.4	11.91

Although the participants with CHARGE syndrome were considerably younger, the Kruskal-Wallis test (used because of heterogeneity of variances) showed the difference in age was not significant, $H(3) = 4.322, p = .229$.

Instrument

The Dutch version (Koot & Dekker, 2001) of the *Developmental Behavior Checklist-Primary Carer* (Einfeld & Tonge, 2002) assesses emotional and behavioral problems in people with an intellectual disability. Parents rate 95 items concerning behavior in the past six months. A total behavior problem score (TBPS) is computed as well as five subscale scores (disruptive/antisocial behavior, self-absorbed behavior, communication disturbance, anxiety, social relating problems). Reliability and validity are satisfactory to good (Koot & Dekker, 2001). To compare the subscale scores, weighed scores have been computed by dividing the subscale scores by the number of items on that particular subscale.

RESULTS

Incidence of Challenging Behavior

The DBC-P cut-off for total problem behavior (Einfeld & Tonge, 2002) showed a considerable amount of participants with a total score within the clinical range in all of the syndromes: 49% in Angelman syndrome, 38% in CHARGE syndrome, 44% in Cornelia de Lange syndrome, and 40% in Prader-Willi syndrome.

Item analysis showed that only a few items were displayed by more than 75% of the participants per syndrome (items scored as *somewhat or sometimes true* and *very true or often true* on DBC-P), especially in CHARGE and Cornelia de Lange syndrome. In Angelman syndrome the following six items were scored for more than 75%: *poor attention span; chews on objects; easily distracted from his/her task; makes non-speech noises; poor sense of danger* and *unusual body movements, posture, or way of walking*. In CHARGE syndrome only *being impatient* was applicable for more than 75% of the participants.

In Cornelia de Lange syndrome only two items were prevalent in more than 75% of the persons, namely *mood changes rapidly for no apparent reason* and *prefers to do things on his/her own, tends to be a loner*. In Prader-Willi syndrome five items passed the criterion being: *arranges objects or routine in a strict order; easily led by others; has temper tantrums; prefers to do things on his/her own, tends to be a loner* and *upset over small changes in routine or environment.*

The items that obtained the highest mean score per syndrome are displayed in Table 2.

Compared to the other syndromes, the mean scores were highest in Angelman syndrome, indicating the similarity in behavior in persons with this syndrome. Most of these items belonged to the self-absorbed subscale. Also in Cornelia de Lange and CHARGE syndrome the items with the highest mean score belonged predominantly to the self-absorbed subscale. In Prader-Willi syndrome the items were scattered across all five subscales. Although the mean scores differed between the syndromes, there was also considerable overlap in items with the highest scores between the syndromes.

In Figure 1 the different subscale profiles are depicted. In Angelman syndrome the mean score on the self-absorbed subscale formed a clear peak in the profile of challenging behavior. In CHARGE syndrome self-absorbed behavior obtained the highest mean, followed by the subscales disruptive/antisocial behavior and social relating problems. In Cornelia de Lange syndrome two peaks were visible with social relating problems as most prevalent, and self-absorbed behavior second. Finally, in Prader-Willi syndrome three subscales obtained almost evenly high means: disruptive/antisocial behavior, communication disturbances and social relating problems.

Table 2. Mean item scores for 12 highest scored DBC-P items per syndrome

Angelman syndrome		CHARGE syndrome	
Item	**Mean**	**Item**	**Mean**
Easily distracted from his/her task*	1.676	Impatient*	1.302
Poor attention span*	1.616	Makes non-speech noises*	1.042
Poor sense of danger*	1.608	Poor attention span*	0.998
Chews or mouths objects*	1.514	Avoids eye contact*	0.958
Unusual body movements, posture or way of walking*	1.486	Has temper tantrums*	0.958
Makes non-speech noises*	1.284	Underreacts to pain*	0.958
Impatient*	1.108	Unusual body movements, posture of walking*	0.958
Laughs for no obvious reason*	1.108	Aloof, in his/her own world*	0.917
Likes to hold unusual object, overly fascinated with something	1.068	Arranges objects or routine in a strict order*	0.917
Overactive, unable to sit still	1.068	Becomes over-excited	0.917
Sleeps too little, disrupted sleep	1.054	Irritable	0.917
Repeated movements of hands, body, head or face	1.041	Overly attention-seeking	0.917

Table 2. (Continued)

Cornelia de Lange syndrome		Prader-Willi syndrome	
Item	**Mean**	**Item**	**Mean**
Makes non-speech noises*	1.206	Arranges objects or routine in a strict order*	1.322
Prefers to do things on his/her own, tends to be a loner*	1.176	Prefers to do things on his/her own, tends to be a loner*	1.167
Poor attention span*	1.088	Upset over small changes in routine or environment	1.153
Mood changes rapidly for no apparent reason	1.059	Scratches or picks at his/her skin	1.133
Avoids eye contact*	1	Easily led by others	1.117
Aloof, in his/her own world*	1	Doesn't mix with his/her own age group	1.083
Impatient*	0.971	Underreacts to pain*	1.083
Poor sense of danger*	0.941	Moves slowly, underactive	1.034
Throws or breaks objects	0.941	Has temper tantrums*	1.033
Chews or mouths objects*	0.912	Easily distracted from his/her task*	1
Easily distracted from his/her task*	0.912	Impatient*	0.9
Laughs for no obvious reason*	0.882	Poor sense of danger*	0.9

* overlapping with one of the other syndromes.

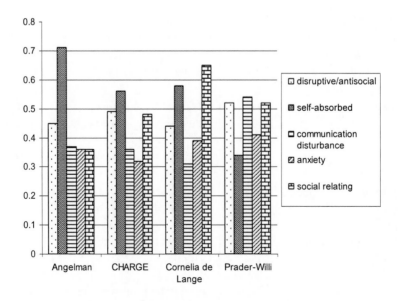

Figure 1. Profile of mean weighed subscale scores on the DBC-P per syndrome.

Comparison of Challenging Behavior between Syndromes

Differences in subscale profiles were found, therefore differences in mean raw subscale scores between the syndromes were tested on significance. Kruskal-Wallis tests were used because of the non-normality of some of the subscale data and heterogeneity of variance in some groups. No differences were found on the total problem behavior scale ($H(3) = 2.450$, $p = .484$), disruptive/antisocial ($H(3) = 2.517$, $p = .472$) and anxiety subscale ($H(3) = 2.322$, $p = .508$). However, significant differences were found on the self-absorbed ($H(3) = 49.432$, $p < .001$), communication disturbance ($H(3) = 17.900$, $p = < .001$) and social relating subscale ($H(3) = 17.230$, $p = .001$). See Table 3 for mean subscale scores on the subscales with significant differences.

Table 3. Mean raw scores and standard deviations for DBC-P subscales with significant differences on Kruskal-Wallis test

	Angelman	CHARGE	Cornelia de Lange	Prader-Willi
Self-absorbed behavior *M*	22.16	17.29	18.06	10.41
SD	8.41	11.66	10.12	5.55
Communication disturbance *M*	4.84	4.63	4.06	6.97
SD	3.33	2.87	3.59	4.04
Social relating problems *M*	3.60	4.83	6.53	5.20
SD	2.49	4.18	3.86	3.22

For the post hoc Mann-Whitney tests an alpha of .001 was used because of the large amount of comparisons. Significant differences were found between Angelman and Cornelia de Lange syndrome on social relating problems ($U = 693.500$, $p < .001$) and between Angelman and Prader-Willi syndrome on self-absorbed behavior ($U = 584.000$, $p < .001$). Furthermore significant differences were found between Cornelia de Lange syndrome and Prader-Willi syndrome on the self-absorbed ($U = 572.500$, $p < .001$) and the communication disturbance subscale ($U = 565.500$, $p < .001$).

DISCUSSION

In the four researched syndromes percentages of persons who showed challenging behavior within the clinical range, range between 38% and 49%. This is only slightly higher than the 41% in a population study of persons with intellectual disability by Einfeld and Tonge (1996).

As such, persons with these syndromes do not seem to be prone to heightened levels of challenging behavior as a whole, as measured by the DBC-P. A more in-depth comparison can be valuable in searching for syndrome-specificity of some behaviors. Keeping the probabilistic view of a behavioral phenotype by Dykens (1995) in mind, very few behaviors appeared to be prevalent in the majority of the persons as item analysis showed. Also in the highest ranked items there were few behaviors high on the list for only one particular syndrome. However, the behaviors that were found to be 'unique' might be seen as characteristic for the description of the particular syndrome.

The comparison of subscale scores made clear that between the syndromes different profiles were present. An important issue that has to be kept in mind though is the large difference in the level of intellectual disability between the four syndromes. Most persons with Angelman syndrome have a severe intellectual disability, and persons with Prader-Willi syndrome will most likely function within the mild range of intellectual disability. In CHARGE and Cornelia de Lange syndrome the levels of functioning range from no intellectual disability to severe intellectual disability. This variability in the researched syndromes will also have its influence on the different behaviors between the syndromes but has not been analyzed yet in this study. A further limitation of the study is the gathering of participants through the Parent Support Groups. It is unclear in which way this influenced the results, e.g. by over-inclusion of children with challenging behavior.

Most research, as well as this project, focused on behaviors in persons with the syndrome itself. The influence of environmental factors such as the family characteristics has been researched far less. Inclusion of this type of variables seems necessary to unravel the specific mechanisms of the genetic disorder and other contributing factors. As a first step we started with projects investigating parenting stress in families with a child with these syndromes and the relation with challenging behavior (Wulffaert, Scholte, Dijkxhoorn, Bergman, Van Ravenswaaij-Arts, & Van Berckelaer-Onnes, submitted; Wulffaert, Van Berckelaer-Onnes, Kroonenberg, Scholte, Bhuiyan, & Hennekam, submitted).

REFERENCES

Dykens, E. (1995). Measuring behavioral phenotypes: Provocations from the "new genetics". *American Journal on Mental Retardation*, 99, 522-532.

Einfeld, S.L., & Tonge, B.J. (1996). Population prevalence of psychopathology in children and adolescents with intellectual disability: II epidemiological findings. *Journal of Intellectual Disability Research*, 40, 99-109.

Einfeld, S.L., & Tonge, B.J. (2002). Manual for the Developmental Behavior Checklist (2nd ed., primary carer version & teacher version). Melbourne, Australia: University of New South Wales and Monash University.

Koot, H.M., & Dekker, M.C. (2001). Handleiding voor de VOG ouder en leerkrachtversie [Manual for the VOG parent and teacher version]. Rotterdam, NL: Afdeling Kinder- en Jeugdpsychiatrie, Erasmus Medisch Centrum, Sophia Kinderziekenhuis/Erasmus Universiteit Rotterdam.

Wulffaert, J., Scholte, E.M., Dijkxhoorn, Y.M., Bergman, J.E.H., Van Ravenswaaij-Arts, C.M.A., & Van Berckelaer-Onnes, I.A. (submitted). Parenting stress in CHARGE syndrome and the relationship with child characteristics.

Wulffaert, J., Van Berckelaer-Onnes, I.A., Kroonenberg, P.M., Scholte, E.M., Bhuiyan, Z.A., & Hennekam, R.C.M. (submitted). Simultaneous analysis of the behavioral phenotype, physical factors, and parenting stress in people with Cornelia de Lange syndrome.

Chapter 21

FETAL ALCOHOL AND FETAL TOBACCO SYNDROMES: A JAPANESE PERSPECTIVE

H. Tanaka

National Institute of Neuroscience, Higashiyamato-shi, Tokyo Japan

AIM AND METHODS

The purpose of this study was to find a means to estimate and prevent the effects of prenatalalcohol and/or tobacco on infant development, especially on the central nervous system (CNS). Therefore, I evaluated the criteria used for the diagnosis of fetal alcohol syndrome (FAS) and fetal tobacco syndrome (FTS), and then demonstrated the concomitant effects of alcohol and tobacco on infant development. Finally, I proposed a new concept based on the Japanese data.

As to the data source, in the 1990s, I collected retrospective information on maternal alcohol or tobacco use and abnormal infants from 3,380 administrative units in Japan. Then, I checked and examined individual cases for the mother's and offspring's conditions before and after pregnancy and birth, respectively. About 500 children who exhibited abnormal findings related to prenatal alcohol and/or tobacco consumption were used a data source. These children are being examined clinically even now.

RESULTS

Alcohol

Fetal Alcohol Syndrome (FAS) and Fetal Alcohol Effects (FAE)

The criteria evaluated for the diagnosis of FAS and FAE were those recommended by the Fetal Alcohol Study Group of the Research Society on Alcoholism (Rosett, 1980). The diagnosis of FAS is made when a history of maternal alcohol abuse can be confirmed and examination reveals that the child meets three criteria, A, B and C. That is, A, prenatal and/or postnatal growth retardation; B, CNS involvement, including signs of neurological abnormality(N), developmental delay(D), and intellectual impairment(I); and C, a characteristic facial dysmorphology. The term FAE is used when a child meets less than three of these criteria.

Maternal Drinking during Pregnancy in FAS and FAE

Using the criteria for the diagnosis of FAS and FAE, 35 cases of FAS and 29 cases of FAE were identified. Then, the relationships between the diagnoses of FAS and FAE, and maternal drinking were evaluated. As to ethanol consumption during pregnancy, drinking group I represents heavy drinking for 5 to 10 years before pregnancy, or alcoholism, group II moderate drinking with continuous daily drinking during pregnancy, and group III light drinking without continuous daily drinking. Children fulfilling the three criteria were born mostly to mothers belonging to drinking group I, but some were also born to ones in drinking group III. Therefore, a mother's alcoholism or heavy drinking is not a differentiating factor for FAS and FAE.

Tobacco

Fetal Tobacco Syndrome (FTS) and Fetal Tobacco Effects (FTE)

The concept of FTS was proposed in 1985 (Nieburg et al, 1985). It is suggested that FTS be applied to an infant when the following four criteria are met.

1. The mother smoked five or more cigarettes a day throughout pregnancy.
2. The mother showed no evidence of hypertension during pregnancy.
3. The newborn exhibited symmetrical growth retardation at term ($\geq$ 37 weeks), with a birth weight of less than 2,500 g.
4. There is no other obvious cause of IUGR.

Therefore, children born to heavy to moderate alcohol drinking mothers were excluded from the diagnosis of FTS. During the past decade, it has become increasingly clear that children born to women who smoke cigarettes during pregnancy exhibit consistent deficits in neurological functioning as well as in physical growth. However, the proposed criteria for FTS do not include maldevelopment of the brain. Furthermore, in my Japanese study of children who exhibited abnormal findings related to prenatal smoking, only 38% satisfied the criteria for FTS.

Regarding FTS family pedigrees, the criteria for FTS are still debatable, because the criterion of a newborn with a birth weight of less than 2,500 g at term does not apply to all abnormal children.

As an example, I present two family pedigrees of FTS, A and B. Neither mothers had a history of alcohol drinking. In both families, the first child, who was born when the mother did not smoke, was normal. The second child in both families, and the fourth one in Family B satisfied the criteria for FTS. However, the third child in both families did not satisfy the criteria for FTS, although both children exhibited D (developmental delay). Therefore, I proposed the term "fetal tobacco effects (FTE)" for when the gestational age is less than 37 weeks (<37).

Maternal Factors in FTS and FTE

The relationships of maternal smoking and other factors to an infant's status being diagnosed as FTS or FTE were evaluated.The daily number of cigarettes during pregnancy and the percentage of mothers who were light drinkers (and also coffee drinkers) were not differentiating factors for FTS and FTE. However, maternal factors during pregnancy or delivery such as anemia, premature rupturing of the membranes, and a placental abnormality (abruptio placentae or placenta previa) exhibited higher percentages for FTE than FTS.

Alcohol and Tobacco

Features of CNS Involvement in FTS, FTE, FAS and FAE

As indicators of maldevelopment of the brain, three abnormalities as signs of CNS involvement for the diagnosis of FAS were examined, D, I and N.

The frequencies of CNS involvement in FTS and FTE were 33% and 46%, respectively. The main feature of CNS involvement in FTS was D, those in FTE being D and I. Therefore, maldevelopment of the brain is not severer in FTS than FTE, to which factors other than smoking causing a reduction in the gestational period, and ones during pregnancy and delivery may contribute. A causal relationship between prenatal smoking and maldevelopment of the brain of offspring should continue to be studied based on the concept of FTE in addition to FTS.

On the other hand, all cases of FAS and FAE exhibited CNS involvement, based on the criterion of at least one of three signs of CNS involvement, D, I and N. FAS showed a severer degree of involvement, as a percentage of D + I + N, and a higher frequency, as a percentage of D + I, than FAE. The most frequent features of CNS involvement were D and I in both FAS and FAE.

Therefore, the diagnostic criteria for FAS or FAE revealed that FAS infants exhibit a severer degree of CNS involvement than FAE ones. Learning difficulties and mental retardation could be key indicators of alcohol exposure *in utero*.

CNS Involvement in the Maternal Drinking and Smoking Groups

The concomitant consumption of alcohol and tobacco by pregnant women, and its effect on fetal growth have been the subject of many studies. A total 58 cases of maternal alcohol and/or tobacco use during pregnancy and abnormal infants could be classified into four groups; nonsmokers and smokers with light to moderate alcoholic intake and heavy intake to alcoholism.

CNS involvement means at least one of the three signs, D, I and N. CNS involvement was shown to increase with increasing consumption of alcohol or tobacco. In the group of heavy drinkers or alcoholics who smoked all cases exhibited CNS involvement with developmental delay, sometimes with intellectual impairment as the most frequent feature. The present data suggest that the concomitant effects of alcohol and tobacco on brain development are additive.

Comparative Effects of Tobacco and Alcohol on Offspring

Based on human observation, the comparative effects of prenatal tobacco and alcohol on child health were examined. As to the period of consumption, smoking prior to pregnancy was related to a decrease in psychomotor development, while pre-pregnancy alcohol consumption was not associated with any of the developmental measures. The birth weight was affected more strongly by smoking than by alcohol drinking. However, the effect of tobacco on body weight reflected postnatal catch-up growth. The effect of tobacco on CNS dysfunction was less than that of alcohol.

Prevalence Rates in Japan

We roughly calculated the prevalence rates of FAS and FAE, and also FTS and FTE in Japan. After several steps, 35 cases of FAS and 29 cases of FAE, and 87 cases of FTS and 35 cases of FTE were conclusively identified. Based on these data, the prevalence rate of FAS and FAE in Japan is less than 0.1 per 1,000 live births, which is a very low compared to those in the USA and European countries. Furthermore, the prevalence rate of FTS and FTE in Japan is almost the same as that of FAS and FAE.

CONCLUSION

1. FAS infants exhibited a severer degree of CNS involvement than FAE ones.
2. Maldevelopment of the brain was not severer in FTS than FTE, to which factors other than smoking causing a reduction in the gestational period, and ones during pregnancy and delivery may contribute.
3. The effects on the CNS of alcohol were more frequent and severer than those of tobacco.
4. CNS involvement was shown to increase with increasing consumption of alcohol and/or tobacco.
5. The prevalence rates of FAS and FAE, and FTS and FTE in Japan are less than 1 per 10,000 live births, respectively.
6. Abstention from both alcohol and tobacco during pregnancy can benefit brain development.

REFERENCES

Nieburg P, Marks JS, McLaren NM, Remington PL. (1985). The fetal tobacco syndrome. *JAMA*, 253: 2998-2999 1985.

Rosett HL. (1980).A clinical perspective of the Fetal Alcohol Syndrome. *Alcohol Clin Exp Res*. 1980 4:119-22.

PART IV. CHALLENGING BEHAVIOR AND OFFENDING

An overlap between intellectual disabilities (ID) and challenging and/or offending behavior has been well established and remains an ongoing concern for a number of services. No moreso than the crminial justice system. *Talbot* reports on an investigation of the experience of prisoners with ID and highlights the need for increased awareness by all staff working within the criminal system, along with the provision of improved resources. *Merrick and colleagues* describe the lack of manpower resources in Israel to manage individuals with ID presenting with challenging behavior. The psychological impact of challenging behavior and associated violence on staff can significantly affect the management of such behaviors. *Rose and Howard* highlight the impact of violence on staff and explore a number of factors which impact on outcome.

Challenging behavior is very much influenced by the environment, and the study of theology and its impact on human behavior remains an interesting area of future research. *Barnhill* discusses an ethological approach to challenging behavior which maybe an additional tool to the understanding and management of challenging behavior in persons with ID. Further, *Barnhill* goes on to discuss the possibility of self injurious behavior being a form of addictive behavior and emphasizes the need for a better understanding of self injurious behavior in this context.

Chapter 22

PEOPLE WITH INTELLECTUAL DISABILITIES IN THE CRIMINAL JUSTICE SYSTEM

J. Talbot
Prison Reform Trust, London, UK

INTRODUCTION

This article presents some of the main findings and recommendations from research undertaken in the UK about the experiences of people with intellectual disabilities (ID) and persons with learning difficulties who come into contact with the criminal justice system as police suspects, defendants and offenders. The programme, entitled *No One Knows,* was led by the Prison Reform Trust and supported by The Diana, Princess of Wales Memorial Fund and Mencap. It was chaired by the Rt Hon Baroness Joyce Quin, former Minister of Prisons for England and Wales.

METHODOLOGY

Empirical research involving 200 prison staff and 173 prisoners was undertaken in 2006 and 2007 and relevant literature and policy documents were reviewed. Participating prisons reflected the levels of security of the prison estates across the UK, the age and gender of prisoners, and mix of public and contracted out establishments.

Research with prison staff took the form of a questionnaire, which included closed and open-ended questions, and explored respondents' perceptions of how prisoners with ID and prisoners with learning difficulties were identified and supported at their prison. Staff from different parts of the prison were invited to participate including from psychology, healthcare, education, residence (the wings or halls where prisoners will often spend most of their time) and prison officers, in particular those responsible for disability liaison.

Research with prisoners took the form of an interview, which included closed and open-ended questions, and explored their experiences of the criminal justice system and aspirations for the future. Prisoners were identified by prison staff and invited to take part. A small number of prisoners without ID or learning difficulties were interviewed so that comparisons could be drawn. Apart from one, all interviews were conducted on a one-to-one basis. Interviewees were also asked to complete:

the LIPS learning disability screening tool[1]
the Glasgow Anxiety Scale for people with an Intellectual Disability[2]
the Glasgow Depression Scale for people with a Learning Disability[3].

SCOPE OF THE RESEARCH

Unusually this research included people with ID and individuals with learning difficulties. This decision was driven by three important factors:

research demonstrating that 'one of the most prevalent vulnerable groups amongst offenders comprises those who do not have ID as formally defined but who have much lower cognitive and adaptive abilities than do either the general population or the offending population.' (McBrien, 2003)
the Disability Discrimination Act, which includes in its scope some people with ID and learning difficulties
the European Convention on Human Rights, in particular article 5 (right to liberty); article 6 (right to a fair hearing) and article 14 (enjoyment of ECHR rights without discrimination).

Thus, the *No One Knows* programme included in its scope people who find some activities that involve thinking and understanding difficult and who need additional help and support in their everyday living. The terms ID or learning difficulties were used in this research to include people who:

experience difficulties in communicating and expressing themselves and understanding ordinary social cues
have unseen or hidden disabilities such as dyslexia
experience difficulties with learning and/or have had disrupted learning experiences that have led them to function at a significantly lower level than the majority of their peers
are on the autistic spectrum, including people with Asperger Syndrome

People with ID are not a homogenous group, neither are those with learning difficulties or those on the autistic spectrum. They are all individuals with a wide range of different life experiences, strengths, weaknesses, and support needs. However many will share common characteristics, which might make them especially vulnerable as they enter and travel through the criminal justice system.

---

1 See Mason, J. and Murphy, G (2002).
2 See Mindham, J. & Espie, C. A.; *Journal of Intellectual Disability Research*, volume 47 part 1, pp22-30, January 2003.
3 See Cuthill, F. M., Espie, Colin A. and Cooper, Sally-Anne; *British Journal of Psychiatry* (2003), 182, 347-353.

PREVALENCE

Research to determine prevalence rates show a wide variability in estimates, which is due to a number of factors. These include which screening or assessment tools were used, whether assessments were undertaken individually or in groups and the level of training of the people administering the assessments (Loucks, 2007).

Recent UK studies show that:

20 – 30% of offenders have learning disabilities or difficulties that interfere with their ability to cope within the criminal justice system (Loucks 2007)

7% of prisoners have an IQ of less than 70 and a further 25% have an IQ of less than 80 (Mottram, 2007)

23% of prisoners under 18 years of age have an IQ of less than 70 (Harrington and Bailey et al, 2005)

20% of the prison population has a 'hidden disability' that 'will affect and undermine their performance in both education and work settings.'(Rack, 2005)

Despite a lack of clarity on prevalence and how best, methodologically, prevalence might be determined, it is clear that high numbers of people with ID are caught up in the criminal justice system.

MAIN FINDINGS

Five overarching themes emerged from the research, which are briefly covered below; some of the recommendations for change are shown.

1. Disability Discrimination and Possible Human Rights Abuses

Evidence suggests that people with ID and persons with learning difficulties are discriminated against personally, systemically and routinely as they enter and travel through the criminal justice system. They experience maltreatment by the police and by prison officers; do not receive the support to which they are entitled during police interview; are unaware of what is happening to them in court and often don't understand the decisions of the court, and are unable to access prison information and regimes routinely. UK criminal justice agencies are failing in their duty to promote disability equality and to eliminate discrimination. In consequence the sense, if not the fact, of injustice prevails.

Recommendation

UK criminal justice agencies should comply with disability discrimination and human rights legislation.

2. Knowing Who Has ID or Learning Difficulties

There is no routine screening or assessment to identify people with ID or learning difficulties at any stage of the criminal justice process. Consequently the particular needs of such people are not recognised let alone met; from the point of arrest through to release from prison the criminal justice system routinely fails them.

Recommendation

People with ID or learning difficulties should be routinely identified at the point of arrest so that appropriate support may be put into place and, where appropriate, diversion from the criminal justice system considered; information sharing between criminal justice agencies and with relevant health, social care and education should be reciprocal and timely.

3. Implications for the Criminal Justice System

The verbal comprehension skills of prisoners with ID or with learning difficulties and lack of appropriate support have potentially very serious implications in particular in regard of the rights of people with ID to a fair hearing (Article 6, ECHR).

Once in prison, poor literacy skills and difficulties expressing themselves made daily living and accessing the prison regime problematic. This can leave prisoners at greater psychological risk as they spend long periods on their own with little to do; many experienced clinically significant depression or anxiety.

Prisoners' exclusion from cognitive behavior treatment programmes (Talbot, 2007; Loucks, 2007) may affect parole and release dates with some prisoners staying in prison longer as a result. In its report, *A Life Like Any Other? Human Rights of Adults with Learning Disabilities* the UK Joint Committee on Human Rights noted, 'This clearly engages Article 5, ECHR (right to liberty) and Article 14 (enjoyment of ECHR rights without discrimination). It is also an area that falls within the Prison Service's responsibility under the Disability Equality Duty.'

Recommendation

Criminal justice information and interventions should be made accessible to all offenders regardless of disability; advocacy support should be routinely available.

4. A Needs Led Approach: Collaborative Multi-Agency Working

Criminal justice agencies do not have the requisite expertise to identify adequately, work with and support people with ID or learning difficulties. Collaboration is required involving the collective efforts of criminal justice agencies, healthcare, social care, education and the full range of local services. Commitment and leadership at the highest level, national standards and mandatory local action are required.

Recommendation

Local multi-agency liaison forums should develop strategies for preventing offending and re-offending by people with ID or with learning difficulties; participation by certain specified local agencies should be mandatory.

5. Workforce Development

Although there were exceptions and some examples of good practice, criminal justice staff do not routinely undertake awareness training in ID and learning difficulties neither do many healthcare and education staff who work with offenders. Such training is important: it alerts staff to the possibility that some prisoners may need support and encourages them to question what might precipitate certain behaviors. Evidence shows that such training can encourage referrals to support services for further investigation (Bryan, 2004).

There are gaps in service provision for this group of offenders and most prison staff said that the quality of existing services was poor and referral procedures were unclear (Talbot, 2007).

Recommendation

All staff in contact with offenders as they enter and travel through the criminal justice system should undertake awareness training in ID and learning difficulties; referral routes and access to expertise in ID and learning difficulties and speech and language therapy should be routinely available.

The full report on which this article is based, entitled *Prisoners' Voices*, can be downloaded from www.prisonreformtrust.org.uk/nok

REFERENCES

Harrington, R. and Bailey, S., with Chitsabesan, P., Kroll, L., Macdonald, W., Sneider, S., Kenning, C., Taylor, G., Byford, S., and Barrett, B. (2005) Mental Health Needs and Effectiveness of Provision for Young Offenders in Custody and in the Community, London: Youth Justice Board for England and Wales.

Joint Committee on Human Rights (2008) A life like any other? Human Rights of Adults with Learning Disabilities. Seventh Report of Session 2007-08. London: TSO.

Loucks, N. (2007) Prisoners with learning difficulties and learning disabilities – review of prevalence and associated needs. London: Prison Reform Trust.

Loucks, N. (2007) Identifying and supporting prisoners with learning difficulties and learning disabilities: the views of prison staff in Scotland. London: Prison Reform Trust.

McBrien, J. (2003) The Intellectually Disabled Offender: Methodological Problems in Identification, *Journal of Applied Research in Intellectual Disabilities,* 16.

Mottram, P. G. (2007) HMP Liverpool, Styal and Hindley Study Report. Liverpool: University of Liverpool.

Rack, J. (2005) The Incidence of Hidden Disabilities in the Prison Population, Egham, Surrey: Dyslexia Institute.

Talbot, J. (2007) Identifying and supporting prisoners with learning difficulties and learning disabilities: the views of prison staff. London: Prison Reform Trust.

Talbot, J. (2008) Prisoners Voices: experiences of the criminal justice system by prisoners with learning disabilities and difficulties. London: Prison Reform Trust.

Chapter 23

MENTAL HEALTH SERVICES FOR PEOPLE WITH INTELLECTUAL DISABILITIES IN RESIDENTIALCARE IN ISRAEL

J. Merrick[1,2], E. Merrick-Kenig[1], I. Kandel[1,3], and M. Morad[1,4]

[1]National Institute of Child Health and Human Development,
Office of the Medical Director, Division for Mental Retardation,
Ministry of Social Affairs, Jerusalem
[2]Kentucky Children's Hospital, University of Kentucky,
Lexington, United States of America
[3]Faculty of Social Sciences, Department of Behavioral Sciences,
Ariel University Center of Samaria, Ariel, Israel
[4]Department of Family Medicine, Faculty of Health Sciences,
Ben Gurion University of the Negev, Beer-Sheva, Israel

INTRODUCTION

Persons with intellectual disabilities (ID) in need of residential care in Israel is provided service according to the law from the Ministry of Social Affairs, Division for Mental Retardation (DMR) in 59 residential care centers (government, private and non-for-profit) around the country. Each residential care center has a medical clinic in operation 24 hours a day staffed by nurses and during day time a physician provides service according to the number of residents. The 2006 profile of the population (6,840 persons) in residential care was 13% between age 0-19 years, 80% between 20-59 years and 7% 60 years and older; 46% severe and profound, 42% moderate and 12% mild ID; 22% nursing patients and 36% with challenging behavior (Merrick, 2007).

Since 1991 there has been severe efforts to recruit psychiatrists to provide consultative service to the general medical clinic in each residential care center. The aim of this chapter was to look at trends over time in the number of psychiatrists recuited, psychiatric medication and hospitalization in this residential care population.

DATA

A questionnaire was developed and pilot tested in 1997 in a few residential care centers, which resulted in a final survey instrument (Merick, 2005). Since 1998 the survey questionnaire with a descriptive letter has been send to each clinic in order for the chief nurse and physician to fill out the questionnaire during the last month of that year and return the questionnaire to the Office of the Medical Director by February of the next year (Merrick, 2005). Data used to fill in the questionnaire at the end of the year has been gathered and registered thorughout the year.

In order to look at trends in the psychiatric service we studied and extracted data from the national survey questionnaires for the 1998-2006 period (100% response rates for each survey).

FINDINGS CONCERNING MENTAL HEALTH SERVICES

The number of psychiatrists recuited over the years 1998-2006, the number of residential care centers with a permanent psychiatric consultant, the rate of psychiatric consultant per 1,000 population and the hours converted to full time positions is shown in table 1. From 1994 the Office of the Medical Director, Division for Mental Retardation, Ministry of Social Affairs, has also employed a parttime psychiatric consultant (40 hours per months) to supervise the psychaitric service/consultants in the residential care centers.. We hope in the near future to increase this to 60 hours per month in order to facilitate more training, supervision and also initiate applied research in the field.

Table 1. Trends in the number of psychiatrists in residential care centers for people with intellectual disability in Israel 1998-2006

Year	Total residents (number of centers)	Number of centers with psychiatrists	Number of psychiatrists per 1,000 residents	Equivalent to full time positions
1998	6,022 (53)	37	6.14	6.49
1999	6,122 (53)	44	7.19	11.96
2000	6,213 (53)	42	6.76	11.55
2001	6,370 (54)	44	6.91	11.77
2002	6,352 (57)	45	7.08	14.05
2003	6,500 (57)	47	7.23	14.48
2004	6,610 (58)	51	7.72	17..53
2005	6,749 (58)	52	7.70	18.83
2006	6,840 (59)	53	7.75	18.07

In table 2 is shown the number of persons with ID in residential care centers receiving chronic medication for any reason (hypertension, diabetes, epilepsy etc), the number of persons treated with anti-epileptic medication due to epilepsy, the number of persons receiving psychiatric medication and the total times SOS medication was given over the year due to challenging or aggressive behavior. In table 3 the trend of psychiatric hospitalization is shown.

Table 2. Trends in medication for persons with intellectual disability in residential care centers in Israel 1998-2006. Number of persons, who received (%)

Year	Chronic medication	AED (anti-epileptic)	Psychotropic Medications	SOS
1998	3,922 (65.13)	1,730 (28.73)	2,741 (45.52)	1,573
1999	4,330 (71.44)	1,816 (29.66)	2,929 (47.84)	5,343
2000	4,785 (77.02)	1,835 (29.53)	2,848 (45.84)	4,735
2001	4,976 (78.12)	1,873 (29.40)	3,240 (50.86)	6,128
2002	5,098 (80.26)	1,967 (30.97)	3,225 (50.77)	6,814
2003	5,233 (80.51)	2,016 (31.02)	3,162 (48.65)	5,632
2004	5.484 (82.95)	1.969 (29.79)	3,473 (52.54)	6,474
2005	5,548 (82.20)	2,043 (30.27)	3,440 (50.97)	6,739
2006	5,890 (86.11)	2,287 (33.44)	3,515 (51.39)	6,297

Table 3. Trends in the number of psychiatric hospitalizations for persons with intellectual disability in residential care centers in Israel 1998-2006

Year	Total hospitalizations	Rate per 1,000	Number of days	Rate per 1,000
1998	33	5.48	548	90.99
1999	44	7.19	609	99.48
2000	43	6.92	785	126.35
2001	46	7.22	808	126.84
2002	31	4.88	452	71.16
2003	34	5.23	565	86.92
2004	33	4.99	569	86.08
2005	33	4.89	655	97.05
2006	53	7.75	782	114.33

DISCUSSION

Recruitment of psychiatrists to work in the field of ID has been a problem in Israel.. One reason has been that it is not attractive to work with this population, but also the fact that psychiatrists have not been trained to handle this special population and a lack of a subspecialty. Since 1991 we have made special efforts to recruit psychiatrists and as can be seen in table 1 these efforts have born fruit and today the manpower is equivalent to 18 full-time positions. We would in fact prefer to convert these positions to full-time, but the infrastructure does not allow us to do it at this moment, but we continue to pursue this idea, because we believe this would be a better solution and getting much more out of the money allocated than having many part-time consultants.

People with ID have a higher prevalence of mental health problems than the general population. In the United Kingdom Birch et al (1970) and Rutter et al (1970) found a prevalence of 40% in this population, Einfeld and Tonge (1996) in Australia found 40%, while Borthwick-Duffy (1994) in a review of 12 studies found 14-80% with a mean of 45%. Reiss and Aman (1997) in their review of 44 published surveys found that 30-50% of residents in large institutions used psychotropic drugs, 25-35% anti-convulsants, while 25-40% used psychotropic drugs in community setting and 20-30% anti-convulsants. In our survey we found that in residential care centers in Israel about 51% of the population used psychotropic and 33% anti-convulsant medication, which is compatable with the above findings. In our annual surveys we do not have specific information on psychiatric diagnosis or psychopathology, but only the number of residents receiving various kinds of medications.

The increase in psychotropic medications over this period could be seen as a result of an increase in psychiatric consultants and further diagnosis, but since we have no data on the specific diagnosis that is just speculation. Our policy has been to decrease poly-pharmacy and try to use more modern drugs with less side effects, which could be another explanation for the increase, while another aspect has been the increase in the number of persons with challenging behavior over the study period (from 27% to 36% (Merrick 2007). We have a problem with the new generation of psychotropic medicine, because these drugs are not designated as drugs for people with ID, but for persons with schizophrenia and the Ministry has not allowed to fund drugs outside of what is accepted to the general population, even though it is known to help also people with ID without schizophrenia.

The data on hospital admissions showed an increase over the study period and compared with the general population a seven times higher rate. Numbers of hospitalization days was less than the general population, maybe due to the fact that the psychiatric service at the centers increased over the same period (Haklai, 2005).

Avaliable psychiatric care for persons with ID in Israel has improved in residential care centers, where more psychiatrists have been employed and willing to work with this special and challenging population. Psychiatrists are needed for this population due to the high prevalence of psychopathology, which cannot be handled by the general medical staff and we hope that in the future we will see further training and a subspecialty emerge.

Unfortunately our data collection does not enable us to differentiate between the psychiatric service provided to each age group, so this paper describes the service for all ages, but 13% of the residents are between 0-19 years of age.

REFERENCES

Birch HG, Richardson SA, Baird D, Horobin G, Illsley R. Mental subnormality in the community: A clinical and epidemiological study. Baltimore, MD: Williams and Wilkins, 1970.

Borthwick-Duffy SA. Epidemiology and prevalence of psychopathology in people with mental retardation. *J Consult Clin Psychol.* 1994;62:17-27.

Einfeld SL, Tonge BJ. Population prevalence of psychopathology in children and adolescents with intellectual disability: II. Epidemiological findings. *J Intellect Disabil Res.* 1996;40(2):99-109.

Haklai Z, Gordon E, Stein N, Shteiman A, Hillel S, Ozeri R, Aburbeh M. Health in Israel. 2005 selected data. Jerusalem, *Min Health*, 2005.

Merrick J. Survey of medical clinics, 2006. Jerusalem: Office Med Dir, *Min Soc Affairs*,2007.

Merrick J. National survey 1998 on medical services for persons with intellectual disability in residential care centers in Israel. *Int J Disabil Hum Dev.* 2005;4(2):139-46.

Merrick J. Trends in challenging behavior of residents with intellectual disability in residential care centers in Israel, 1998-2006. Jerusalem: Office Med Director, *Min Soc Affairs*, 2007.

Reiss S, Aman MG. The international consensus process on psychopharmacology and intellectual disability. *J Intellect Disabil Res.* 1997;41(6):448-55.

Rutter M, Graham P, Yule W. A neuropsychiatric study of childhood. London: *Spastics Int Med Publ.* 1970.

Chapter 24

THE PSYCHOLOGICAL IMPACT OF VIOLENCE ON STAFF

J.L. Rose[1] and R. Howard[2]

[1]School of Psychology, The University of Birmingham, Birmingham, UK
[2]Community Learning Disabilities Team, Crewe, UK

INTRODUCTION

Staff working in intellectual disability services are in a powerful position with regards to shaping the behavior of people in their care (Hastings, 1997). Staff responses to violent behaviors, often examined under the umbrella term 'challenging behavior', may play a key role in shaping behavior (Hastings & Remington, 1993; Hastings & Remington, 1994).

The term 'challenging behavior' is used to describe "culturally abnormal behavior of such intensity, frequency or duration that the physical safety of the person or others is likely to be placed in serious jeopardy, or behavior that is likely to seriously limit or delay access to and use of ordinary community facilities" (Emerson et al, 1987). This definition includes violent behaviors but also behaviors such as stereotypy and self-injurious behavior.

A number of studies have explored staff emotional reactions to challenging behavior. The findings suggest that different topographies of behavior produce different emotional reactions (Bromley & Emerson, 1995). Given these findings, it seems unusual that the literature tends to explore staff reactions to challenging behavior as a whole, rather than to specific topographies of challenging behavior.

The term 'challenging behavior' may create difficulty within research due to its subjective nature (Clegg, 1994; Heyman et al, 1998). Within stress research, this term may create 'circular arguments', as individuals experiencing greater stress may perceive behaviors as more challenging (Lazarus & Folkman, 1986). Whilst the term 'violence' is somewhat subjective (Farrell, 1997), clearer definitions exist (e.g. 'Any incident in which a person is verbally abused, threatened or assaulted by a service user': Health and Safety Commission, 1997 pp.1). Varying definitions may account for the inconsistent relationship found between challenging behavior and stress within the research. For instance, Chung and Corbett (1998) found that burnout was more strongly associated with job variables than challenging behavior. However, Jenkins et al (1997) found that challenging behavior was associated with psychological wellbeing.

High levels of violent behavior have been reported within some intellectual disability services (Reed et al, 2004; Sigafoos et al, 1994). The links between stress and violence found in other research areas, e.g. psychiatric nursing (Poster, 1996; Rippon, 2000), the potential impact upon service users (Rose et al, 1998), and the clearer definition of violence, suggest that research considering these areas is timely.

STRESS IN STAFF WORKING IN INTELLECTUAL DISABILITY SETTINGS

Stress is defined as, 'a reaction to personal harms and threats of various kinds that emerge out of the person-environment relationship' (Lazarus, 1993, pp. 7). Health care research often refers to 'burnout', which is an emotional state thought to result from persistently high levels of staff stress: characterised by emotional exhaustion, depersonalisation of service users, and a reduced sense of personal accomplishment (Maslach & Jackson, 1993). The terms burnout and stress are used interchangeably in the literature. This paper will generally use the term stress, as this is a more generic term, encompassing a wider area of psychological well-being and allowing a broader view of the literature.

Early concepts of stress were based upon the stimulus-response model (Holmes & Rahe, 1967). Later research views stress as the result of primary and secondary appraisals, rather than the stimulus itself. Primary appraisals are appraisals of the stimuli in relation to personal goals, beliefs about self and the world, values, and situational intentions. Secondary appraisals involve appraisals of personal resources and ability to cope (Lazarus & Folkman, 1984).

While levels of stress or burnout reported by staff in intellectual disability services are not necessarily high (Hatton and Lobban, 2007; Skirrow and Hatton, 2007), levels of stress are variable and can be a problem for some staff. Numerous sources of stress, or 'stressors', have been identified for staff working in intellectual disability settings; including work overload (Male & May, 1997), team climate (Rose & Schelewa-Davies, 1996), role conflict (Dyer & Quine, 1998) staff support (Rose, 1997), coping strategies (Mitchell & Hastings, 2001), expectations of clients (Stevens & O'Neil, 1983) client characteristics (Stenfert Kroese & Fleming, 1992), personality (Rose et al, 2003), and organisational culture (Dyer & Quine, 1998). Staff stress may impact negatively on services in a number of ways such as increased absenteeism (Lawson & O'Brien, 1994), high turnover (Hatton & Emerson, 1993) and reduced interaction with service-users (Rose et al., 1998).

STAFF STRESS AND VIOLENCE IN SERVICES FOR PEOPLE WITH INTELLECTUAL DISABILITIES

Previous research has demonstrated that experiencing physical injury from violence is not a necessary condition for negative psychological reactions to develop: it is sufficient that somebody is exposed to the threat of violence (Budd, 1999). A similar definition of violence is offered by Winstanley and Whittington (2002) who defined assault as aggressive physical contact from a service user towards staff, irrespective of injury. Threats include verbal threats and physically threatening violence through gesture or behavior. The literature uses the term aggressive behavior interchangeably with the term violent behavior, the current paper also adopts these terms. Research suggests that workplace violence impacts negatively on psychological and physical well-being (Budd, 1999; Caldwell, 1992; Flannery, 1996).

Relatively few papers exist that specifically identify a link between violence and stress in Intellectual disability services. Mitchell and Hastings (2001) suggest that a relationship between violence and burnout exists, although methodological issues limit the certainty of their findings. In this study, the greatest predictors of increased burnout, were the emotional reactions of depression and anger. Rose et al. (2004) provided support for these findings, in a replication with participants working with challenging behavior. Unfortunately, the levels of aggressive behavior experienced by participants were not established.

Murray et al. (1999) engaged in a more direct investigation of the stress/violence relationship, by examining reported staff sickness and client assault levels over an 18 month period, in an intellectual disability service for adults with challenging behaviors. Assaults were defined clearly as verbal threats of physical assaults, attempted physical assaults and actual physical assaults. No relationship was found between assault levels and staff sickness. Murray et al. (1999) conclude that participant training for managing aggressive behavior may have reduced the impact of aggression. However, although staff sickness levels appear to be related to stress (Callaghan et al, 2000; Lawson & O'Brien, 1994), they may not accurately reflect stress (Fletcher, 1991). Furthermore, other organisational variables which may influence stress were not measured.

Hatton et al. (1995) suggested that other organisational variables lost significance in predicting high levels of perceived work stress, when violence entered the analysis. The relationship between a range of variables and stress in residential staff, working in intellectual disability services, was explored. Violent behavior was defined as damage to self, others, or property. All participants rated service user violent behavior, among the five most stressful elements of their work.

Rose and Rose (2005) surveyed community staff working with adults with ID. Service managers completed the Aberrant Behavior Checklist for aggression, for each service user. Staff were either assigned to a low incidence of aggression group (26%), or a high incident of aggression group (28%). No differences in burnout and the general health questionnaire (GHQ), a measure of stress, were identified between these groups. This would suggest that burnout and stress are not related to the experience of violence. However, lack of variability within the sample may have limited these findings, as all participants worked with service users with significant levels of reported aggression.

Lundstrom et al (2007) explored the relationship between the personality of staff, violence, and staff strain. They found an association between personality and strain and the risk of burnout in that certain staff exposed to violence felt more emotionally exhausted than staff who were not exposed. This suggests that certain staff may need special support to help them cope with violence.

In a qualitative study, Hellzen et al. (2004) provide a rich insight into the wellbeing of nurses, working with one adult with ID displaying sexual, physical, and verbally, aggressive behavior. Twenty-two interviews, with eight participants, were analysed. Participants described numerous symptoms associated with stress, including exhaustion and feeling 'burnt out'. Some participants also reported that their experience had undermined their view of themselves as 'good nurses', which was associated with feelings of guilt. The qualitative nature of this research means that it cannot be generalised and is contextual (Denzin & Lincoln, 1994), presenting difficulties in clinical application. However, the descriptions highlight the potentially enormous impact of one individual upon staff psychological wellbeing.

Howard et al (In Press) explored levels of violence, fear of violence, burnout, self-efficacy, staff support, and coping by direct care staff working both a medium secure setting with a high incidence of violence, and a community settings with a low incidence of violence. Participants working in the medium secure setting reported very similar levels of burnout to those in the community setting. However those working in the medium secure setting reported significantly lower fear of violence and higher self-efficacy compared to community participants. Self-efficacy demonstrated a significant moderator relationship with levels of violence and burnout. Higher threats of violence significantly correlated with lower fear of violence. This finding suggests that services that expect to manage violence may be better placed to support staff experiencing violence. Fear of violence may decrease in line with exposure to violence, perhaps due to increased self-efficacy. Training and support for staff may also increase self-efficacy, thus reducing burnout. As a result this research starts to provide an insight into the complex relationship between violence and burnout.

To understand the relationship between violence and staff stress we need to look for a range of variables that may be impacting upon this relationship. A number of factors that may moderate or mediate the stress/violence relationship have been suggested. For instance, attributions (Cottle et al. 1995; Wanless & Jahoda, 2002) coping strategies (Hastings, 1995; Hastings & Brown, 2002a; Mitchell & Hastings, 2001; Whittington & Burns, 2005), training (Allen & Tynan, 2000; Grey et al., 2002), emotional intelligence (Gerits et al., 2004), experience (Hastings, et al., 1995; Hastings & Remington, 1995; Kiely & Pankhurst, 1998), characteristics of violence (Howard & Hegarty, 2003), and self-efficacy (Hastings & Brown, 2002b). Understanding these relationships could lead to significant improvements in service design and delivery.

ACKNOWLEDGMENT

An expanded version of this article is published elsewhere (Howard et al, In Press).

REFERENCES

Allen, D., & Tynan, H. (2000). Responding to aggressive behavior: Impact of training on staff member's knowledge and confidence. *Mental Retardation,* Vol. 38, No. 2, pp. 97-104.

Bromley, J., & Emerson, E. (1995). Beliefs and emotional reactions of care staff working with people with challenging behavior. *Journal of Intellectual Disabilities Research,* Vol. 39, No. 4, pp.341-352.

Budd, T. (1999). *Violence at work: Findings from the British Crime Survey.* Health and Safety Executive, London.

Caldwell, M.F. (1992). Incidence of PTSD among staff victims of patient violence. *Hospital and Community Psychiatry, Vol. 43, No. 8, pp. 838-839.*

Callaghan, P., Tak-Ying, S A., & Wyatt, P.A. (2000). Factors related to stress and coping among Chinese nurses in Hong Kong. *Journal of Advanced Nursing,* Vol. 31, No. 6, pp. 1518-1527.

Chung, M.C., & Corbett, J. (1998). The burnout of nursing staff working with challenging behavior clients in hospital-based bungalows and a community unit. *International Journal of Nursing Studies,* Vol. 35, pp. 56-64.

Clegg, J.A. (1994). Epistemology and learning disabilities: Invited commentary on Hastings and Remington. *British Journal of Clinical Psychology,* Vol. 33, pp. 439-444.

Cottle, M., Kuipers, L., Murphy, G., & Oakes, P. (1995). Expressed emotion, attributions and coping in staff who have been victims of violent incidents. *Mental Handicap Research,* Vol. 8, No. 3, pp. 168-184.

Denzin, N.K., & Lincoln, Y.S. (1994). Entering the field of qualitative research. In Denzin, N.K., & Lincoln, Y.S. (Eds). (1994). *Handbook of Qualitative Research.* Sage Publications, London.

Dyer, S., & Quine, L. (1998). Predictors of job satisfaction and burnout among the direct care staff of a community learning disability service. *Journal of Applied Research in Intellectual Disabilities, Vol. 84, No. 6, pp. 874-884.*

Emerson, E., Barrett, S., Bell., C., Cummings, R., McCool, C., Toogood., A., & Mansell, J. (1987). *Developing services for people with severe learning difficulties and challenging behaviors.* Institute of Social and Applied Psychology, University of Kent, Canterbury.

Farrell, G.A. (1997). Aggression in clinical settings: Nurses views. *Journal of Advanced Nursing, Vol. 25, pp. 501-508.*

Flannery, R.B. (1996). Violence in the workplace, 1970-1995: A review of the literature. *Aggression & Violent Behavior, Vol. 1, pp. 57-68.*

Fletcher, B.C. (1991). *Work, stress, disease and life expectancy.* Wiley, Chicester.

Gerits, L., Derksen, J.L., & Verbruggen, A.B. (2004). Emotional intelligence and adaptive success of nurses caring for people with mental retardation and severe behavior problems. *Mental Retardation, Vol. 42, No. 2, pp.106-121.*

Grey, I. M., McClean, B., & Barnes-Holmes, D. (2002). Staff attributions about the causes of challenging behaviors. *Journal of Learning Disabilities, Vol.6, No. 3, pp. 297-312.*

Hastings, R.P. (1995). Understanding factors that influence staff responses to challenging behaviors: An exploratory interview study. *Mental Handicap Research,* Vol. 8, No. 4, 196-320.

Hastings, R.P. (1997). Staff beliefs about the challenging behaviors of children and adults with mental retardation. *Clinical Psychology Review,* Vol. 17, No 7, pp. 775-790.

Hastings, R. P., & Brown, T. (2002a). Coping strategies and the impact of challenging behavior on special educators' burnout. *Mental Retardation,* Vol. 40, pp.148-156.

Hastings, R.P., & Brown, T. (2002b). Behavioral knowledge, causal beliefs and self-efficacy as predictors of special educators' emotional reactions to challenging behaviors. *Journal of Intellectual Disability Research,* Vol. 46, Part 2, pp. 144-150.

Hastings, R., & Remington, B. (1993). Is there anything on ....Why 'good' behavioral programmes fail?' A brief review. *Clinical Psychology Forum,* No.55, pp.9-11.

Hastings, R.P., & Remington, B. (1994). Staff behavior and its implications for people with learning disabilities and challenging behaviors. *British Journal of Clinical Psychology,* Vol. 33, pp. 423-438

Hastings, R.P., & Remington, B. (1995). The emotional dimension of working with challenging behaviors. *Clinical Psychology Forum,* No. 79, pp. 11-16.

Hastings, R.P., Remington, B., & Hopper, G.M. (1995). Experienced and inexperienced health care workers' beliefs about challenging behaviors. *Journal of Intellectual Disability Research,* Vol. 39, No. 4, pp. 474-483.

Hatton, C., Brown, R., Caine, A., & Emerson, E. (1995). Stressors, coping strategies and stress-related outcomes among direct care staff in staffed houses for people with learning disabilities. *Mental Handicap Research,* Vol. 8, No. 4, 1995.

Hatton, C., & Emerson, E. (1993). Organizational predictors of staff stress, satisfaction and intended turnover in a service for people with multiple disabilities. *Mental Retardation,* Vol. 31, No. 6, pp. 388-395.

Hatton, C. and Lobban, F. (2007) Staff Supporting people with Intellectual Disabilities and Mental Health problems. In Bouras, N. and Holt, G (Eds.) *Psychiatric and behavioral disorders in Intellectual and Developmental Disabilities* (2nd Ed). Pp. 388-399. New York: Cambridge.

Health and Safety Commission. (1997). *Violence and Aggression to Staff in Health Services.* HSE, London.

Hellzen, O., Asplund, K., Sandman, P., & Norberg, A. (2004). The meaning of caring as described by nurses caring for a person who acts provokingly: An interview study. *Scandinavian Journal of Caring Sciences,* Vol. 18, pp. 3-11.

Heyman, B., Swain, J., & Gillman, M. (1998). A risk management dilemma: How day center staff understand challenging behavior. *Disability & Society,* Vol. 13, No. 2, pp. 163-182.

Holmes, T.H., & Rahe, R.H. (1967). The social readjustment rating scale. *Journal of Psychosomatic Research,* Vol. 11, pp. 213-218.

Howard, R., & Hegarty, J.R. (2003). Violent incidents and staff stress. *The British Journal of Developmental Disabilities,* Vol. 49, Part 1, No. 96, pp. 3-21.

Howard, R., Rose, J. and Levinson, V. (In Press) The Psychological Impact of Violence on Staff Working with Adults with Intellectual Disabilities. *Journal of Applied Research in Intellectual Disabilities.*

Jenkins, R., Rose, J., & Lovell, C. (1997). Psychological well-being of staff working with people who have challenging behavior. *Journal of Intellectual Disability Research,* Vol. 41, No. 6, pp. 502-511.

Kiely, J., & Pankhurst, H. (1998). Violence faced by staff in a learning disability service. *Disability and Rehabilitation,* Vol. 20, No.3, pp. 81-89.

Lawson, D.A., & O'Brien, R.M. (1994). Behavioral and self-report measures of burnout in developmental disabilities. *Journal of Organizational Behavior Management,* Vol. 14, pp.37-44.

Lazarus, R.S. (1993). From psychological stress to the emotions: A history of changing outlooks. *Annual Review of Psychology,* Vol. 44, pp. 1-21.

Lazarus, R.S., & Folkman, S. (1984). *Stress, Appraisal and Coping.* Springer, New York.

Lazarus, R.S., & Folkman, S. (1986). Cognitive theories of stress and the issue of circularity. In: Appley, M.H., & Trumbull, R. (1986). *Dynamics of Stress.* Plenum Press, New York.

Lundstrom, M., Graneheim, U., Eisemanm, M., Richter, J. and Astrom, S. (2007) Personality Impact on experiences of strain among staff exposed to violence in care of people with intellectual disabilities. *Journal of Policy and Practice in Intellectual Disabilities*, 4, 1, 30 -39.

Male, D.B., & May, D.S. (1997). Burnout and workload in teachers of children with severe learning difficulties. *British Journal of Learning Disabilities,* Vol. 25, pp. 117-121.

Maslach, C., & Jackson, S.E. (1993). Maslach Burnout Inventory. Manual. (2nd Edition). Consulting Psychologists Press, Inc., U.S.A.

Mitchell, G., & Hastings, R.P. (2001). Coping, burnout and emotion in staff working in community settings for people with challenging behavior. *American Journal of Mental Retardation, Vol. 107, pp. 252-260.*

Murray, G.C., Sinclair, B., Kidd, G.R., & Quigley, A. (1999). The relationship between staff sickness and client assault levels in a health service unit for people with an intellectual disability and severely challenging behavior. *Journal of Applied Research in Intellectual Disabilities*, Vol. 12, No. 3, pp. 263-268.

Poster, E.C. (1996). A multinational study of psychiatric nursing staffs' beliefs and concerns about work safety and patient assault. *Archives of Psychiatric Nursing*, Vol. 10, No. 6, pp. 365-373.

Reed, S., Russell, A., Xenitidis, K., & Murphy, D. (2004). People with learning disabilities in a low secure in-patient unit: Comparison of offenders and non-offenders. *British Journal of Psychiatry*, 185, pp. 499-405.

Rippon, T.J. (2000). Aggression and violence in health care professionals. *Journal of Advanced Nursing,* Vol. 31, No. 2, pp. 452-460.

Rose, D., Horne, S., Rose, J.L., & Hastings, R.P. (2004). Negative emotional reactions to challenging behavior and staff burnout: two replication studies. *Journal of Applied Research in Intellectual Disabilities*, Vol. 17, pp. 219-223.

Rose, D., & Rose, J. (2005). Staff in services for people with intellectual disabilities: The impact of stress on attributions of challenging behavior. *Journal of Intellectual Disability Research*, Vol. 49, No. 11, pp. 827-838.

Rose, J. (1997). Stress and stress management training. *Tizard Learning Disability Review*, Vol. 2, pp. 8-15.

Rose, J., David, G., & Jones, C. (2003). Staff who work with people who have intellectual disabilities: The importance of personality. *Journal of Applied Research in Intellectual Disabilities*, Vol. 16, pp. 267-277.

Rose, J., Jones, F., & Fletcher, B. (1998). Investigating the relationship between stress and worker behavior. *Journal of Intellectual Disability Research*, Vol. 42, No. 2, pp. 163-172.

Rose, J., & Schelewa-Davies, D. (1996). The relationship between staff stress and team climate in residential services. *Journal of Learning Disabilities for Nursing, Health and Social Care,* Vol. 1, No.1, pp. 19-24.

Sigafoos, J., Elkins, J., Kerr, M., & Attwood, T. (1994). A survey of aggressive behavior among a population of persons with intellectual disability in Queensland. *Journal of Intellectual Disability Research, Vol. 38,* 369-381.

Skirrow, P. and Hatton, C. (2007) "Burnout" Amongst direct care workers in services for adults with Intellectual disabilities: A systematic review of research findings and initial normative data. *Journal of Applied Research in Intellectual Disabilities,* 20, 1, 131 – 144.

Stenfert Kroese, B., & Fleming, I. (1992). Staffs' attitudes and working conditions in community-based group homes of people with mental handicaps. *Mental Handicap Research,* Vol.5, pp. 82-91.

Stevens, G.B., & O'Neil, P. (1983). Expectation and burnout in the developmental disabilities field. *American Journal of Community Psychology,* Vol. 11, No. 6, pp. 615 – 627.

Wanless, L.K., & Jahoda, A. (2002). Responses of staff towards people with mild to moderate intellectual disability who behave aggressively: A cognitive emotional analysis. *Journal of Intellectual Disability Research,* Vol. 46, No. 6, pp. 507-516.

Whittington, R., & Burns, J. (2005). The dilemmas of residential care staff working with the challenging behavior of people with learning disabilities. *British Journal of Clinical Psychology,* Vol. 44, No. 1, pp. 59-77.

Winstanley, S., & Whittington, R. (2002). Anxiety, burnout and coping styles in general hospital staff exposed to workplace aggression: A cyclical model of burnout and vulnerability to aggression. *Work & Stress,* Vol. 16, No. 4, pp. 302-315.

Chapter 25

ETHOLOGY AND NEUROPHARMACOLOGY OF AGGRESSIVE BEHAVIORS IN INDIVIDUALS WITH INTELLECTUAL DISABILITIES

J. Barnhill

Developmental Neuropharmacology Clinic, University of North Carolina School of Medicine, USA.

INTRODUCTION

Ethology is the study of animal behavior in naturalistic settings. When applied to primates by researchers such as Goodall and Fosse, field studies provide valuable insights and revolutionized our understanding of social behaviors among chimpanzees and mountain gorillas (Alcock 1993; Boyd, 1993; Relethford 1997; Stein 1998). Combining their data with the behavioral neurosciences (neuro-ethology) we can define many of the neurobiological substrates of social behaviors. Adding functional neuro-imaging studies of human psychopathology to the mix aids in understanding of social- emotional perception and attachment behaviors (childhood anxiety disorders) (Serra, 1998); relationship between fixed action patterns released by territorial or dominance conflicts with obsessive compulsive and stereotypic behaviors; alliance formation and subtypes of aggressive behavior (Arnold, 1990:, Oliver, et al, 2002; Barnhill, 2007).

AGGRESSION IN SEVERE AND PROFOUND INTELLECTUAL DISABILITIES

The assessment of aggressive behavior in individuals with severe or profound intellectual disabilities (ID) is affected by severe deficits in language, increased sensitivity to environmental disruption, deficits in adaptive behaviors; and problems with the social ecology (Menolascino, 1986; Szymanski et al 1997; Coccaro et al, 2002). In addition, persons with severe or profound intellectual disabilities have an increased prevalence of epilepsy (Ettinger et al, 2001), cerebral palsy, metabolic disorders, and other neurological syndromes (Damasio et al 1995; Gardner et al 2004; Sugden et al 2006). As a result of severe brain dysfunction, there is an increased risk for both mental disorders and nonspecific behaviors such as stereotypies (Schroeder et al 1989), self-injurious behaviors, aggression, and sensitivity to environmental changes (Craig et al 1994, Ishikawa et al 2003, Harris 2006).

In social settings clinicians may observe aggression characterized by explosive outbursts. This subtype of aggressive behavior is usually associated with intense sympathetic arousal (flight or fight systems) and is occasionally described by direct care staff as "fighting as if his life depended on it."(Charney et al, 1996) A subset of explosive aggression appears defensive in nature. Often in retrospect, there is a degree of stimulus selectivity (responses to specific events, settings or individuals). The individuals may engage in a similar pattern of warning behaviors that antecede these defensive outbursts- occasionally giving everyone an opportunity to react (Coccaro et al 2002; Barnhill 2007). One exception may be due to extreme forms of fear conditioning perhaps linked to previous physical or sexual abuse. In this context-specific stimuli (resemblance to abuser) or setting (in a bathtub) may serve as a conditioned stimulus and fear may be the only clue that the outburst is about to occur (Charney et al 1996; Parson et al 1994). For individuals with psychotic disorders, paranoia presents a similar hypersensitivity to a misperceived though often specific contextual or specific trigger social stimulus (Coccaro et al 2002, Ishikawa et al 2003; Shelley, 2008).

The most common form of reported aggression is affective or explosive in nature. It occurs in reaction to a range of nonsocial, ecologically driven factors. In contrast to defensive aggressive, affective-explosive aggressive behaviors appear far more impulsive and unpredictable, frequently involving less clear-cut warning signals (Gardner et al, 2004). There seems to be limited ritualization or displaced aggression (turning over furniture) suggesting less neuro-regulation. On the other hand many explosive-aggressive behaviors do occur in a social context and evoke social consequences, blurring the boundary between defensive and impulsive subtypes (Ishikawa et al 2003). As such, the communicative nature of these impulsive behaviors can still be conceptualized and approached from an ethological frame of reference. Unfortunately the extremely short latency may obscure connections to specific social or communicative functions (Barnhill 2007).

From this clinical perspective, an ethological analysis is a useful adjunct to the differential diagnosis of aggressive behaviors among nonverbal individuals with severe or profound intellectual disabilities. To be successful however we need to take additional steps in the assessment. Temperamental factors, life experiences (conditioning and learning) and individual variability (personality) require integration with our observational data collection (Gardner et al 2004; Witwer et al 2008; Ursano et al 2008). This level of complexity should remind us not to become over reliant on one-tract treatments: psychopharmacological treatments based on single neurotransmitter models or overly simplified chains of antecedent-behavior-consequences (Gardner et al 2004; Bostic et al, 2006). Both interventions should focus instead on the multidirectional impact of brain dysfunction on behavior. In short, we should routinely design treatment programs grounded in a thorough functional behavioral analyses and neuropsychiatric assessment. For purposes of this paper, it is helpful to move beyond the "laboratory" of psychiatric diagnosis and behavioral assessments towards direct "field observations" within ecological settings (Harris, 1995; Barnhill, 2007).

ETHOLOGY, SEVERE AND PROFOUND INTELLECTUAL DISABILITIES AND AGGRESSIVE BEHAVIOR

From an ethological perspective aggression is best characterized based on the qualitative state of threat perception, intensity of emotional reactions, impulse control, threshold for behaviors, planning and goal directedness (Sugden et al, 2006). Social aggression is modulated by social context, cultural values and sanctions, qualities of attachment behaviors, intensity and expression of social drives (motivation), state of affective arousal (sympathetic and neuroendocrine activation), frustration tolerance, and top-down regulation of ritualized expressions of aggressive behaviors by higher cortical centers (Siever et al, 1985; Ratey et al 1996; Ishikawa et al 2003). Aggression can be defensive in response to perceived threat; instrumental to obtain preferred objects or social contact or avoid unpleasant tasks (goal directed); predatory (well planned, low arousal) or as an outgrowth of territorial and dominance disputes between members of a stable social group (Oliver et al 2002; Barnhill 2007).

Compared to nonhuman primates, social and cultural conventions help modulate but do not eliminate aggressive behavior in humans, especially those involving conflicts over mate selection, territorial disputes between groups or intra-group dominance/social hierarchy (Relethford et al 1997, Rose et al 2004). Top-down regulation (prefrontal cortex) and increased use of language/social communication help this process. The linguistic/social communication and prefrontal modulation of limbic activity also permit greater behavioral flexibility and modification of pre-potent, automatic behaviors (Augustyn et al 1998; Coccaro et al 2002). As a result fixed action patterns and ritualistic behaviors are less obvious in humans but present nonetheless as we adapt and cope with some complex social environments (Cohen et al 1997; Dodman et al, 1999).

The expansion and rewiring of fronto-temporal-limbic interconnections allows for extensive integration of cognitive, memory and affective inputs (Ishikawa et al 2003). For many individual with severe developmental disorders, deficits exist in the capacity for top down regulation and cognitive override of limbic activation. In addition, the capacity to use language to regulate and communicate is affected. As a result, the individual is more apt to rely on nonverbal communication and motor action as a means of expression (Harris, 2006; Barnhill, 2007). From a behavioral frame of reference, associatively conditioned events may trigger arousal state (stress responses) and drive patterns of repetitive, ritualized, and conditioned motor behaviors (including aggressive behaviors). For many, behaviors may also be intrinsically re-enforced, especially if they relieve internal distress, perceived threat or conflict, or sense of incompleteness (threat perception is not "turned off"). As we noted earlier, these behaviors can also represent a form of nonlinguistic, social communication. Unfortunately understanding this action-language largely depends on others who can decipher their intent and meaning. Ethological understanding may help with interpreting these ambiguous communications (Winslow & Insel, 1991; Rose et al 2004; Barnhill 2007).

The addition of an ethological perspective can also be a useful tool for deciphering the social contexts of these behaviors. Knowledge of social and attachment behaviors broaden our understanding of some challenging behaviors, especially those dependent on perception of emotional cues and social context (Gardner et al, 2004; Barnhill 2007). For example, some forms of property destruction, clothes tearing, or tantrums may be a reaction to a disruption of expected social interactions. These behaviors may include ritualized behaviors that are a part of dominance or territorial displays that often include dramatic affective or threat displays, vocalizations, and vocal warnings or posturing. A careful analysis of this form of social aggression may clarify dominance hierarchies based on proximity of seating and patterns of sharing, as well as the forms of social interaction, friendships, and allies during times of distress, comforters, and supporters. For example, aggression may be displaced onto objects or other individuals at the lower end of the group's dominance hierarchy- "pecking order". Over time the rates of aggressive behaviors may diminish as disrupted dominance and/or territorial claims are resolved (Oliver et al, 2002; Barnhill, 2007).

CONCLUSION

The ethological approach to clinical problems such as aggressive behavior can provide a useful tool for understanding and treating challenging behaviors. Neuro-ethological studies can provide insights into the brain-social behavioral substrates of clinical psychopathology individuals with severe or profound intellectual disabilities (Barnhill, 2007). Using an ethological model we can look for the impact of mood disorders on attachment behaviors, territorial or dominance displays, and conflict-triggered ritualistic or displacement behaviors. But we must always remember that no classification or single model ever completely captures the complexity of aggressive behavior. As we have seen the combination of functional behavioral analysis and neurobiological approaches may help subtype aggressive behavior but still cannot completely resolve the problems created by the considerable overlap between and dimensional nature of these clinical categories (Oliver et al, 2002; Ishikawa et al 2003; Barnhill 2007).

Although speculative, this paper explored ethological approaches as a partial solution to clinical obstacles in the differential diagnosis and treatment of aggressive behaviors in nonverbal individuals with severe or profound intellectual disabilities. The goal human ethological investigation is to combine our understanding of species-specific behaviors with existing assessment tools. Finally, a reminder that attempts to develop treatment models based on an ethological data does not undermine, replace or challenge the need for individualized programs. The use of charts depicting these nature and extent of social relationships (ethograms) provides another tool integrating various modalities of assessment and treatment planning. Taking such an approach does not dehumanize nor does it debase challenging behaviors among individuals with severe or profound intellectual disabilities to unregulated instinct.

REFERENCES

Alcock, J (1993). The ecology of social behavior. In: *Animal Behavior* (ed Alcock, J), pp 501-40, Sunderland, Massachusetts: Sinauer Assoc.

Alcock, J (1993). An evolutionary approach to human behavior. In: *Animal Behavior*, (ed Alcock, J, pp541-69, Sunderland: Sinauer Assoc.

Arnold, S.J. (1990). Inheritance and the evolution of behavioral ontogenies. In: *Developmental Behavior Genetics* (eds Hahn, M.E., Hewitt, J.K., Henderson, N.D., and Benno R), pp167-90, New York: Oxford University.

Augustyn, M. and Zuckerman, B (1998). Normal behavioral development. In:, *Textbook of Pediatric Neuropsychiatry*, (eds Coffey, C.E. and Brumback, R.A), pp117-138,Washington, DC: American Psychiatric Assoc. Press.

Barnhill J (2007) Ethological Approach to Individuals with Intellectual and Developmental Disabilities. *Mental Health Aspects of Developmental Disabilities,* 10, 53-63.

Bostic JQ et al (2006). Target Symptom Psychopharmacology. *Child Adol Psychiatric Clin North America* 15, 289-302.

Boyd, R. and Richerson, P.J. (1993). Culture and human evolution. In: *The Origin and Evolution of Humans and Humanness* (ed Rasmussen, D.T), pp119-131, Boston: Jones and Bartlett Pub.

Charney, D.S.; Nagy, I., Bremer, D., Goddard, A.W., Yehuda, R., and Southwich, S.(1996). Neurobiologic mechanisms of human anxiety. In: *Neuropsychiatry*, (eds Fogel, B.S.; Schiffer, R.B.; and Rao, S.M), pp 257-78, Baltimore: Williams and Wilkins.

Coccaro EF, Siever, L (2002). Pathophysiology and Treatment of Aggression. In:, *Neuropsychopharmacology: The Fifth Generation of Progress,* (eds Davis KL, Charney D, Coyle JT, Nemeroff C), 1709-24, Philadelphia: Lippincott, Williams & Wilkins.

Cohen, L.J., Stein, D, Galynker, I., and Hollander, E. (1997). Towards an integration of psychological and biological models of obsessive-compulsive disorder: phylogenetic considerations. *CNS Spectrums,* 2, 26-44.

Craig, K.J., Brown, K.J., and Baum, A. (1994).Environmental factors in the etiology of anxiety disorders. In: *Psychopharmacology: The Fourth_Generation of Progress* (eds Bloom, FE, Kupfer, D.J. (Eds), pp1325-40. New York: Raven Press.

Damasio A.R. (1995). Towards a neurobiology of emotion and feeling: operational concepts and hypotheses. *The Neuroscientist,* 1, 19-25.

Dodman, N.H. and Oliver, B. (1999). In search of animal models for OCD. *CNS Spectrums* 1, 10-16.

Ettinger AB Kanner A (2001). Psychiatric Issues in Patients with Epilepsy and Mental Retardation; In: *Psychiatric Issues in Epilepsy: A Practical Guide to Diagnosis and Treatment* (eds Ettinger AB Kanner A) Philadelphia:: Lippincott, Williams &Wilkins.

Gardner WI Griffiths D (2004). *Treatment of Aggressive and Related Disruptive Behaviors in Persons with Intellectual Disabilities and Mental Health Issues.* Vol 1. Kingston NY: NADD Press.

Harris J. (1995). Developmental Neuropsychiatry vol 1 (pp169-91). New York: Oxford University Press.

Harris J (2006). Intellectual Disability: Understanding Its Development, Causes, Classification, Evaluation, and Treatment. New York, NY: Oxford University Press.

Ishikawa SS, Raine A (2003). The Neuropsychiatry of Aggression. In: Neuropsychiatry: Second Edition (eds Schiffer RB, Rao SM, Fogel BS), pp 660-78, Philadelphia: Lippincott, Williams & Wilkins.

Menolascino, F.J., Levitas, A. and Greiner, C. (1986). The nature and types of mental illness in the mentally retarded. *Psychopharmacology Bulletin,* 22, 1060-71.

Oliver B, Siever L (2202). Animal Models of Aggression. In: *Neuropsychopharmacology: The Fifth Generation of Progress.* (eds Davis KL, Charney D, Coyle JT, Nemeroff C), pp1709-4, Philadelphia: Lippincott, Williams & Wilkins.

Parsons, J.A., May, J.G., and Menolascino, F.J. (1984). The nature and incidence of mental illness in mentally retarded individuals. In: *Handbook of Mental Illness in the Mentally Retarded* (Menolascino, F.J. and Stark J.A.Eds), pp3-44, New York: Plenum.

Ratey, J.J. and Dynek, M.P. (1996). Neuropsychiatry of mental retardation and cerebral Palsy. In:). *Neuropsychiatry* (eds Fogel, B.S., Schiffer, R.B., and Rao, S.M. Eds), pp549-70, Baltimore: Williams and Wilkins.

Relethford J.H. (1997). The biology and behavior of living primates. In: *The Human Species,* pp170-203. Mountain View, CA: Mayfield Publishers.

Rose R, Maughan B, Wortham CM, Costello EJ, Angold A (2004). Testosterone, antisocial behavior, social dominance: Pubertal Development and Biosocial interaction. *Biol Psychiatry* 55, 546-52.

Serra, M; Jackson, E; vanGreet, LC and Mindeerva, RB (1998). Interpretation of Facial Expression, Postures, and Gestures in Children with a Pervasive Developmental Disorder Not Otherwise Specified *J Autism and Dev Dis* 28, 257-64.

Shelley B Trimble M, Boutros NN (2008). Electroencephalographic Cerebral Dysrythmic Abnormalities in the Trinity of Nonepileptic General Population, Neuropsychiatric and Neurobehavioral Disorders. *J Neuropsychiatry Clin Neuroscience.* 21, 7-22.

Schroeder, S.R. (1989). Abnormal stereotyped behaviors. *Treatments of Psychiatric Disorders: A Task Force Report.* Washington, DC: American Psychiatric Press.

Siever, L.W., Klar, H., Coccaro, E. (1985). Psychobiological substrates of personality. In: *Biological Response Styles: Clinical Implications* (eds Klar, H.A. and Siever, L.J.(Eds), 37-66. Washington, DC: American Psychiatric Association Press.

Stein, MB (1998)"Neurobiological Perspectives on Social Phobia: From Affiliation to Zoology" *Biol Psychiatry* 44, 1277-85.

Sugden SG, Kile SJ, Hendren RL (2006) Neurodevelopmental pathways to aggression: a model to understand and target treatment in youth. *J Neuropsychiatry and Clinical Neurosciences* 16, 320-17

Szymanski, L.S. and Kaplan, L.C. (1997). Mental Retardation. In: *Textbook of Child and Adolescent* (ed Weiner, JM), pp183-215. Washington, DC: American Psychiatric Association Press.

Winslow J.T. and Insel, T. (1991). Neuro-ethological models of obsessive-compulsive disorder. In:. *The Psychobiology of Obsessive-Compulsive Disorder* (eds Zohar, J., Insel, T., Rasmussen, S), pp208-220. New York: Springer Publishing.

Witwer AN, Lecavalier L (2008). Psychopathology in Children with Intellectual Disability. *J Mental Health Research in Intellectual Disabilities.* 1, 75-96.

Ursano AM, Kartheiser P, Barnhill LJ (2008). Disorders Usually First Diagnosed in Infancy, Childhood, and Adolescence. In: *Textbook of Psychiatry: Fifth Edition* (eds Hales RE Yudovsky S, Gabbard DO), pp 861-920, Washington: American Psychiatric Association Press.

Chapter 26

IS SELF-INJURIOUS BEHAVIOR RELATED TO ADDICTION BEHAVIORS?

J. Barnhill

Developmental Neuropharmacology Clinic, University of North Carolina School of Medicine, USA.

INTRODUCTION

Self-injurious behavior (SIB) affects between 10-15% of individuals with severe intellectual disabilities (ID) (Romanczyk, 1989; Schroeder et al, 2001). Because of the considerable heterogeneity of both individuals with ID and the typology of SIB clinicians tend to divide it into subtypes. The critical points of this subdivision are based on observable and quantifiable differences among ecological factors (setting-events), triggers (antecedents); severity/intensity, typology, topography of the behaviors and factors that maintain self-injury (patterns of reinforcement) (Romanczyk 1989; Barnhill, 2004). In an attempt to create some order to our understanding, SIB is currently classified as Stereotypic Movement Disorder (SMD) in both the DSM-IV-TR (APA, 2000) and Diagnostic Manual- Intellectual Disability (DM-ID) (Fletcher et al, 2007). Both systems rely on a descriptive, phenomenological approach that minimizes subtyping and avoids classification based on etiology-based or endophenotype models.

Even though categorized as a subtype of Stereotypic Movement Disorder (SMD) SIB can vary due to etiological or causative factors (Fletcher et al, 2007). SIB can occur in response to pain; antecedent irritability due to interictal states in epilepsy; cortical dysfunction or cerebral palsy; premenstrual behavioral changes or frustration due to an inability to verbally communicate needs or distress (Gedeye, 1992; Herpetz, 1995; Mace and Mauk, 1995). The intensity or frequency of SIB can also increase during the course of a primary psychiatric disorder -e.g. baseline exaggeration at the onset of mood or anxiety disorders. In fact it is uncertain whether an increase in SIB is related to subsyndromal forms of mood disorders or a specific endophenotype of a mood disorder among some individuals with severe or profound intellectual disabilities (Barnhill, 2004; Fletcher et al 2007). In the strictest sense, none of these clinical scenarios routinely associated with self-injury are major or defining criteria for

SMD, leaving many forms of SIB in the realm of challenging behaviors that may or may not be related to other psychiatric disorders (Fletcher, et al 2007).

This paper addresses the intrinsic heterogeneity of self-injury by attempting to define a particular subset of SIB- one characterized by episodic, compulsive and severe tissue damaging self-injury and addiction behaviors. Our goal is to search for qualities of severe SIB that might help define a specific endophenotype that shares a common neurobiological and behavioral pharmacological substrate with other forms of self-destructive behaviors (Barnhill, 2000; Barnhill, 2004. Narrowing the focus further, we will explore the relationship between addiction/addiction behaviors (out of control binge drug use) Kupferman et al 2000), obsessive-spectrum disorders (Hollander et al 1996), and the metamorphosis of factors affecting the development of escape-related repetitive behaviors (Guess et al, 1991; Hall et al, 2001). One underlying characteristic of each of these patterns of repetitive behaviors is a tendency to persist in spite of dire physical or emotional consequences. This plus other characteristics suggest that episodic, severe, compulsive self-mutilating SIB among individuals with severe or profound intellectual disabilities can be conceptualized as similar in selected ways to addiction behaviors in normo-cognitive populations (Barnhill, 2004).

SIB, DRUG ADDICTION AND ADDICTION BEHAVIORS

Drug addiction is a complex behavior that involves the compulsive search for and use of the substance irrespective of potentially life-threatening medical consequences, worsening of psychiatric disorders, high rates suicidal behavior and adverse health and mental health outcomes (Goldstein, 2001). Genetic vulnerability to addiction is grounded in temperamental differences noted during childhood; (Cloninger et al 1993), sensitivity to drug effects (Koob et al, 1999) or altered brain responses to the drug (Kupferman et al, 2000). Addiction behaviors represent a larger group of repetitive, self-defeating or potentially self-destructive behaviors characterized by an increasing psychological tension or urge to act. Once engaged in the behavior the individual continues until the urge is resolved (Kupferman et al, 2000; Barnhill, 2004). The temporary sense of relief or mild euphoria ("high" or reduced tension) afforded by this action makes it similar to other self-reinforcing behaviors (London et al, 1995). This pattern of repetitive behaviors is included among obsessive-compulsive spectrum disorders (Hollander et al 1996).

In each of these conditions, some genetically vulnerable individuals develop apparent tolerance to the tension-reducing sense of relief and pleasure from these actions (London et al, 1995). This decline in the strength of intrinsic reinforcement contributes to an increased frequency (extinction spurt) or intensification of negative emotional consequences (autonomic arousal or intense dysphoria of withdrawal). This state is can also be associated with a sense of incompleteness and an increasing urge (craving) to re-engage and repeat it. Once "addicted" to this pattern of behavior, the individual experiences significant craving or increased motivation to escape from increasingly unpleasant withdrawal states (Kandel, 2000; Kupferman et al 2000). During this process genetically vulnerable individuals "cross the wall" as these patterns of increasingly destructive behaviors become "ingrained" (conditioned escape responses) and even replace other sources of enjoyment and pleasure (Hollander et al, 1996; Koob et al, 1999; Kupferman et al, 2000). In addition, conditioned environmental or context cues now trigger appetitive behaviors (craving and drug seeking) or affect symptoms of withdrawal (cues to escape conditions associate with withdrawal states). Thwarting craving behaviors seem to intensify it as if the capacity for extinction is also temporarily out of commission (Becker, 1999; Koob, 1999, Swift, 1999).

SIB AND SENSITIZATION

In contrast to tolerance, sensitization represents an increased sensitivity to the drug. Cocaine addiction best illustrates this point. Chronic cocaine abuse leads to the development of tolerance to its euphorigenic effects. Tolerance to drug-induced changes in multiple neurotransmitter systems pushes the individual from continuous use into a pattern of discontinuous use (bingeing) interrupted by withdrawal states (urges or craving and drug seeking). Over time, high dose bingeing-withdrawal result in stereotypies-ritualistic behaviors (punding), tactile hallucinosis, excoriation to eliminate the cocaine "bugs", increasing paranoia and risk for psychosis (Alper, 1999; Goldstein, 2001). These changes resemble kindling of seizure activity by repeated chemical or electrical induction (Nestler, 1999; Kraus, 2000). In kindling models, the intensity of the initiating stimulus for a seizure declines with repeated seizure induction. Eventually, threshold for induction decreases to the point that spontaneous seizure occurs (Kraus, 2000).

Some forms of compulsive severe SIB evolve towards this outcome (Becker, 1999). For example, during childhood, milder forms of SIB (high frequency/low intensity) overlap stereotypies, complex tics (Barnhill, 2000) and other intrinsic or self-reinforced repetitive behaviors (Guess et al, 1991: Hall et al 2001). These milder forms of self-injury appear analogous to early drug use behavior. The drug-induced "high" resembles self-stimulation and contributes to a positive affective state and intrinsic reinforcement. For most, the process stops here. For others tolerance and sensitization or kindling create a situation where the more the individual self-injures, the more likely he or she is to continue that behavior (Becker, 1999. Barnhill, 2004).

In addition, antecedents for self-injury are obscured by both a secondary conditioning hierarchy of context stimuli and/or changing thresholds and intensities of arousal and motivational states (Kraus, 2000; Troften, 2008). Thus both learning experiences and temperamental sensitivities complicate our understanding of specific triggers critical to initiating periods of compulsive SIB (Barnhill, 2004). In a similar light, episodes of autonomic arousal (distress or anxiety) related to interruption of routines or pleasurable experiences may also trigger an episode of severe self-injury- analogous to withdrawal states. This pattern of conditioned responses play an increasingly critical role in triggering, sensitizing and maintaining SIB as withdrawal states do for drug seeking and bingeing (Guess et al, 1991; Mace et al, 1995; Barnhill, 2004).

By the time an individual reaches this stage, we can anticipate that tissue-damaging self-injury is increasingly resistant to single intervention strategies. Likewise once SIB starts, it is likely to continue until the individual is exhausted or restraint is applied. Even intense pain may not terminate the self-injury (Russ et al 1992; Barnhill, 2000; Schroeder et al, 2001). In short, there is a lowered threshold for self-injury and an increased probability that once started the self-injury continues until exhausted or interrupted.

CONCLUSION

Individuals genetically (Comings, 1996) or temperamentally vulnerable to addiction (Cloninger, 1993) quickly move beyond intrinsically reinforcing patterns of behavior. The trend towards escape motivated self-stimulatory behaviors begin to dominate the picture. Embedded in this process is the development of tolerance, sensitization and increased level of associative conditioning between negative emotional effects of drug use and/or SIB in response to growing list of adverse emotional and environmental events. The genetic risk for this transformation may be the common linkage between addiction and the tendency among some individuals towards this subset of severe SIB (Becker, 1999; Alper, 1999; Krauss, 2000, Barnhill, 2004).

Clinicians treating severe self-injury may need to borrow a page from modern treatment of addictions (Russ, 1992; Barnhill, 2004). This approach to treatment incorporates the role of comorbid mental disorders and the addiction process. Biological treatment models focus on modifying endorphins/peptide (Gianoulakis, 1996), glutamate/GABA and catecholamine networks (Decaria et al 1998) that involve learning, resistance to extinction and sensitization (Trafton et al, 2008). The use of addiction-modifying interventions such as odansetron (Falda, 1991), acamprosate, dopamine antagonists, glutamate modulators, and long acting mixed opiate agonists/antagonsts is changing the face of addiction treatment (Garbutt, 1999). Unfortunately naltrexone is not always effective as currently used and not routinely used for severe SIB (Barnhill, 2004). These pharmacological strategies are most effective when augmented by combination with behavioral programs that emphasize extinction of both associative and operant conditioned experiences and searching for alternative forms of social reinforcement (Swift, 1999).

REFERENCES

Alper KR (1999). The EEG and Cocaine Sensitization: A Hypothesis. *J. Neuropsychiatry and Clin Neuroscience*, 11, 209-20.

American Psychiatric Association. *Diagnostic and Statistical Manual of Mental Disorders, Fourth Edition, Revised*. DSM-IV-TR. Washington, DC: American Psychiatric Association, 2000.

Barnhill J (2000). Behavioral Phenotypes: A Glimpse into the Neuropsychiatry of Genes- Part I: Lesch-Nyhan Syndrome and Subtypes of Self-Injurious Behaviors. *NADD Bull*, 3, 66-69.

Barnhill J (2004), Addiction and self-injurious behavior (SIB): A common ground. *Journal of Intellectual Disability Research*, 48:293.

Becker HC (1999). Alcohol Withdrawal: Neuroadaptation and Sensitization *CNS Spectrums*, 4, 38-43.

Cloninger CR, Svrakic DS and Przybeck T (1993). A Psychobiological Model of Temperament and Character. *Arch Gen Psychiatry*, 50, 075-90.

Commings DA (1996). Genetic Factors in Drug Abuse and Dependence. In: Gordon HW and Glantz MD (Eds) *NIDA Research Monograph Series*, 159, 16-39.

Decaria CM, Begaz T and Hollander E (1998). Serotonergic and Noradrenergic Function in Pathological Gambling. *CNS Spectrums,* 3, 38-47.

Falda F, Garau B, Marchei F, Colombo G, Gessa GI (1991). MDL 72222 A Selective 5-HT-3 Receptor Antagonist suppresses voluntary Alcohol Consumption in Alcohol Preferring Rats. *Alcohol Alcohol,* 26, 107-110.

Fletcher R Loeschen E, Stavrakaki C, First M (Eds) (2007). *Diagnostic Manual- Intellectual Disability: Textbook of Diagnosis of Mental Disorders in Persons with Intellectual Disability.* Kingston NY: NADD Press.

Garbutt JC, West SL, Carey TS, Lohr KN and Crews FT (1999). Psychopharmacological Treatment of Alcohol Dependency: A Review of the Evidence. *JAMA,* 281, 1318-25.

Gedeye, A (1992) "Anatomy of Self-injurious, Stereotypic, and Aggressive Movements: Evidence for an Involuntary Mechanism. *Am J Mental Retardation,* 48, 766-78

Gianoulakis C (1996). Implications of Endogenous Opiates and Dopamine in Alcoholism: Human and Basic Science. *Alcohol Alcoholism Supp* 1, 33-42.

Goldstein A (2001). *Addiction: From Biology to Policy* 2nd Edition. New York: Oxford University Press. New York.

Guess D and Carr E (1991) "Emergence and Maintenance of Stereotypy and Self-injury" *Am J Mental Retardation,* 96, 299-319.

Hall S, Oliver C and Murphy G (2001). Early Development of Self-Injurious Behavior: An Empirical Study. *Am J Ment Retard,* 106, 189-99.

Herpetz, S (1995) "Self-Injurious Behavior: Psychopathological and Nosological Characteristics of Subtypes of Self-injurers" *Acta Psychiatr Scan,* 91, 57-68.

Hollander E and Benzaquen SD (1996) "Is There a Distinct OCD Spectrum?" *CNS Spectrums,* 1, 17-26.

Koob GF and Roberts AJ (1999). Brain Reward Circuits in Alcoholism. *CNS Spectrums,* 4, 23-37.

Kandel E (2000). Cellular Mechanisms of Learning and the Biological Basis of Individuality. In: *Principles of Neural Science* (eds Kandel ER, Schwartz JH and Jessel TM) McGraw Hill: New York: 1247-77.

Kraus JE (2000). Sensitization Phenomena in Psychiatric Illness: Lessons from the Kindling Model. *J Neuropsychiatry and Clin Neurosciences,* 12, 228-43.

Kupferman, Kandel ER and Iverson S (2000). Motivational and Addictive States. In: *Principles of Neural Science,* (eds Kandel SR, Schwartz JH and Jessell TM. New York: McGraw-Hill, pp998-1012.

London ED, Grant SJ, Morgan MJ and Zukin SR (1995). Neurobiology of Drug Abuse. In: *Neuropsychiatry* (Eds Fogel BS, Schiffer RB and Rao SM) Baltimore: Williams and Wilkins, pp 635-75.

Mace FC and Mauk JE (1995) "Bio-Behavioral Diagnosis and Treatment of Self-injury" *Ment Retard and Dev Disabilities Research Rev,* 1, 104-11.

Romanczyk, R (1989). A Review of the Literature on Self-Injurious Behavior: Factors that Should Affect critical Decision-Making. *Treatment of Destructive Behaviors in Persons with Developmental Disorder.* NIH Consensus Conference. US Dept of Health and Human Services, 52-57.

Russ MJ, Roth SD, Lerman A, Kakuma T, Harrison K, Shindledecker RD, Hull J and Mattis S (1992). "Pain Perception in Self-injurious Patients with Borderline Personality disorder" *Biol Psychiatry,* 32, 501-11.

Schroeder SR, Hammock RG, Mulick JA, Rojahn J, Walson P, Ferrald W, Meinhold P and
    Shephere G (1995). Clinical Trial of DA1 and DA2 dopamine Modulating Drugs in Self-
    Injury in Mental Retardation and Developmental Disability. *Mental Retardation and Dev
    Disabilities Research Rev,* 1, 120-9.

Schroeder SR et al (2001). Self-Injurious Behavior: Gene-Brain-Behavior Relationship*s.
    Mental Retardation and Dev Disabilities Research Rev*, 7, 3-13.

Swift RW (1999). Medications and Alcohol Craving. *Alcohol Res Health,* 23, 207-13.

Trafton JA, Gifford EV (2008). Behavioral Reactivity of Addiction: The Application of
    Behavioral Response and Reward Opportunities, *J Neuropsychiatry Beh Neuroscience*
    20, 23-35.

PART V. COMMUNICATION AND SOCIAL ISSUES

By definition all individuals with intellectual disabilities (ID) have impairment of cognition, communication and social skills. Greater the severity of ID, greater the impairment in communication. Good communication is dependent on numerous factors, including the underlying cognitive deficits, associated psychiatric morbidity, the environment, personality traits, use of additional support and empathy of carers. *Mophosho and Wenke* and *Lyng* and *Esposito and colleagues* stress important cognitive, communication and social issues affecting individuals with autism spectrum disorder. The importance of crying, movement and autonomy in autism are areas where our understanding is still limited. Other areas, such as the importance of a multi-disciplinary approach, including the involvement of specially trained speech-language therapist is now more mainstream.

Bunning highlights the potential role and meaningful contribution that total communication can make to the lives of people with ID. *Porter and Daniels* report on the value of non-directive methods of information collection in schools.

Chapter 27

THE PERCEPTIONS OF PROFESSIONALS ON THE PROTOCOLS OF THE SLTS IN THE DIAGNOSIS OF CHILDREN WITH AUTISM SPECTRUM DISORDERS

M. Mophosho[1] and A. Wenke[1]

[1]Department of Speech Pathology & Audiology, University of Witwatersrand. South Africa

INTRODUCTION

The purpose of this study was to investigate (i) what the protocol in the Johannesburg region of South Africa is, by Professionals (Neurologists, Paediatricians and Child Psychiatrists), for diagnosing a child with autism. (ii) Whether a multidisciplinary team is involved was questioned and (iii) the perceptions of the professionals working with autistic children on the role of the Speech-Language Therapist (SLT) as part of the multidisciplinary team.

Speech pathology and audiology is an area of professional specialization which is concerned with the process of communication in individuals. The American Speech-Language-Hearing Association (ASHA) (2006) has recommended that SLTs working within this scope of practice are able to diagnose and provide appropriate intervention for children with autism. In ASHA's official document (2006), it outlines the knowledge, skills, roles and responsibilities of SLTs in order to diagnose, assess and treat children on the autistic spectrum (ASHA, 2006). Therefore the SLTs working in this field need to be appropriately trained, experienced and engaged in continual research in order to understand and enhance the child's communication. Early identification and treatment of autism is documented widely as a critical issue in need of attention (Canadian Best Practice Guidelines).

METHODOLOGY

Professionals

Sixteen Professionals were interviewed at one public hospital and within the private sector. Nine were paediatricians from the public sector and five were from the private sector. One child psychiatrist from the public sector participated in this research project and one child psychiatrist, one psychiatrist and one clinical psychologist from the private sector participated. Only one neurologist from the public sector and two neurologists from the private sector participated. The one child psychiatrist that participated worked within both the government and private sector and was therefore interviewed in this respect.

Research Design

An exploratory, descriptive survey design within the qualitative and quantitative framework of research design was selected. The analysis was based on quantitative and qualitative data as information was obtained form a variety of sources. Open ended questions were asked.

Content of the Questions with Rationale

The questionnaire was divided into three sections. In the first section professional information of the participants was required. The second section, made up of one question, professionals were required to describe the protocol he / she used when diagnosing a child with autism. This was asked to establish if there are specific guidelines that professionals needed to follow in order to diagnose children with autism in South Africa as well as to establish if the SLT assesses the child's communication before a diagnosis of autism is made. The third section constituted the participant describing their practice experience in terms of referals and perceptions of role of SLT.

RESULTS AND DISCUSSION

Experiences in the Field of Autism

The Professionals had varying number of years in the field of autism, from one to forty years of experience. The amount of children diagnosed by professionals each month ranged from 1 to 6.

From the research it was interesting to note that on average more children are being diagnosed in the public sector than the private sector and Neuro-Developmental Paediatricians are the Professionals diagnosing most children with autism. Most Professionals in the private sector are diagnosing 1-2 children each year with autism while in the public sector that amount of children are being diagnosed on average each month.

The Protocol of the Professionals when Diagnosing Autism

Detailed Case History

Only eight of the sixteen professionals mentioned how vital a detailed case history needs to be performed when diagnosing a child with autism.

DSM IV Criteria

It is evident though that the DSM-IV criteria is widely used among all professionals as nine of the sixteen participants described criteria from the DSM-IV to diagnose a child with autism.

Neurological Impairment

Six of the professionals noted that a neurological investigation is important especially for differential diagnosis. A child who meets the DSM-IV criteria should undergo a thorough medical examination (Karande, 2006).

Psychological Impairment

Only the neurologist from the government sector and the clinical psychologist from the private sector noted that children with autism often have multiple complications such as psychological impairment. This needs to be differentiated and noted.

Observe Behavior

Three Neuro-Developmental Paediatricians mentioned the importance of observing the child's behavior. A diagnostic evaluation should be based on the observation of the child's skills in all areas, especially in communication, interaction with others and developmental skills level (Karande, 2006).

Play

Only one Neuro-Developmental Paediatricians indicated the importance of watching a child play before making the diagnosis of autism. This is significant as play is one of the criteria from the DSM-IV described as the child has a lack of varied spontaneous make-believe play or social imitative play appropriate to developmental level (Lord & Risi, 1998).

Standard Scoring

One government Neuro-Developmental Paediatrician suggested the use of standard scoring tests such as the Childhood Autism Rating Scale (CARS) which one can use when diagnosing a child with autism.

General Examination

Only two professionals, a psychiatrist from the private sector and a neuro-developmental paediatrician from the government sector, reported conducting a general examination as part of their protocol when diagnosing a child with autism. A child who meets the DSM-IV criteria should undergo a thorough medical examination which would involve a physical examination to identify neurocutaneous markers for tuberous sclerosis and dysmorphic features for fragile X syndrome. A complete blood count and peripheral blood smear examination should be done (Karande, 2006).

Referrals

Five professionals reported the importance of referring children to other professionals as part of their protocol when diagnosing a child with autism. It is important to mention this was only done by professionals in the private sector. These professionals indicated that they often refer children suspected as having autism to occupational therapists, SLTs, physical therapists, psychologists, audiologists, educators and general practitioners. Two paediatricians noted that they refer children to developmental clinics already established at some government hospitals as well as to schools.

From these results no definite protocol is evident in diagnosing autism in the Johannesburg region of South Africa. It was also important to note that paediatricians are not the professionals who diagnosed autism but rather specialized pediatricians such as Neuro-Developmental Paediatricians should have been the sample group as a diagnosis of autism is often provided by Developmental Paediatricians, Psychologists, Child Psychiatrists or Neurologists (Autism and Autism Spectrum Disorders).

From these answers it is evident that most professionals attempt to work within a multidisciplinary team however due to a lack of resources and limited professionals available in each setting, this was not always possible. In developing countries like South Africa, a multidisciplinary team is often challenged by lack of resources, the fragmentation of the health care system and inadequate referrals (Ross, 2004).

Of the information provided by the participants only 20.7% were that the speech-language plays an important role in the team and they need to be included. Therefore the SLT must be and should be included in terms of assessing communication impairment as well as providing intervention for the needs of the child.

Three participants reported not having worked in conjunction with a SLT and therefore they were unable to note if they found the SLT to be beneficial. Two professionals working in the private sector which made it difficult to find professionals with whom to work.

The last question to each participant within this sub-aim was on rating the importance of communication in a child with autism. It was ranked on a scale from 1-10 with 1 being not important at all, 5 being important and 10 vitally important. Once again fourteen of the sixteen professionals indicated that communication is vitally important in children with autism and everyone for that matter. One private neurologist said that communication should be rated at five, being important, as activities of daily living are vitally important along with behavioral modification. The clinical psychologist noted that it all depends on the age of the child. If the child was 8-9 years of age, then communication would be vitally important. However, if the child was younger they would first need to learn social interaction which will be needed in order to learn communication.

REFERRAL OF CHILDREN BY NEUROLOGISTS, PAEDIATRICIANS AND CHILD PSYCHIATRISTS TO A SLT FOR INTERVENTION ONCE THE DIAGNOSIS OF AUTISM IS MADE

Fifteen of the sixteen professionals refer children to a SLT for intervention once the diagnosis of autism is made. The reasons being, children need to communicate either verbally or non-verbally; that communication is a lifelong difficulty that needs to be maintained; and that the SLT is the most active member of the team. The one professional, a private paediatrician who does not refer children to a SLT, stated that he only referred children to specialists. He also further explained that he was not the right person to ask as he does not work with autistic children on a daily basis.

THE UNDERSTANDING AND KNOWLEDGE BY PROFESSIONALS OF THE ROLES AND RESPONSIBILITIES OF SLTS

The professionals were asked whether they are familiar with the roles and responsibilities of a SLT. Of the sixteen professionals, only seven said they know what the roles and responsibilities of a SLT are. Three stated that they think they know what the roles of a SLT are and the remaining four participants know they have a role, but they not entirely sure what it is.

CONCLUSION

This research aimed to investigate what the role of a SLT is as perceived by professionals, before and after a diagnosis of autism is made in the Johannesburg region of South Africa.

There is evidence of a lack of referral from the results which suggests that the children with autism are most affected. Perhaps there should be training of professionals at a university level, so that they are aware of the roles and responsibilities are of a SLT as well as other professionals. The results of the study suggest that it is important to improve collaboration and communication between diverse professionals who are working with children with autism.

Assessment and diagnosis of Autism in young children requires well-trained and experienced professionals. This research has shown that children with autism in the region of Johannesburg South Africa are not being assessed by a multidisciplinary team.There also appears to be a lack of resources and professionals which is a common occurrence in developing countries. We need to find a strategy in professional training that will help professionals to work within a transdisciplinary or multidisciplinary team. The research suggests it is more possible to refer children with autism to other professionals within the public sector.

REFERENCES

American Speech-Language-Hearing Association. (2006). Guidelines for speech- language pathologists for diagnosis, assessment, and treatment of autism spectrum disorders across the life span. Available from http://www.asha.org/members/deskref-journal/deskref/default

American Speech-Language-Hearing Association. (2006). Knowledge and skills needed by speech-language pathologists for diagnosis, assessment, and treatment of autism spectrum disorders across the life span. Available from http://www.asha.org/members/deskref-journal/deskref/default

American Speech-Language-Hearing Association. (2006). Roles and Responsibilities of speech-language pathologists in diagnosis, assessment, and treatment of autism spectrum disorders across the life span: Position statement. Available from http://www.asha.org/members/deskref-journal/deskref/default

Karande, S. (2006). Autism: A Review for Family Physicians. *Indian Journal of Medical Science,* 60(5).

Lord, C. & Risi, S. (1998). Frameworks and Methods in Diagnosing Autism Spectrum Disorders. *Mental Retardation and Developmental Disabilities,* 4, 90-96.

Ross, E., & Deverell, A. (2004). Psychosocial Approaches to Health, Illness and Disability: A Reader for Health Care Professionals. Hatfield: van Schaik.Publishers.

Chapter 28

AUTONOMY AS EXPLAINED BY AUTISM DIAGNOSIS, AGE COHORT, LANGUAGE SKILLS AND BEHAVIOR

K. Lyng
Molde University College, Molde, Norway

BACKGROUND

The acquisition of language skills are considered as basic to development of humans and also basic for humans' ability to control their own behavior and establishing independent functioning (Vygotsky, 1978).

Inferior language skills, as well as intellectual disability and challenging behavior are considered cardinal features in Autism spectrum disorders (ASD) (Bailey et al, 1996). On the other side, teaching language skills has, in modern approaches towards educating people with ASD, been seen as a key to obtain better quality of life and participation in society for individuals with ASD and for people with intellectual disability in general (Bailey et al, 1996). Hence larger autonomy and self-determination should be associated with better language skills as well as a better ability to control your own behavior. Younger age cohorts with ASD would also be expected to have better language skills than older age cohorts due to more adequate training.

In general, autonomy among individuals with ASD is lower than in other persons with intellectual disability (Hatton et al., 2004; Ward & Meyer, 1999; Wehmeyer & Garner, 2003). To what extent is autonomy and self-determination associated with level of language skills, the presence of ASD, age cohort and challenging behavior?

METHOD

Sample

The data presented here is from Tøssebro's (2001) evaluation of the transition of the care and services to people with intellectual disability in Norway from the responsibility of the county to the level of the municipality. A randomized and stratified sample of Norwegian municipalities (N=515), representing 11.2% of the population of Norway, were drawn. Participation was based on presence of intellectual disability, age between 20 and 67 years old, living at their own (not in family) in their own housing, community homes or collective living. For further descriptions of the sample see Tøssebro (2001).

Materials

The information given was based of the proxies' knowledge of the person, their preferences, skills and living conditions. The information about the participants was based on a subjective evaluation. The material contained information on age, autism diagnosis (yes/no), autistic features (yes/no), expressive- and receptive language, the presence of challenging behavior and degree of self-determination. See appendix for details of response categories and construction of autonomy score.

Procedure

Participation was asked for through the person's conservator. A questionnaire containing x questions were filled in by the proxies of the individuals in the sample. Data were collected in 2001. The response rate was 55.7%. Systematic biases in the sample have not been observed (Tossebro, 2002).

Statistical Analysis

Multiple stepwise linear regression analysis with the autonomy variable as dependent variable was conducted using SPSS 11 for Mac. The subjects were divided into two age cohorts, those born before and after 1971. This division is made because the training and educational regime for the younger population born after 1970 would be different regarding language and social training. Interactions were computed for:

1. Autism x age cohort
2. Autism x receptive language
3. Autism x expressive language
4. Age cohort x receptive language
5. Age cohort x expressive language
6. Receptive language x expressive language
7. Receptive language x expressive language x Autism
8. Age cohort x expressive language x Age cohort
9. Receptive language x expressive language x Autism x age cohort
10. Receptive language x Autism x age cohort
11. Expressive language x Autism x age cohort

RESULTS AND DISCUSSION

Table 1 shows that the best predictor of autonomy is the interaction between receptive and expressive language, explaining 36% of the variance in autonomy scores. The interaction between autism and receptive language, receptive language skills, challenging behavior, and birth cohort adds significantly to the explained variance, explaining 44.7% of the variance. Good language skills, absence of autism and good receptive language skills, absence of challenging behavior, and belonging to a younger birth cohort all increases the likelihood of self-determination.

That both receptive and expressive language skills as perceived by the staff were the best predictor of autonomy, is not surprising as language is fundamental to managing ones owns life and is an important vehicle for the participation in social life through communication. Language skills are associated with general intelligence and more independence and self-help skills.

Autism alone does not alone contribute to the explanation of the variance in the dependent variable. Autism only contributes in interaction with receptive language skills. Although the interaction adds significantly to the explained variance (F=37.46), the explained variance is low (4.3%). Absence of autism and good receptive language increases the autonomy score and may reflect the general association between language skills and autism; that good receptive language skills and lack of autism or autism-like features are likely to increase self-determination. In addition challenging behavior and age cohort adds significantly to the explained variance.

Only two of the possible interactions between variables computed had an impact on the dependent variable. Those were the interaction between receptive and expressive language, the second was the interaction between autism diagnosis and receptive language. The strongest contribution to degree of self-determination was the interaction between the two measures of language skills (R=. 598). The next strongest contribution comes from the interaction between autism and receptive language.

Basically, the data presented here indicates that autism in it self is not a strong predictor of the level of autonomy unless associated with the level of receptive language. With increasing level of receptive language, autonomy is increasing independent of the presence of autism.

The measures of language skills as well as the measures of challenging behavior used here is the staffs' evaluation of the participants skills and behavior, not linguistic measures of language skills. However, measured by the evaluation of the staff in practical daily life would give a measure close to real life performance from someone that knew the person well.

CONCLUSION

About 46% of the variance in autonomy scores is explained by autism diagnosis, language skills, age cohort and the interaction between challenging behavior and receptive language skills as measured in this study.Autism in itself does not turn out as the main factor explaining autonomy. Language skills and in particular receptive skills seem to be the stronger predictors of autonomy, together with age cohort and challenging behavior.

ACKNOWLEDGMENT

Thanks to Professor Jan Tøssebro, Technical University of Trondheim, Norway, for making data from the national evaluation of the Reform of the Care for people with intellectual disability in Norway available for this paper.

REFERENCES

Bailey, A., Phillips, W., & Rutter, M. (1996). Autism: Towards an Intergration of Clinical, Genetic, Neuropsychological and Neurobiological Perspectives. *Journal of Child Psychiatry, 37*(1), 89-126.

Hatton, C., Emerson, E., Robertson, J., Gregory, N., Kessissoglou, S., & Walsh, P. N. (2004). The Resident Choice Scale: A measure to assess opportunities for self-determination in residential settings. *Journal of Intellectual Disability Research, 48*(2), 103-113.

Vygotsky, L. S. (1978). *Mind in Society: The Development of Higher Psychological Processes*. Cambridge, Massachusetts: Harvard University Press.

Ward, M. J., & Meyer, R. N. (1999). Self-determination for people with developmental disabilities and autism: Two self-advocates' perspectives. *Focus on Autism and Other Developmental Disabilities, 14*(3), 133-139.

Wehmeyer, M. L., & Garner, N. W. (2003). The Impact of Personal Characteristics of People with Intellectual and Developmental Disability on Self-determination and Autonomous Functioning. *Journal of Applied Research in ID, 16*(4), 255-265.

Chapter 29

MAKING CONNECTIONS: EVALUATION OF A TOTAL COMMUNICATION TRAINING CASCADE IN ADULT SERVICES IN A RURAL PART OF THE U.K.

K. Bunning

School of Allied Health Professions, University of East Anglia

BACKGROUND TO STUDY

Total Communication (TC) involves the flexible use of communication across the range of modalities (Bradshaw, 2002; Jones, 2000; Lawson and Fawcus, 1999; Pound et al, 2000). Communication is viewed as having multiple representations that move beyond conventional linguistic code (e.g. the spoken and written word), and include the use of facial, vocal and body gesture, writing, drawing and objects, pictures and environmental points of reference, specific communication devices.

A TC strategy was developed in response to the challenge of addressing communication needs in a service for adults with intellectual disability in a rural setting of the United Kingdom, which involved a training cascade populated by staff members with particular responsibilities for TC. The aim was to provide information about the communication abilities of individuals and to focus on practical approaches to communication support. The post of Communication Development Worker (CDW) was established, to which four people, with experience of the population and an interest in communication, were appointed. The CDWs were trained by the Speech & Language Therapists to deliver the TC strategy via a system of cascade training. Each CDW was responsible for rolling out the strategy across service in a particular geographical area. The next level in the cascade was occupied by a number of Communication Co-ordinators (CC) who, as key members of a support staff team, assumed particular responsibility for dissemination of instruction to their colleagues amongst the frontline staff. The CCs received 2 separate weeks of specialist training from the CDWs, delivered a month apart. After this, the CCs, in negotiation with the team leader of their staff group, engaged in the development of a TC plan for local implementation. Ongoing support was provided from CDWs through individual meetings and telephone contact as required.

Table 1. Characteristics of participants

Designation	Participants (n)	Employed in Organisation (years)	Work Exper-ience (years)	Examples of Specialist Training Undertaken (excl. mandatory training)
Speech & Language Therapists (SLTs)	4	2 - 8	2 - 9	Degree in SLT/HPC registered; Signalong, dementia, Makaton; dysphagia; negotiation skills; motivational interviewing and leadership courses
Multi-disciplinary Team Members (excluding SLTs)	5	7 - 30	11 – 30	Psychology, Nursing, Management and short courses – a wide range: manual handling, sign along, mental health, ethnicity, adult protection, care management
Communi-cation Develop-ment Worker (CDW)	4	5 - 28	8 - 28	Total Communication (provided by SLTs); Signalong, presentation skills; facilitating groups; health psychology
Communi-cation Co-ordinators (CC)	7	1 - 16	3 - 18	Total Communication (provided by CDWs); person-centerd planning; Picture Exchange Communication System' Signalong; bereavement; visual impairment; autism
Managers	6	3 - 20	10 - 32	Person-centerd planning; advocacy autism awareness; recruitment and management courses; REACT; disability awareness
Support Staff (SS)	6	1 - 8	1 - 11	Person centerd planning; autism awareness; REACT,

Bi-monthly meetings were held to provide the opportunity for peer support amongst the CCs, which might include the mutual exchange of ideas, problem-solving and sharing of resources. At the start of the study it was reported that 194 support staff had been trained on the TC strategy (personal communication from CDW, 12.12.06).

STUDY AIM

The aim of the study was to explore and evaluate the impact of the TC training cascade on staff employed at different levels within four different services.

METHOD

Thirty-two staff-participants were recruited from four sites, which were already involved in the TC training cascade. They were all of White British ethnic origin with English as the first language. The characteristics of the staff-participants are given in Table 1.

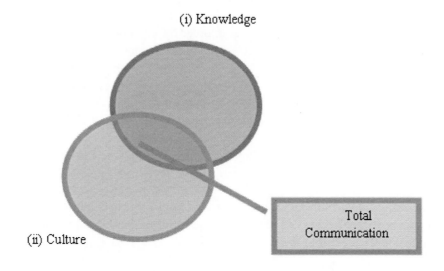

Figure 1. Critical Themes Centerd on Total Communication.

Semi-structured interviews were carried out with the staff-participants. Three main topics were addressed by the interviewer. Firstly, the informant was asked to describe his/her role within the service; secondly, about his/her role in the TC strategy and personal experience of training and support in TC; thirdly, about the impact of the TC strategy in terms of working with service users, participation in communication opportunities and the emission of challenging behavior. The informant was also invited to talk about an individual service user in relation to the TC work. Finally, they were asked to talk about any difficulties encountered and their ideas for improving the TC strategy. All the interviews were conducted in situ and recorded with digital audio equipment. The interviews were transcribed.

Two over-arching themes emerged from the combined data set that centerd on Total Communication: knowledge and culture. *Knowledge* was defined as information about TC held by the staff participants. *Culture* was expressed routine communication practice characterised by opportunities and TC techniques

FINDINGS

Knowledge of TC appeared to reach all levels of service provision. Whilst there was a degree of variation across the staff group, and in particular between the different levels of the cascade training structure, there was general agreement about the importance of a deliberate approach to communication and the potential benefits of TC to service users. For communication to be relevant and responsive to the needs of individuals, there first needs to be a certain conscious awareness of the prevailing issues as a natural precursor to the successful adoption of new practices.

> ...everybody thinks more about communication

There was a general understanding that in order for communication to be accessible and meaningful for people with intellectual disability, specific adaptations or approaches would need to be invoked. The training on TC appears to have prompted consideration of other possibilities for social communication: A range of techniques were identified by the participants demonstrating not only awareness of the range of possible techniques that may be relevant when communicating with service users, but also the reasons underpinning their use.

> ...don't overload people with information and give them time to process that info as well...

Some staff were encouraged to search out the reasons that may underpin a service user's idiosyncratic or particular ways of responding and to seek a more complete understanding of the individual in the context of their communication skills and needs.

> ... I felt that a lot of her challenging behavior might arise from a situation where she made a communication that wasn't picked up on and then she's getting quite frustrated and her needs aren't being met...

Integral to the emergent theme of 'knowledge' was the perceived 'expertise' of individual staff members - their sense of their own skills in addressing the TC needs of the service users. Generally positive value was attributed to developing competencies around TC, with some being encouraged sufficiently to develop new approaches to practice or to change existing practice as a result of training received.

> ...one of the first things ...when I finished my communication training was to change around the service users meetings.....

The concept of 'ownership' resonated throughout the interview data. Some of the participants made reference to past roles that had fallen within their remit; however, TC was seen as the precinct of no one profession or staff team in particular. There was a real sense of shared commitment to and collective rights over TC.

> ... communication in a sense (is) "everybody's business"

For some, the establishment of the CDW posts was critical to the general perception of what communication was all about in relation to the learning difficulties service. There was also a sense of CDWs serving as well placed conduits between the frontline of service provision, e.g. in residential homes and day services, and the professional members of the multi-disciplinary team. The role of the CDW was developed as a post in its own right – not requiring any particular professional affiliation. This in itself, has brought communication into general arena of service provision for everyone. This has helped to facilitate the sharing of responsibility for TC and its implementation. However, the implementation of TC was not without its difficulties. Differences in knowledge were identified as a source of tension by some, particularly in the working relationship between CC and support staff. Naturally within a cascade training system there will be different levels of knowledge at any one point in time. Knowledge transfer occurs as a result of training that is passed down the line, which requires skills in disseminating information and training others.

> it can make for slightly rocky relationships with your co-workers who haven't had the training and maybe don't have the depth of insight that you do....

Whilst it is acknowledged that TC has undoubtedly helped to raise the general level of expertise amongst staff, the scope and limitations of that expertise was expressed as an altogether vaguer concept. It was clear from some of the interviews that there was a fair amount of confusion regarding the roles of assessment and clinical decision-making. In some cases this has led to courses of action that may not have been recommended had a comprehensive assessment of communication need taken place. This is an important issue and one which requires close attention if service users are to really benefit from the strategy. The dedication and hard work of CCs is clearly evident; however there is an inherent risk that critical issues may be missed and wrong decisions taken if scope of practice is not defined.

> there is a danger of communication co-ordinators seeing themselves as or being seen as "font of all knowledge" ...

TC brings with it some key concepts that inform practices. Not surprisingly, the interviews revealed a strong sense of the form taken by communication, including signing, facial expression, objects of reference, photographs and symbols. Informants talked about the various ways of presenting information to service users. Pictorial display was by far the most frequently mentioned mode of communication. Practices ranged from wall-mounted staff photo display boards to individually tailored communication books. \

> he's got his photos and also we've put little symbols in the kitchen for where various things are kept

Although the predominant view of communication focused on the forms it takes, the relevance of linguistic input and listener inference was considered in places. Modification of language to enable service user understanding was a concern for one participant:

> they won't understand what you're trying to say and they may take it the wrong way and again get anxious about that. .....I'll just try and explain it in a different way

Some of the more subtle or non-conventional ways of communicating that may be relevant to the person with more severe or profound intellectual disability received more limited notice. One or two participants made reference in their accounts of service user communication, but generally there was no reflection on what it means to the communication of the staff member.

The prevailing *culture* of the services demonstrated the influence of TC. Davis and Watson (2002) argue that it is the underlying values held by individuals and groups that serve to minimise difference. Byng et al (2002) go further and suggest that values are a critical variable in the intervention process and the potential for success. The values espoused by many of the participants indicated a strong belief in the power of TC and this was related to unlocking the potential of individuals. Mutually held beliefs concerning TC were enormously important to the uptake of TC within the service and the adoption of new practices. This resonated throughout the data and was a view expressed at every level within the service provider organisations.

> the presence of "common thought processes" around communication (and shared values) makes TC effective in a location and/or for an individual

The interviews highlighted the value staff placed on communication artefacts in the environment. Photographic resources had been accumulated in most research sites for use as prompts for activities and/or in reminiscence work with service users. Walls displays of photographs had various purposes including depicting members of the whole staff team or just those ones on duty.

> our main thing here is the communication board which we've got up on the wall because all our guys can recognise photographs and we've taken photographs of absolutely everything......

Various viewpoints were expressed with regard to the place TC occupies in the context of daily practice. It was not automatically seen as part and parcel of support work.

> People often see communication as something they bring into their job or add on to it rather than it actually being their job

Sometimes the general routine of the residential home was based on the over-arching needs of the residents. For instance routine was considered very important to working with service users on the autistic spectrum, which, in itself, brought potential benefits to service user understanding. Sometimes the individual needs of a service user translated into particular routines with obvious benefits to the individual.

I think the total communication has helped by showing her pictures, sort of recognition things like that I think ...

One interesting comment challenged what was felt to be the perceived emphasis on *image* over *process*. Of course, this is only one view; however, the data generally revealed a major focus on communicative form, in particular the visible artefacts of TC, and the nature of transaction (e.g. exchanging information – making choices). Does this indicate a need to explore some of the more invisible forms of TC, such as vocalisation, use of eye gaze and social interaction (e.g. playing with sound and turn-taking for fun and the social experience)?

....too much emphasis placed on "what we look like" as opposed to "what we're actually doing"

CONCLUSION

The emerging culture and growing knowledge base of TC shows the potential for making a relevant and meaningful contribution to the lives of people with intellectual disability. A real sense of momentum resonated throughout the data set, which provides a rich and fertile basis for ongoing development of the TC strategy. The cascade training structure, whilst providing the means for disseminating knowledge across the hierarchical levels of the organisation, also needs to make deliberate consideration of a bi-directional flow of information whereby staff at the bottom of the cascade, e.g. in this case the frontline support staff, are able to influence the upper layers of management and specialist communication workers in the same way that the upper layer operates.

REFERENCES

Bradshaw, J. (2002). The management of challenging behavior within a communication framework. In S. Aburdarham & A. Hurd (eds) *Management of Communication Needs in People with a Learning Disability.* London: Whurr Publishers Ltd. pp 246-75.

Byng, S., Cairns D., Duchan, J (2002). Values in practice and practising values. J Commun Disord 35, 89-106.

Davis, J. M. & Watson, N. (2001). Where are the children's experiences? Analysing social and cultural exclusion in 'special' and 'mainstream' schools. *Disability & Society* 16: 671-87.

Jones, J. (2000). A total communication approach to meeting the communication needs of people with learning disabilities. *Tizard Learning Disability Review* 5, 1, 20-26.

Lawson, R. & Fawcus, M. (1999). Increasing effective communication using a total communication approach. In: S. Byng, K. Swinburn & C. Pound, (eds) *The Aphasia Therapy File.* Hove: Psychology Press. pp 61-71.

Pound, C., Parr, S., Lindsay, J. & Woolf, C. (2000). *Beyond Aphasia: Therapies for Living with Communication Disability.* Buckinghamshire UK: Winslow Press.

Chapter 30

EXPRESSION OF DISTRESS IN CHILDREN WITH AUTISM SPECTRUM DISORDER IN THE FIRST TWO YEARS OF LIKE

G. Esposito[1], S. de Falco[1] and P. Venuti[1]

[1]Department of Cognitive Science, University of Trento, Italy

INTRODUCTION

Crying is part of a first communicative system infants use to express their needs and communicate with their environment (Irwin, 2003) and it elicits specific physiological reactions in adults (Fleming et al, 2002). Such physiological reactions activate those listening to cries to take measures to eliminate the cause of the uneasiness. Many studies have examined cries of infants with specific medical conditions demonstrating an association between crying and neurological status. While many researches have concentrated on cry of children with brain damage, Down syndrome, hypothyroidism, Krabbe's Disease, Meningitis, and Asphyxia (LaGasse et al., 2005) very few studies have investigated the specificity of cry in infants with Autism Spectrum Disorder (ASD). Since ASD afflicts individuals by compromising their communicative and social skills, and crying can be viewed as both part of a first communicative system and an early social structure in human development, the aim of this commentary is to present some of our studies that have investigated how in children with ASD, as opposed to Typically Developing (TD) children and children with other Developmental Disability (DD), crying is expressed and perceived. These studies have employed different methodologies, such as: (i) survey for parents; (ii) experimental set-up, (iii) observational methodology.

SURVEY FOR PARENTS

Participants of this study were 120 parents with children from 3 to 5 years of age (50 TD, 35 ASD and 35 DD). The survey included items on parental perception of the morphology of the episodes of crying and on their adequacy to the social context. Moreover, parents were asked to judge how relevant the role of specific stimuli were in the provocation of a crying and the feelings experienced by parents during their child's crying episodes. The answers of parents with ASD children followed a pattern; the episode of crying was characterized by screaming, a near to total absence of tears, often provoked by unexpected and inexplicable causes. However, these crying episodes were described mostly as unexpected and were often associated with frustration on the part of the parent. Statistical differences in the emotional state during crying episodes were also noted. In particular, parents of children with ASD expressed many more negative emotions relative to controls. This result could be interpreted as a mnemonic bias. Because of this bias parents of children with ASD referred to the global behavior of the child more than to a specific episode of crying. However, parents of children with DD do not express such negative states as the parents of children with ASD (Esposito & Venuti, 2008).

EXPERIMENTAL STUDY

Starting from the results of the survey study, we wanted to understand through an experimental procedure whether the atypical structure of crying episodes of children with ASD could bias parents' perception. Using a "Listen-and-Response" experiment a total of 40 women (25-35 year-old) participated to this study. Twelwe episodes (audio file) of crying at different ages (13 and 20 months) were selected from retrospective home video of children with ASD, DD and TD. Participants were asked to listen to the stimuli, randomly presented, and then answer three questions. (1) To guess the age of the child who was crying; (2) to guess the reasons which led them to cry; (3) to describe what they felt in hearing the episode of cries. The results showed some specificity of ASD crying episodes. In particular, when listening to ASD crying episodes, participants felt more negative states. In contrast, more positive mental states were felt when listening to crying episodes of TD children. Nevertheless, participants assigned younger ages to ASD cries. These different patterns may be interpreted as resulting from an incorrect decoding of the acoustic stimulus. In particular, because of the acoustic characteristics (few peaks, small modulation and absence of turn-taking), the crying episodes of the children with ASD are difficult to interpret and for this reason may evoke mental states of uneasiness (Esposito & Venuti, 2008). This suggestion is supported by Zeskind and Marshall (1988) who found that shorter pauses were perceived to be more aversive.

OBSERVATIONAL STUDY

Although the results of our experimental study were challenging, they were limited to an experimental set up. For this reason we decided to analyze, using observational methods, the mother child interaction during an episode of cry in a real scenario. Forty-eight mother-infant interactions, during episodes of crying were coded using the Cry Observation Codes (COC, Esposito et al., 2008). The COC is composed of 3 codes that analyzed infant and mother behaviors during an episode of crying. COC1 was an exhaustive and mutually exclusive code that analyzed the infant cry morphology. Its categories were: (i) scream, (ii) moan, (iii) aspiration/expiration and (iv) pause. COC2 was an exhaustive and mutually exclusive code as well, and it analyzed the presence of stereotypy (mechanical repetition of a movement). COC3, analyzed the maternal response to infant crying. It was an exhaustive but not mutually exclusive code (it means that more than one category could occur at the same time). Its categories were: (a) tactile or vestibular stimulation, (b) object presentation, (c) verbal production and (d) no action. We found that at one year of age children with ASD of our sample showed a different pattern of cry compared to the matching control group (specifically, ASD episodes of cry had less waveform modulation and more dysphonation). Maternal reactions to ASD cries were qualitatively different from the responses to cries of the other children of the same age (fewer tactile or vestibular stimulation and more verbal production).

CONCLUSION

Healthy parent–child interaction is as fundamental to the development of special needs children as it is for typically developing children (Trevarthen et al., 1998). In our studies, it emerged that parents of infants with ASD have problems with understanding the causes of crying episodes. Such misunderstandings can initiate a vicious cycle where because the mother fails to recognize the child's needs, she gives an inadequate feedback to the child. We argue that this circle play a role in the difficulties in sharing feelings and developing inter-subjectivity processes in ASD.

REFERENCES

Esposito, G. & Venuti P. (2008). How is crying perceived in children with Autistic Spectrum Disorder? *Research in Autism Spectrum Disorders*. 2(2), 371-384.

Esposito, G. de Falco, S. & Venuti P. (2008) Early communication signals in children with Autistic Spectrum Disorder. *Journal of Intellectual Disability Research*, 52(8):677.

LaGasse, L., Neal, A.R. & Lester, B.M. (2005). Assessment of Infant Cry: acoustic Cry analysis and parental perception. *Mental Retardation and Development disabilities: Research Review*. 11, 83-93.

Fleming, A.S., Corter, C., Stallings, J. & Steiner, M. (2002). Testosterone and prolactin are associated with emotional responses to infant cries in new fathers. *Hormones & Behavior*. 42, 399-413.

Irwin, J.R. (2003). Parent and Non-parent Perception of the Multimodal Infant Cry. *Infancy*. 4, 503-516.

Trevarthen, C., Aitken, K., Papoudi, D. & Robarts, J. (1998). *Children with autism: Diagnosis and interventions to meet their needs*. London: Jessica Kingsley .

Zeskind, P.S. & Marshall, T.R. (1988). The Relation between Variations in Pitch and Maternal Perceptions of Infant Crying. *Child Development*. 59(1), 193-196.

Chapter 31

MOVEMENT DEVELOPMENT IN AUTISM SPECTRUM DISORDER: EVIDENCES FOR EARLY DIAGNOSIS

G. Esposito[1], S. de Falco[1] and P. Venuti[1]

[1]Department of Cognitive Science, University of Trento, Italy

INTRODUCTION

Autism is a lifelong developmental condition characterised by impaired social interaction and communication as well as repetitive behaviors and restricted interests (American Psychatric Association, 1994). The manifestation of autism varies in severity, and it is generally agreed that there is a spectrum of disorders (Autism Spectrum Disorder, ASD). Many studies have highlighted that early intensive treatments can lead to a substantial improvement in the life conditions of children with autism. These studies have shown that children with autism, diagnosed within the second year of life, have been able to reach a satisfactory living standard and to perform cognitive skills with competency (Osterling, et al., 2002). According to these evidences, early diagnosis and the study of predictors of the syndrome are extremely important. Movement has gained much attention in the last decades as early indicator of ASD. Movement disorders are considered one of the first signs which probably precede social or linguistic abnormalities (Esposito & Venuti, 2008a). In particular, authors have focused their work on: fine and general movements, walking and spinning (see for a review Esposito & Venuti, 2008b).

Damasio and Maurer (1978) showed that children with ASD between three and ten years of age walk somewhat like Parkinsonian adults (more slowly and with shorter steps). Nonetheless, the existence of such a Parkinsonian-type disturbance was disputed by Hallett et al. (1993) that identified movement abnormalities, in ASD people, such as a decreased range of motion of the ankle, slightly decreased knee flexion in early stance and gait irregularity. They thus proposed that this clinical picture is suggestive of a disturbance of the cerebellum. In 1998, Teitelbaum and colleagues have used the Eshkol-Wachman Movement Notation (EWMN, for reference see Eshkol and Harris, 2001) for studying the major motor milestones in the child's development namely, lying, righting, sitting, crawling, standing, and walking. The children with ASD of their sample displayed asymmetric patterns of movement. In another work, Teitelbaum and colleagues (2004) found that almost all the movement disturbances in autism may be interpreted as infantile reflexes "gone astray"; for instance, some reflexes are not inhibited at the appropriate age in development, whereas others fail to appear when they should, thy also referred to the importance of the dopaminergic system.

Based on the hypothesis that suggests movement as an early indicator of ASD, the purpose of this short commentary is to describe some recent studies we have carried out to study early motor development in children with ASD as opposed to children with Developmental Delay (DD) or Typically Developing (TD) children. In particular, in two different studies, using observational tools we have analyzed movement development at 5 and 20 months. Since we were interested in investigating an age prior of the age of an actual diagnosis of ASD we used retrospective video analysis. Retrospective video analysis appears to be an excellent option for accessing very early periods in development, months or years before a child with ASD is diagnosed.

ANALYSIS OF SYMMETRY IN EARLY ASD

This study aimed to verify the possibility of distinguishing infants with ASD from infants with TD or with DD through the analysis of postural symmetry during lying at five months of age. Analysis of static and dynamical symmetry during lying, was carried out to retrospective home videos, regarding the first five months of life, of children with ASD (n=18), TD (n=18), or with DD (n=12). From Retrospective home videos, various scenes of the same child were edited and assembled into a video compilation. When the video was ready, it was split in frames with a rates of 4 frames for second. Each frame of the slideshow was coded from 2 coders with a specific tool: the Positional Pattern for Symmetry during Lying (PPSL). The general framework for the building of the PPSL was the same used from Teitelbaum and collegues: the EWMN; the EWMN assumes one general form that will stand conceptually for all bodies. In that form, each limb is reduced to its longitudinal axis, an imaginary straight line of unchanging length. Results showed significant differences between ASD and the two control groups (p<.05). Data also highlight differences within ASD group, revealing two types of infants with ASD characterised by high or low levels of symmetry. This study suggested that different pattern of motor functioning probably relate to different pathways to ASD. It was hypothesised that the low levels of symmetry since the first months of life could be related to the loss of the Purkinje cells described in ASD.

ANALYSIS OF GAIT AFTER SIX MONTHS OF INDEPENDENT WALKING

To analyze gait in toddlers it was used the Walking Observation Scale (WOS) which includes 11 items that analyze gait through three axes: foot movements, arm movements and global movements. Significant differences in the average scores on the three axes of the WOS among the groups of toddlers with ASD as opposed to those with TD or with DD were hypothesized. In particular, it was expected to find more atypical gait patterns and more asymmetric posture while walking in children with ASD because due to a specific cerebellar deficit (Kern, 2003). Data showed different distributions (p <.05) for the three groups. The ASD group differed both from TD and DD group, both for the whole WOS and for each respective axis. The results also highlighted that after six months of independent walking, different patterns in gait among the groups were evident. These results are in agreement with the evidence that acknowledge the importance of movement as an early indicator for the diagnosis of ASD. Furthermore, these results agree with the idea of a Purkinje cells disruption in ASD. Indeed a general agreement exists that the microscopic anatomic pathology of ASD involves Purkinje cell loss and neuron size reductions in the cerebellar hemispheres and neocerebellar vermis. As well a report by Kern (2003) implies the possibility of some children becoming ASD from neuronal cell death or brain damage occurring postnatally owing to injuries. Purkinje cells in the cerebellum can be selectively vulnerable to certain types of insult such as ischaemia, hypoxia, excitotoxicity, viral infections, heavy metals, and toxins such as ethanol (Welsh et al., 2002) and they may play a role in motor disturbances in children with ASD.

REFERENCES

American Psychiatric Association (1994) *Diagnostic and statistical manual of mental disorders*. (4th ed.). Washington, DC.

Damasio, A. R., & Maurer, R. G. (1978) A neurological model for childhood autism. *Archives of Neurology*, 35, 777-786.

Eshkol, N., & Harris, J. (2001) *Eshkol Wacheman Movement Notation Part 1*. Holon Israel: The Movement Notation Society.

Esposito, G., Venuti, P.,Maestro, S. & Muratori F. (2008a) Movement in infants with Autism Spectrum Disorder: The Analysis of Lying. *Brain and Development.*

Esposito, G., & Venuti, P. (2008b) Movement and Autistic Disorder: the analysis of gait after 6 months of independent walking. *Perceptual and Motor Skills*, 106: 259-269.

Hallett, M., Lebiedowska, M. K., Thomas, S. L., Stanhope, S. J., Denckla, M. B., & Rumsey, J. (1993) Locomotion of autistic adults. *Archives of Neurology*, 50,1304-08.

Kern, K. J. (2003) Purkinje cell vulnerability and autism: a possible etiological connection. *Brain and Development*, 25, 377–82

Osterling, J., Dawson, G., & Munson, J. (2002) Early recognition of 1-year-old infants with autism spectrum disorder versus mental retardation. *Development and Psychopathology*, 14, 239-251.

Teitelbaum, O., Benton, T., Shah, P. K., Prince, A., Kelly, J. L., & Teitelbaum, P. (2004) Eshkol-Wachman Movement Notation in diagnosis: the early detection of Asperger's syndrome. *Proceedings of the National Academy of Sciences*, 101, 11909-11914.

Teitelbaum, P., Teitelbaum, O., Nye, J., Fryman, J., & Maurer, R. (1998) Movement analysis in infancy may be useful for early diagnosis of autism. *Proceedings of the National Academy of Sciences*, 95, 13982-13987.

Welsh JP, Yuen G, Placantonakis DG et al (2002). Why do Purkinje cells die so easily after global brain ischemia? Aldose C, EAAT4, and the cerebellar contribution to posthypoxic myoclonus. *Adv Neurol*. 89, 331-359.

Chapter 32

USING NON-DIRECTIVE RESEARCH METHODS TO EXPLORE THE BARRIERS AND SUPPORTS TO LEARNING

J. Porter[1] and H. Daniels[1]
[1]Department of Education, University of Bath. UK

INTRODUCTION

This paper draws on research that was undertaken as part of a government sponsored national initiative to develop methods for collecting disability data in order to support schools in complying with legislation to promote equality of opportunity for disabled people. The research drew on an interactional model of disability (Shakespeare 2005) where need is defined in the context of readily available supports. Thus individual and social elements were both seen as integral to a definition of disability which recognizes the complexity of factors and the ways in which they interact and are experienced by different people (Lowe 2001; Rhodes et al 2008). As Shakespeare (2005) has written:

"The experience of a disabled person results from the relationship between factors intrinsic to the individual, and extrinsic factors arising from the wider context in which she finds herself. Among the intrinsic issues are factors such as the nature and severity of her impairment, her own attitudes to it, her personal qualities and abilities, and her personality. Among the contextual factors are: the attitudes and reactions of others, the extent to which the environment is enabling or disabling, and wider cultural, social and economic issues relevant to disability in that society." p55-56

In this way the definition reflected the heterogeneity of experiences of disability.

Despite guidance from the World Health Organisation (WHO, 2007), census surveys concerning children with disabilities often seek to collect data that understands the nature of their difficulties through placing them within categories thereby reducing the child's experiences to be ones that originate with the child rather than seeking to explore them within the context of the mediating environment. This data is usually collected by proxy, either from parents or professionals or both, with few national models of children being asked to supply the data. It is limited therefore in the extent to which it provides insight into a child's actual experience of the world, and places this experience within an account of their particular setting. Social and environmental barriers constitute a major problem for many disabled children, and removing such obstacles is a major priority. We need to find out what these obstacles are and the prime source of this information are pupils themselves. In an educational context we need therefore to collect data from pupils about things that help or hinder learning.

Research on forensic interviewing of children makes a strong case for using open forms of questioning without repetition to elicit accurate and stable information (Cederburg et al 2000; Lamb & Fauchier 2001; Krachenbuhl & Blades 2006). Disability can however be a variable experience both with respect to temporal and contextual factors. Moreover open questions can be very difficult for less articulate people to respond to which can lead staff to support people through situating the questions to make them more accessible but also in a way that ultimately constrains or predetermine the types of response young people make (Porter in press: Antataki et al 2002). Booth and Booth (1996) specifically argue for the place of closed questions and the importance of listening to silence- an unusual plea for researchers to make and a challenge to the data collection process.

This research sought to develop tools which would enable schools to gain an understanding of the supports and barriers experienced as well as the categories invoked.

METHOD

45 schools, 24, primary, 9 secondary and 12 special schools volunteered to take part in this part of the project. The target population were pupils both with and without a known disability aged 5-6; 9-10; and 12-13 years.,

A range of 6 tools were developed, which reflected the heterogeneity of need and the challenges of communicating with young people who may have alternative or idiosyncratic patterns of communication. The tools included ones that teachers could customise, and use in a range of contexts depending on whether individual or group methods were preferred. Guidance was provided to all schools in the project, without pre-judging the appropriateness of any particular method (and can be found on the web-site www.bath.ac.uk/research/pdes). In brief, and in the order in the tools might be considered directive they were:

Focus Groups: These drew on nominal group technique, a structured method for group-work that encourages contributions from everyone which through discussion are narrowed down prior to every member of the group ranking them through a voting system (Van de Ven & Delbecq 1972). This method is seen to have the advantage over interviews where people's responses "are often continuously tailored to the reactions of the interviewer" (p388) and where language barriers may intrude as researchers fail to find the argot of the interviewees-both particular issues for school based studies. This method has the strength of providing an open forum for a wide range of views to emerge which are then prioritised by the group, thus removing contamination of researcher coding.

Point to Point. This tool is based around counselling techniques and provides a concrete approach focusing on specific events that the child identifies as good or bad. Pupils represent these events with a mark on paper and position themselves on a visual scale drawing a line between the best and worst events indicating where they feel they are today. This activity provides a vehicle for then exploring the barriers that contributed to the worst event and the positive supports that contributed to the best. Research has shown that children with learning difficulties often find it easier to discuss their views about specific events (Connors & Stalker 2002) rather than respond to more general questions. However with this method the event that is discussed originates with the child.

Semi-structured Interviews. These were designed to be undertaken either individually or in a small group and explore children's favourite things about school as well as those aspects they don't like doing and asks what would make these activities easier. It explored with children aspects that they might find difficult about different lessons, places, people, moving around or getting to school. Photographs either collected by the children or staff could be used to support this activity.

Online questionnaire. Following a brief introductory explanation of the project a series of simple questions were presented asking children to rate their experiences during lessons, during break, during lunch times and on special event days using a 5 point smiley face scale. Children were also invited to "tell us a bit more, what helps at different times" and "what makes things more difficult". In a similar way information was sought about different places in the school, different ways of working and different types of lessons.Towards the end of the questionnaire children were also asked whether they had a disability or difficulty and if it had gone on for a long time and again what helps and what makes it more difficult

Talking Mats: This symbol led system was originally developed to enable people with learning disabilities to engage in decision-making around important issues in their lives (Cameron & Murphy 2002). It is particularly well suited to using with individuals who have limited formal systems of communication, although it does assume that individuals have an understanding of representation i.e. that a symbol or picture or a photograph is representative of the thing it depicts. Using this material a facilitator asks children to indicate their like or dislike for particular activities and contexts for learning by placing personalised photographs alongside a symbol representation of like, dislike and a middle position of "so-so".

Symbol questionnaire. This had 11 closed questions exploring good and bad things about school. It included a disability question and asked if the child experienced difficulties. Children were also asked what would make school better and whether they had enjoyed completing the questionnaire. It was only available in hard form. As with all the other tools this was an activity that could be undertaken in a group or individually, with or without support.

RESULTS AND DISCUSSION

As table 1 shows some methods proved to be more popular than others with more schools choosing to opt for questionnaires (either symbol or online) than other more flexible tools. The online questionnaire in particular was used with a large number of pupils, often in hard copy form. Although this was originally designed for pupils in secondary schools, its visual format made it attractive to younger pupils but those with ID may have found the linguistic demands of open questions challenging. Schools therefore in some instances had to provide one to one support changing the dynamics of the way views were collected. The majority of special schools opted to use the symbol questionnaire, reducing the literacy demands of the task. However some children still found the negative questions difficult and because it was only available in hard copy it could not be adapted or individualised in the same way that other tools could. Talking mats were used only rarely in special schools to collect data on pupil views of learning but was used more extensively in primary schools.

Table 1. Schools' use of the tools

	Primary	Secondary	Special	Total
Talking Mats - Number of Schools N(pupils participating)	8 (238)	0	1 (2)	9 (240)
Symbol Questionnaire Number of Schools N(pupils participating)	8 (124)	1 (15)	11 (158)	20 (297)
Online Questionnaire Number of Schools N(pupils participating)	16 (832)	8 (849)	1 (7)	25 (1688)
Interview schedule Number of Schools N(pupils participating)	9 (259)	2 (128)	5 (30)	16 (417)
Focus group Number of Schools N(pupils participating)	4 (131)	0	0	4 (131)
Point to point Number of Schools N(pupils participating)	2 (6)	0	0	2 (6)
Total schools using at least one flexible tool (no. using 2+ tools)	24 (12)	9 (1)	12 (5)	45 (18)
Total pupils participating	1529	992	197	**2774**

Noticeably the methods that provided the most open forums for pupils to express their views, focus groups and point to point, were selected by relatively few schools and used only with primary aged pupils. These however are methods which schools are less familiar with and coupled with the less directive nature of the data collection may have been viewed hesitantly by teachers given the other options.

Feedback from staff suggested that they had often chosen tools that they were more familiar with and that required little by way of preparation or customisation. These also proved less time intensive to administer to children. However 40% of schools tried out more than one type of tool for data collection, with some schools using four different tools. A greater range of tools was employed in the primary and special schools – reflecting the wider range of communication needs.

Despite our earlier argument about the contextualised nature of the difficulties pupils experience, some broad general messages emerged from the data.

many pupils found peer support particularly helpful

others found problematic peer relationships made learning difficult

pupils often wanted further teacher input both generically to the whole class in the form of clearer explanations, and individually

noise and overcrowding were the main issues in physical environment

there were a number of pupils, with and without disability, who were struggling with aspects of school life

In particular the most reflective comments emerged from open questions that were non-directive. For example:

"If you had a magic wand, what is the one thing you would like to change about school?"

I would crack down hard on bullying

To get rid of kids who slow me and others down and get rid of older kids being nasty.

to alway have someone to talk to about your problems

not having stressy teachers, you feel you cannot talk to them

CONCLUSION

Schools opted to choose structured methods to collect data from children even where they were not best suited to the needs of the children. In consequence they had to provide additional one to one support that removed the anonymity of those tools and changed the dynamics of the data collection. Schools have a number of pressures on them which shape the ways in which they collect pupil views but in choosing and adapting methods they need to be alert to the way in which this can constrain the messages that are shared with staff. Institutions mediate the ways in which views are heard- and thereby the degree to which meanings are negotiated and understood. The risk is that the methods used can compound the experience of disability as only certain barriers within the environment are acknowledged. This emphasises the importance of non-directive methods and personalised approaches to those with the most significant needs if their voices are to be heard. While schools may be committed to collecting pupil views they need to direct energy to considering the strengths and limitations of particular ways of doing so in order to avoid compounding the experience of disability.

REFERENCES

Antaki C., Young N., & Finlay M. (2002) Shaping Clients' Answers: departures from neutrality in care-staff interviews with people with a learning disability. *Disability & Society*, 17, 4, 435-455

Booth, T., & Booth W., (1996) Sounds of Silence: narrative research with inarticulate subjects. *Disability & Society*, 11, 1, 55-69.

Cameron, L., & Murphy J., (2002) Enabling young people with a learning disability to makechoices at a time of transition. *British Journal of Learning Disabilities*, 30, 105-112.

Cederburg, A-C., Orbach Y., Sterberg K., & Lamb M. (2000) Invesitagive Interviews of child witnesses in Sweden, *Child Abuse and Neglect*, 24, 10, 1355-1361.

Connors, C., & Stalker K., (2002) *Children's Experiences of Disability: A Positive Outlook.* Interchange 75. Edinburgh: Scottish Executive.

Krahenbuhl S., & Blades M. (2006) The effect of question repetition within interviews on young children's eyewitness recall. *Journal of Experimental Child Psychology*, 94, 57-67.

Lamb M.E. & Fauchier A. (2001) The Effects of Question Type on Self-Contradictions by Children in the Course of Forensic Interviews. *Applied Cognitive Psychology*, 15, 483-491.

Lowe, C., (2001) Controversial Speech by British Activist: Have Disability Rights Gone Too Far ? Disability World, 7 http://www.disabilityworld.org/03-04_01/news/low.shtml

PorterJ., (in press) Missing Out ? Challenges to Hearing the Views of All Children on the Barriers and Supports to Learning. *Education 3-13*.

Rhodes P., Nocon A., Small N., & Wright J., (2008) Disability and Identity: the challenge of epilepsy. *Disability & Society*, 23, 4, 385-395.

Shakespeare, T (2005) *Disability Rights and Wrongs*. London: Routledge.

Van de Ven A.H. & Delbecq A.L. (1972) The Nominal group as a research Instrument for Exploratory Health Studies. *A.J.P.H* February 1972 pgs 337-342.

World Health Organisation (2007) *International classification of functioning, disability and health. (ICF-CY)* Geneva: WHO.

PART VI. EMPOWERMENT, RIGHTS AND ETHICS

In this section *Burns* highlights a number of issues specifically related to women with intellectual disabilities (ID). Their place in history from 1800s to 2000s is documented. More modern-day concerns of safeguarding reproductive rights of women and understanding female-female sex relationships are discussed. *Blyth and Carson* go onto talk about male-male sexual relationships. Many issues are non-gender specific and are issues previously experienced by the gay and bisexual general population. The empowerment and expression of one's right always causes disquiet when individuals with ID are victims of abuse; particularly sexual abuse. *Koopman and Roux* report on sexual assaults on individuals with ID in South Africa. They endorse the need for proactive intervention for persons with ID to receive justice. Being able to 'speak for one's self' is an essential part of empowerment. *Grove and colleagues* demonstate that storysharing, where there is a narrative recall of personal experience, can promote friendships and better social integration even for children and adults with severe ID.

Chapter 33

WOMEN WITH INTELLECTUAL DISABILITIES: THEIR PLACE IN HISTORY 1800'S-2000'S

J. Burns

Department of Applied Social and Psychological Development,
Canterbury Christ Church University

INTRODUCTION

The place of people with intellectual disabilities (ID) within society in the Western world has a fascinating history; however, this narrative has largely been gender blind (Carpenter, 2001). Looking at this history through the lens of gender allows the history of women with ID to be traced alongside the evolving role of women in our society, and provides us with some insight to understand their position today. Within this chapter some of the key milestones along this journey will be highlighted.

In England the establishment of both the County Asylums Acts of 1808 and 1828 and the Poor Law of 1834 resulted in the building of large institutions to care for both people with mental health problems and ID. During this time we saw the establishment of the segregation of the sexes, even in the workhouses, where whole families were admitted, and therapeutic emphasis was given to work, but strictly along gendered divisions of labour (Scheerenberger, 1983; Atkinson et al, 1997).

This is well illustrated through the work of Dr John Langdon Down whose pioneering work on Down syndrome (DS) was carried out in the 'Royal Earlswood Asylum for Idiots' in Surrey (Ward, 1998). Photography had come of an age and Dr Langdon Down carefully logged the characteristics of men, women and children with DS. The influence of the Victorian scientific movement of 'moral management' can clearly be seen through these portraits, encouraging strict regimes, the adherence to Victorian values and stringent gendered codes of behavior (Showalter, 1987). Other prevailing attitudes also influenced his work, including the imperialist attitude to racial categorisation, biological determinism, enacted through the 'sciences' of physiognomy and phrenology, and a colonial belief in Anglo- Saxon racial supremacy (Rimke & Hunt, 2002; Bigby & Fyffe, 2006).

At this time, although the British Empire had a woman at its helm, generally women were not held to have the same moral and intellectual aptitudes as men. Hence, those carrying out the research, devising and implementing social policy were men (Carpenter, 2001). For those women who were deemed 'idiots' their degeneration into immorality and the potential corruption of others was seen as inevitable. They were seen in terms of more primitive development, again aligned to racial divides, and to have no agency in their own civilisation, another Victorian preoccupation. It was clear to those in power that the way out of this degeneration was to take control and give people the privilege of taking up the roles and tasks associated with good Victorian citizens, cut off of course at the point of marriage and procreation. Hence, in the pictures of the women under the care of Dr Langdon Down we see Victorian ladies, clean, modestly dressed, clearly engaged in roles of domesticity[1]

This issue of sexuality was becoming an increasing problem, and with women being seen as the morally weaker gender was a preoccupying concern for the protectorates of the female 'feeble minded' (McDonagh, 2001). Science was starting to reveal the secrets of genetics, although genetic inheritance was imbued with a power never realized, and control of breeding was seen as a solution to some of these problems.

> 'They intermarry with the hitherto untainted and normal member of the community, and in doing so constantly drag fresh blood into the vortex of disease...... to check this evil, three methods have been proposed 1) Asexualisation; 2) compulsory segregation during the reproductive age; and 3) the regulation of marriage.' p457, (Tredgold, 1908).

The rise of the science of eugenics brought forth two classic case studies in the history of women with ID. The first is that of the Kallikak family written up by Robert Goddard in 1912, the then principle of the Vineland school for the 'feebleminded' in the US. Martin Kallikak returning from the US civil war had a liaison with a 'feeble minded' barmaid, but went on to marry a 'respectable' woman and father more children. Goddard traced the genealogy of both lines claiming evidence for a 'feeble-minded' and a 'normal' strain, descending through the two mothers, clearly placing the defective genetic inheritance within the maternal line (Goddard, 1912; Tucker, 1987; Block, 2000).

The second case study occurred later in history and again in the US. This was the case of Carrie Buck who was compulsory detained in the 'Virginia Colony for Epileptics and Feeble-Minded' after becoming pregnant through a family rape, and subsequently forcibly sterilised in 1927. Again the social, moral and intellectual inheritance of the Buck family was investigated and in the court case leading to the implementation of sterilisation laws within the state of Virginia, Supreme Court Justice, Oliver Wendall Jones, Jr, commented 'Three generations of imbeciles are enough.' (Block, 2000). The Virginia Statute was not revoked until 2001. Such examples culminated in the UK in 1934 in the Brock Commission which recommended a regime of 'voluntary' sterilisation of the 'mentally handicapped', and cited ten countries that had already brought in such laws (Scheerenberger, 1983).

The decades between the 1940-1950's brought their own problems with two world wars, but the 60's and 70s heralded new perspectives with the arrival of Normalisation (Wolfensberger, 1972), the increasing economic cost of care based on an infra structure of large institutions and a number of scandals involving abuse in such hospitals. The experience

---

[1] See http://www.intellectualdisability.info/values/history_DS.htm for examples of such photographs.

of the plight of people within these institutions in the US is well captured in the photographs of Blatt and Kaplan in Christmas in Purgatory (1974). These pictures illustrate the changes that had come about for women living in these circumstances, where the regime had moved onto that of medication, neurosurgery, and occasionally training. For those with ID the more medically orientated therapeutic approaches of the time provided little help and these places became ones of containment, starved of resources and sharing little hope. Institutionalisation became a problem in of itself (Blatt & Kaplan, 1974).

For women in living in such hospitals, contrary to the time of therapeutic optimism, their gendered roles were lost, subsumed under titles such as 'the mentally handicapped' or 'the mentally retarded'. Within Blatt and Kaplan's (1974) photo montage we can see young women, hardly dressed, sitting in bare corridors, or clutching a baby doll as the only possession within an otherwise bare environment[2]. The struggle for these women became that of regaining their gender, and being seen to belong to a more mainstream community. These dynamics are superbly illustrated through the work of the photographer Diane Arbus whose work 'Untitled' was published posthumously in 1995, but was carried out in 1971-72 (Arbus, 1995). Here she shows women symbolising both their own struggle to be women first and handicapped second through their handbags and their bonnets. It also demonstrates the projections of the outside world through the frequent images of women with ID dressed as clowns, with masks on, and appearing child like within adult bodies.

So history has both enforced gendered roles and stripped them from women with ID. As women's roles and presence within large society has developed and advanced so has that for women with ID, although inevitably with some time lag. Publications now document the experience of women with ID and some of this history (Burns, 1993; Atkinson et al., 2000; Trausdottir & Johnson, 2000; Scior, 2003). They describe a more delicate negotiation between attaining and maintaining the identity of 'woman' whilst managing and resisting some of the restrictions and inequalities that can accompany that role. Such work also describes how some women may choose to offset some of the more negative and abusive aspects of womanhood, just to escape that other role of 'ID'. However, the important aspect of this time is the word choice; in the history of women with ID we are now only beginning to hear what they would choose for themselves and work with their responses.

REFERENCES

Arbus, D. (1995). *Untitled*. New York: Aperture.

Atkinson, D., Jackson, M., & Walmsley , J. (Eds.). (1997). *Forgotten lives: exploring the history of learning disability*. Kidderminster: British Institute of Learning Disabilities.

Atkinson, D., McCarthy, M., Walmsley, J., Cooper, M., Rolph, S., Aspis, S., et al (Eds.). (2000). *Good times, bad times: women with learning difficulties telling their stories*. Kidderminster: British Institute of Learning Disabilities.

Bigby, C., & Fyffe, C. (2006). Tensions between institutional closure and deinstitutionalisation: What can be learned from victoria's institutional redevelopment? *Disability & Society, 21*(6), 567-581.

---

2 Some of these photographs can be viewed at this site http://www.disabilitymuseum.org/lib/docs/

Blatt, B., & Kaplan, F. (1974). *Christmas in purgatory: A photographic essay on mental retardation*. Syracuse: Human Policy Press.

Block, P. (2000). Sexuality, fertility and danger: Twentieth-century images of women with cognitive disabilities. *Sexuality and Disability. Special Issue: Disability, Sexuality, and Culture: Societal and Experiential Perspectives on Multiple Identities .Part II, 18*(4), 239-239.

Burns, J. (1993). Invisible women - women who have learning disabilities. *The Psychologist, 6,* 102-105.

Carpenter, P. (2001). The role of victorian women in the care of "idiots" and the "feebleminded.". *Journal on Developmental Disabilities, 8*(2), 31-31.

Goddard, H. H. (1912). *The story of Deborah*. New York, NY, US: MacMillan Co.

McDonagh, P. (2001). "Only an almost": Helen MacMurchy, feeble minds, and the evidence of literature. *Journal on Developmental Disabilities, 8*(2), 61-61.

Rimke, H., & Hunt, A. (2002). From sinners to degenerates: The medicalization of morality in the 19th century. *History of the Human Sciences, 15*(1), 59-59.

Scheerenberger,R.(1983). *A history of mental retardation*. Baltimore: Paul Brookes.

Scior, K. (2003). Using discourse analysis to study the experiences of women with learning disabilities. *Disability & Society, 18*(6), 779-779.

Showalter, E. (1987). *The female malady: Women, madness and english culture, 1830-1980*. London: Virago.

Tredgold, A. (1908). *Mental deficiency (amentia)*. New York: Wood.

Trausdottir, R. & Johnson, K. (2000). *Women with Intellectual Disabilities: Finding a Place in the World*. London: Jessica Kingsley

Tucker, W. H. (1987). The Kallikaks revisited: A trip worth taking. *PsycCRITIQUES, 32*(3), 288.

Ward, O. C. (1998). *John langdon down 1828-1896, a caring pioneer*. London: Royal Society of Medicine.

Wolfensberger, W., National Institute on Mental Retardation, & Canadian Association for the Mentally Retarded. (1972). *The principle of normalization in human services*. Toronto: Published by National Institute on Mental Retardation through L. Crainford.

Chapter 34

Safeguarding the Reproductive Rights of Women with Intellectual Disabilities

J. Burns
Canterbury Christ Church University, UK

Introduction

The position of women with intellectual disabilities (ID) in relation to their reproductive rights has undergone many changes and remains variable across the world. In the Western world it has shifted from that of denial to a dialogue of acceptance and promotion of rights along side protection, both of the adult and the child. However, these developments have not been in isolation, they have occurred in a context of the changing expression of women's sexuality and reproductive rights in the world at large. Even today the position of women with ID has to be understood in relation to the position held generally by women within that culture. History has dictated that the promotion of the reproductive rights for women with ID cannot be in advance of the position of women in the main, but tends to lag behind it, and even then the attainment of such rights might be a hard fought battle. It must also be recognised that the expression of these 'rights' is not always clear cut. The rights of the mother or parents compared to the rights of the child is a challenging area, strewn with ethical and moral dilemmas, bringing into play individual, cultural and constitutional value bases. Whilst mainstream approaches to these issues can be helpful the specific features of ID bring unique aspects to these dilemmas.

Mapping the Existing Territory

Even in the most 'advanced' societies the expression of the reproductive rights by women with ID remains contested (Parish, 2002). Historically, we have seen these rights resisted through three main mechanisms: removal, denial and suppression. Early in the history of our treatment of people with ID we saw people incarcerated in large institutions, often in same sex wards, denied any opportunity to express their sexuality, never mind their reproductive rights (Block, 2000). These individuals were physically removed from society into an alternative life where all the usual human rights were suspended. Later in history we saw a more medical solution to the possibility of people with ID expressing their reproductive rights, through both 'voluntary' and compulsory sterilisation. Such regimes occurred in Europe right up until the 1970's (Armstrong, 1997) and the countries which introduced such laws included: the US, Canada, German, Sweden, Japan, China and India (Kempton & Kahn, 1991). In the UK Winston Churchill advocated for such procedures but failed to get them accepted:

> "The unnatural and increasingly rapid growth of the feeble minded and insane classes, coupled as it is with a steady restriction among all the thrifty, energetic and superior stocks, constitutes a national and race danger which it is impossible to exaggerate...I feel that the source from which the stream of madness is fed should be cut off and sealed up before another year has passed."

Churchill to Prime Minister Asquith, 1910

A more subtle resistance towards the expression of reproductive rights comes through the denial of services to support people express these ambitions. That people with ID tend to receive less than adequate health, social and educational services, throughout both the developed and less developed nations has been well documented (WHO, 2007). In the opening line in the Independent Inquiry into Access to Healthcare for People with Learning Disabilities (Department of Health, 2008) in the UK, Sir Jonathan Michael wrote:

> 'The health and strength of a society can be measured by how well it cares for its most vulnerable members.' p7

Even in the UK, which aspires to 'world leading healthcare' and a legislative system supposedly holding equality at its heart, the inquiry went on to state that it found:

> '....convincing evidence that people with learning disabilities have higher levels of unmet need and receive less effective treatment, despite the fact that the Disability Discrimination Act and Mental Capacity Act set out a clear legal framework for the delivery of equal treatment.' p7

A third form of resistance is that of suppression by restricting opportunities and encouragement to express these rights. This can be through continuing same-sex services, lack of sex education, contraception and pregnancy advice not being available or accessible, observation and undue controls leading to lack of privacy. The impact of such controls can easily be seen from this quote taken from some research asking a young woman about herself:

> I: ...and is he still your boyfriend?
> B: on a Wednesday night and Friday mornings...at the club,... yeah, on the minibus coming home on a Friday afternoon.

(Webb, 2004)

Mapping the Future Territory

With the advancement of science we face even more ethically and medically sophisticated challenges within this area, demonstrated through well publicised test cases. Such cases firmly place these issues under the general gaze and comment of the public at large. No longer are they the concerns of just the individuals, families and professionals involved, but they challenge constitutional attitudes, family values and our economic priorities. As such the views of the general voting public now take on a much greater relevance than previously and what was once the private battle for one woman's reproductive rights now becomes a very public contest mediated by the popular media.

By researching these media accounts we can gain an insight into the dominant discourses that may influence social change and the potential outcomes for women with ID. A case in point is that of a young, severely disabled woman, aged 15, in the UK whose mother wished her to have a hysterectomy to avoid the discomfort and possible fear attached to menstruation. As the young woman was unable to consent and there was no medical reason for such an intervention the case was taken to the courts to debate and found itself under the media spotlight.

The ensuing debate highlighted a range of discourses including a largely parental backlash to the perceived increasing professional domination of parental rights. The following quotes are taken from a survey of 200 comments posted on the websites of 4 UK national daily papers, resulting from the coverage of this case.

> 'Like Mrs-----, and all parents, I want only what is right for my daughter - not what suits the politically correct health professionals, charities and activists who are so obsessed with our children's "rights" that all too often they perpetrate the most terrible wrongs.'

> The Sun

Interestingly the sanctity of motherhood was also brought into play, being used to both exclude and subjugate other views.

> 'Either the mother has charge over the child and is considered to be a fit person with the child's best welfare at heart or she does not. If she has, then her decision must be paramount. '

> The Mail

Whilst at the same time as promoting the special place of motherhood the denial of this young woman's opportunities to share in such experiences does not even enter the debate. However, not all parents took a similar position:

> 'My daughter Z is 20, who also has cerebral palsy, is similar to X, especially as she too doesn't talk, but communicates non-verbally. But when Z came of age, we celebrated with a special meal welcoming her into womanhood - not major surgery. '

> Preethi Manuel columnist in The Guardian (October, 2007)

A third discourse which dominated this debate was that of the confidence in the medical model and where ordinary biological and developmental events are depicted as serious medical problems

> 'For all parents of handicapped children, the issue of sex and reproduction is a source of constant anxiety.'

> Meg Henderson, columnist in The Mail, (October, 2007)

> 'Unable to cope with her sexual feelings, she had a breakdown and was hospitalised.'

> The Sun

Some comments also illustrated the consequences of earlier advancements not being recognised and understood within the wider public view, to the extent that the voice of the individual with ID is not expected to be represented at all, and the problems surrounding the expression of sexuality firmly located within the individual themselves.

> 'I also know of 2 girls with Down's Syndrome, and 1 with severe retardation that have also been sterilised to make sure that they cannot get pregnant if they are abused, as all 3 are "obedient", and will do as they are told. Is that wrong?'

> The Mail

SUMMARY

Whilst the expressions of the reproductive rights of women with ID have a come a long way there is still yet further to go. We now have a good understanding and evidence base of the structural restrictions that both deny and do not actively promote such rights and much work is being accomplished to rectify these wrongs. However, what we are being faced with now are a much more sophisticated set of ethical and moral issues, playing off one set of rights against another. This is also taking place much more under the public gaze which highlights an increasing need for public awareness and education in some of the complexities surrounding these issues.

REFERENCES

Armstrong, C. (1997). Thousands of women sterilised in Sweden without consent. *British Medical Journal*, 315, 563-568

Block, P. (2000). Sexuality, Fertility, and Danger: Twentieth-Century Images of Women with Cognitive Disabilities. *Sexuality and Disability*, Vol. 18, (4), 239-254.

Kempton, W. & Kahn, E. (1991). Sexuality and People with Intellectual Disabilities: A Historical Perspective. *Sexuality and Disability*, Vol. 9, (2), 93-111.

Parish, S. (2002). Parenting. In P. Noonan Walsh & T. Heller (Eds.). *Health of Women with Intellectual Disabilities* (p103-p120). Oxford: Blackwell.

Webb, K. (2004). Life transitions: the impact on identity for women with learning disabilities. Unpublished thesis, Canterbury Christ Church University.

World Health Organisation, (2007). Atlas: Global Resources for Person with Intellectual Disabilities. Geneva: WHO.

Chapter 35

WOMEN WITH INTELLECTUAL DISABILITIES: UNDERSTANDING SAME-SEX RELATIONSHIPS

J. Burns

Department of Social and Psychological Development,
Canterbury Christ Church University

INTRODUCTION

Whilst there is increasing international recognition and acceptance in the western world of people expressing their sexuality in different ways, this is not always the case for women with intellectual disabilities (ID). The battle to be able to express one's sexuality in any positive way as an individual with ID has been an ongoing and now well recorded contest (Servais, 2006). The positioning of sexuality for women with ID can be traced back to the 1800s, even then illustrating debate and contradiction starting from a position of complete denial through the personification of the 'holy innocent' and at the same time the contradictory stance of the highly fertile, highly promiscuous individual. The debate has moved on over the years to a position of fighting for equal rights to both express one's sexuality whilst at the same time receive appropriate support and protection as a potentially vulnerable person. What has been absent throughout these discussions, due to the entire topic in itself being a contested subject, is that of the expression of more minority sexualities, in this case women who form sexual relationships with other women, the 'minority within the minority' Basson (1998, p.360).

In terms of the information that we have available to us about women with ID engaged in same sex relationships, it seems to be one of the least openly expressed forms of sexuality within this group (McCarthy, 1999; Abbott & Howarth, 2005; Lofgren-Mayenrtenson, 2009). In terms of people with ID knowing about different forms of sexuality, whilst there has been a growth of accessible and comprehensive sex education material (Grieveo et al, 2007) within this area there is evidence that the actual impact on the knowledge base of people with ID about homosexuality remains limited (Lumley & Scotti, 2001; Murphy & O'Callaghan,

2004). Indeed, there is evidence that some people with ID hold more conservative views towards same sex relationships and sexual activity than the ordinary population (Lunsky & Konstantareas, 1998; Thompson et al, 2001; Lofgren-Mayenrtenson, 2009).

Indeed, if we turn to the history of ID and some of the prevailing ideologies over this time we can perhaps see why this may be. Brown and others have well documented some of the problems surrounding the regulation of sexuality through the ideology of normalization (Burns, 1992; Brown, 1994; 1996). Within this 'meta theory', as Wolfensberger (1972) termed it, the use of social dynamics which have resulting in people with ID finding themselves at the bottom of the pecking order are attempted to be put in reverse and the very same dynamics used to promote a more valued identity. Hence, attempts should be made if one is to increase the social standing of devalued people to attach signifiers of valued identities, not at just at an acceptable level but at a higher level. This is clearly problematic in two ways, one being that it does not directly challenge practices which result in social inequality, and two it even further disenfranchises identities that are not valued within wider society, such as being lesbian or gay.

Whilst normalization received both acceptance and criticism in western societies it did have a prevailing influence, which we can see in the discourses of many of the social policies today. One of the positives that such ideologies did bring was an acceptance that we live in a gendered world, and as such men and women with ID must be accepted as such and not treated as 'other' (Burns, 1993; Scior, 2003). Seeing people with ID under the 'people' label and not as men and women automatically de-sexes them, making their sexuality a redundant concept. It is only when we recognize that women with ID have the right to express their sexuality that we can then take the next step in recognizing the range of sexualities that they also have the right to express.

A second area is that of how the person with the ID manages their identity, which is now recognized as a highly complex and skilled navigation (Rapley, 2004). Edgerton in his groundbreaking ethnographic studies of people's attempts at 'passing' clearly illustrated the sensitivities to understanding 'spoiled identities' and the herculean attempts people go through to present a more positive identity (Edgerton, 1967; Edgerton & Bercovici, 1976; Edgerton et al, 1984). Whilst people may not always be able to articulate these processes they do enact them on a day to day basis through the choices they make and the actions they may attempt to suppress. Given that the majority of people live within societies where homophobia, heterosexism and heteronormativity exist it is not surprising that people with ID might internalize such negative attitudes themselves or at least steer well clear of acquiring another identity which provides a further obstacle to social inclusion and acceptance (Thompson, 2003; Bennett & Coyle, 2007). However, despite very clear obstacles some women with ID do manage to express their minority sexuality, as demonstrated in the most extensive research that exists on this topic so far; the 'Secret Loves, Hidden Lives' project carried out in the UK (Abbott & Howarth, 2005). This study documents the views of gay, lesbian and bisexual people and staff working with them about their experiences of trying to express their sexuality. It documents the prejudice, discrimination and struggles that people have gone through, the need for support, but also stories of resistance, resilience and ultimately love.

Even for those people supported within both their intellectual disability and lesbian or gay identities penetrating and gaining acceptance within such communities is difficult. Firstly, people need to know where and how to access such communities and whilst gay men and the pink pound have influenced the visibility of such communities this remains less so for lesbians (Hennessy, 1994). Considering just the media portrayals of openly gay men and women, where many ongoing TV soaps have incorporated a gay man at some point they are much less likely to have included a woman. Obvious, 'out' lesbian role models within popular culture are few and far between (Diamond & Butterworth, 2008). For women with ID who wish to engage in same sex relationships and access such a community, a relationship which acts as a 'go between' similar to that described in Edgerton's early studies, that of the 'benevolent benefactor', might be vital. Such a need was poignantly articulated by a participant in the UK 'Secret Loves, Hidden Lives' study (Abbott & Burns, 2007).

> "I nearly walked there the other day. It was so sunny and all these people were out there under the umbrellas with the tables, and a part of me wanted to go there and a part of me was two steps back. I will try and get there, but...I know it's scary, very scary". *p32*

In other contexts, for paid carers to take on such a role would be a perfectly orthodox part of their role, i.e. to facilitate access to a social grouping. However, as the exisiting studies have identified (Thompson, 2003; Abbott & Howarth, 2006) this is simply not the case. It is likely that the range of prevailing attitudes towards homosexuality operating within wider society also operate at a personal level within paid care staff. For example, in a study examining the implementation of human rights by care staff, Clarke & Finnegan (2005) found 76% of staff said they would support heterosexual relationship for people with ID, but only 41% said they would support same sex relationships. The complexity of this role is well described in the study 'Secret Loves, Hidden Lives' (Abbott and Howarth, 2006), where they uncovered the delicate path needing to be negotiated around this topic, and described staff trying hard not to be overly intrusive into other peoples personal lives, holding fears about the interpretations of their actions, lacking training and guidance and anxious of attack by the reactions of others such as parents. They also found a frequently expressed view was that:

> "...the sexual contact that men and women with intellectual disabilities initiated, or experienced, was not related to sexual identity, but was an expression of sexual need in an environment which offered limited choices." *p120*

This could easily be interpreted as an expression of the myths surrounding homosexuality in relation to opportunity and developmental stage (Thompson et al, 2001), but it also does raise an important issue, as it is easy to fall into a strict categorical view of sexuality; heterosexual, bisexual or homosexual. Research tells us that the expression of sexuality is much more variable than this and can vary over time for the individual (Dickson et al, 2003). Whilst recognizing same sex relationships we must also be accepting of variations within that theme, and acknowledge that even whilst people are engaged in these relationships they may not use or accept the terminology and identity that goes along side it. Hence, it is entirely possible for a woman with ID to have an intimate relationship with another woman but not identify as a lesbian, or a bisexual woman, as indeed some women in mainstream society also position themselves (Diamond & Butterworth, 2008).

CONCLUSION

In conclusion, supporting women with ID who wish to engage in same sex relationships cannot be seen in isolation from the position of women with the same desires in mainstream society, and as a consequence is not only an individual issue but a political one. In his paper on supporting gay men with ID Thompson (2003) points to a number of practical supportive strategies that professional staff can take, but also calls for a 'subversive and political praxis' aimed at addressing the 'social structures that both subscribe and produce those 'needs' in the first place' p734. Having staff that are enabled to take this role is a clear lynch pin for progress and reflecting back to Edgerton's identification of the 'benevolent benefactor' as a key relationship to successful 'community' living, such benefactors may still be important but also need to be enabled as agents of political and social change. Nevertheless, for the 'minority within the minority', women with ID who want to engage in same sex relationships, the visibility of such an option clearly needs to be highlighted, through whatever means we have at our disposal.

REFERENCES

Abbott, D., & Howarth, J. (2005). Love - A human rights issue? The experiences of gay, lesbian, and bisexual people with intellectual disabilities. *Culture Health & Sexuality, 7*, S1-S1.

Abbott, D., & Howarth, J. (2006). *Secret loves, hidden lives? exploring issues for people with learning disabilities who are gay, lesbian and bisexual*. Bristol: The Policy Press.

Abbott, D., & Burns, J. (2007). What's love got to do with it?: Experiences of lesbian, gay, and bisexual people with intellectual disabilities in the united kingdom and views of the staff who support them. *Sexuality Research & Social Policy: A Journal of the NSRC, 4*(1), 27-39.

Basson, R. (1998). Sexual health of women with disabilities. Canadian Medical Association Journal, 4, 359-362

Bennett, C., & Coyle, A. (2007). A minority within a minority: Experiences of gay men with intellectual disabilities. In V. Clarke, & E. Peel (Eds.), *Out in psychology: Lesbian, gay, bisexual, trans and queer perspectives*. (pp. 125-145). New York, NY, US: John Wiley & Sons Ltd.

Brown, H. (1994). "An ordinary sexual life?": A review of the normalisation principle as it applies to the sexual options of people with learning disabilities. *Disability & Society, 9*(2), 123-123.

Brown, H. (1996). Ordinary women: Issues for women with learning disabilities: A keynote review. *British Journal of Learning Disabilities, 24*(2), 47-47.

Burns, J. (1992). Normalisation through the looking glass. *Clinical Psychoogy Forum, 39*, 22-24.

Burns, J. (1993). Invisible women - women who have learning disabilities. *The Psychologist, 6*, 102-105.

Clarke, S., & Finnegan, P. (2005). One law for all? the impact of the human rights act on people with learning disabilities. London: Values into Action.

Diamond, L. M., & Butterworth, M. (2008). Questioning gender and sexual identity: Dynamic links over time. *Sex Roles, 59*(5-6), 365-376.

Dickson, N., Paul, C., & Herbison, P. (2003). Same-sex attraction in a birth cohort: Prevalence and persistence in early adulthood. *Social Science & Medicine, 56*(8), 1607.

Edgerton, R. B. (1967). *The cloak of competence; stigma in the lives of the mentally retarded.* Berkeley: University of California Press.

Edgerton, R. B., & Bercovici, S. M. (1976). The cloak of competence: Years later. *American Journal of Mental Deficiency, 80*(5), 485-497.

Edgerton, R. B., Bollinger, M., & Herr, B. (1984). The cloak of competence: After two decades. *American Journal of Mental Deficiency, 88*(4), 345-345.

Grieveo, A., McLaren, S., & Lindsay, W. R. (2007). An evaluation of research and training resources for the sex education of people with moderate to severe learning disabilities. *British Journal of Learning Disabilities, 35*(1), 30-37.

Hennessy, R. (1994). Queer visibility in commodity culture. *Cultural Critique,* (29), 31-76.

Lofgren-Mayenrtenson, L. (2009). The invisibility of young homosexual women and men with intellectual disabilities. *Sexuality and Disability, 27*(1), 21-26.

Lumley, V., & Scotti, J. (2001). Supporting the sexuality of adults with mental retardation. *Journal of Positive Behavior Intervention, 3*(2), 109-119.

Lunsky, Y., & Konstantareas, M. M. (1998). The attitudes of individuals with autism and mental retardation towards sexuality. *Education and Training in Mental Retardation and Developmental Disabilities, 33*(1), 24-33.

McCarthy, M. (1999). *Sexuality and women with learning disabilities.* Philadelphia: Jessica Kingsley.

Murphy, G. H., & O'Callaghan, A. (2004). Capacity of adults with intellectual disabilities to consent to sexual relationships. *Psychol.Med., 34*(7), 1347-1357.

Rapley, M. (2004). *The social construction of intellectual disability.* New York, NY, US: Cambridge University Press.

Scior, K. (2003). Using discourse analysis to study the experiences of women with learning disabilities. *Disability & Society, 18*(6), 779-779.

Servais, L. (2006). Sexual health care in persons with intellectual disabilities. *Mental Retardation and Developmental Disabilities Research Reviews, 12*(1), 48-56.

Thompson, S. A., Bryson, M., & de Castell, S. (2001). Prospects for identity formation for lesbian, gay, or bisexual persons with developmental disabilities. *International Journal of Disability, Development and Education, 48*(1).

Thompson, S. A. (2003). Subversive political praxis: Supporting choice, power and control for people with learning difficulties. *Disability & Society, 18*(6), 719-736.

Wolfensberger, W. (1972). The principle of normalization in human services. Toronto: National Institute on Mental Retardation.

Chapter 36

"Who'd Want Him!" Barriers to Gay Men with Intellectual Disabilities Developing Sexual Identities

C. Blyth[1] and I. Carson[1]

[1]School of Education, University of Manchester, Manchester UK.

Introduction

This chapter is based upon an amalgam of two research projects that focused upon the developing identities of young men with intellectual disabilities (ID) who identify as being gay: one of these projects was undertaken in two mainstream schools in England (Iain Carson), and the other in Manchester's gay village (Craig Blyth). A qualitative approach was adopted in relation to both projects and data were collected via a combination of overt observation and narrative accounts.

The Research

The title of this chapter comes from a statement made by a school teacher about a young man with ID in his class. Simon was educated in a mainstream school in England and thus, was supposedly receiving an 'inclusive' education. When asked why Simon was being excluded from aspects of the sex education his class was receiving, the teacher responded: 'look at him, who'd want him anyway'. We cannot be certain what the teacher was implying; Simon was a very personable, attractive young man who identified as being gay and was keen to make friends and develop his emerging sexuality. We refer elsewhere (Blyth & Carson, 2007) to the 'certainties' that exist in the minds of some about what it means to be disabled, i.e. because Simon had ID, it was a 'certainty' that 'not only would he not have an active sex life, but also that he was not entitled to one' (Carson, 2002). This is reinforced by Grieve *et al* (2009) who cite a number of sources that suggest that there is a significant level of negative attitude toward the sexuality of people with ID amongst the general population. The issues identified above relate to sexuality generally; when one extends this beyond the heteronormativity that dominates much of our society, the negativity towards people with ID who identify as gay seems to increase. An example of such is highlighted by Löfgren-Mårtenson (2009) who, when interviewing a female care worker about the sexuality of the people with intellectual disability she supported, was given the following response: 'I have a real hard time imagining two fags here at the day-center' (p 23). Another female member of staff seemed to believe that gay people with ID would find it too difficult to express their sexuality……. 'since they are so vulnerable, it would be difficult for them to demonstrate their sexual orientation' (p 23). We ask, if such homophobia and heteronormative assumptions exist amongst those who support people with ID, what discriminatory barriers are people like Simon likely to encounter within the wider community?

In addition to the disablist comments made by Simon's teacher, his learning support assistant informed him (in a sex education class) that he couldn't be gay 'because it wasn't nice' and that he didn't need to worry about condoms, because he didn't need them. In addition to being seriously misinformed (he believed that he must be physiologically different to other boys), Simon left school 'with an imposed negative status and stigma in relation to how he perceived himself' (Carson, 2002).

It was evident throughout the research that teachers and learning support staff were not alone in terms of the 'certainties' that exist in relation to the sexuality and sexual identity of young people with ID; it was not unusual for similar views to be held by parents. Nathan, the father of a young man who identified as being gay, whilst acknowledging that his son had a right and a need to express himself sexually, felt very strongly that this must take place within 'normal' relationships only. Following a discussion with Nathan, my analysis of his stance is that he firmly believes that his son's intellectual disability caused him to make the 'wrong' choices regarding his sexual identity and thus, his intervention was required in order to put him on the 'right' path. Orchestrated attempts to 'normalise' his son's sexual behavior included installing a female prostitute in a hotel bedroom for a weekend and sending his son to stay there. Nathan believed that 'it was enough for his son to cope with ID without adding unnecessary additional 'abnormalities' to his situation'.

Nathan is not alone in his beliefs; whilst discussing the view of intellectual disability care workers, Löfgren-Mårtenson (2009) suggests that 'they are often concerned that the young people do not do anything that is an "unnecessary deviation". They are worried that the intellectual disability is already enough of a deviation from "the normal"' (p 25).

The second part of the paper presented to the Congress focused on the experiences of Fred. Fred lives in a Local Authority supported housing scheme. Part-way through the project Fred's flat-mate moved to another supported housing scheme and Fred found himself living alone. The Local Authority made several attempts to allocate the vacant room to another person and therefore spent several months 'showing' other people Fred's flat.

Fred explained that, often, prior to these visits certain members of his support staff would inform him that he needed to remove 'gay' items (such as rainbow flags) from around his flat. On one occasion Fred was told to remove posters of men that he had on the wall and replace them with posters of women because, as one member of staff 'explained' 'that's what men have on their walls'.

It is clear from Fred's experience, that for many members of staff it was a 'certainty' that Fred should want to look at pictures of women and not other men. Additionally, it is evident that the staff were concerned that if Fred failed to conform to this heteronormative certainty he would 'put-off' other people wanting to move into the flat. Whilst the actions of those staff could be seen as simply mirroring the heterosexist attitudes that are prevalent in wider society (Valentine and Skelton 2003) , it is telling that when Fred attempted to talk to a number of the same members of staff about issues directly connected to sexuality and specifically actual sex he was informed that he should not be thinking about such things; on one occasion being told that he didn't need to know about sex and he should 'stop being dirty and shut up'. When considering these responses, we want to suggest that, for Fred, the certainties held by those members of staff amount to the construction of a somewhat contradictory sexual identity that we term 'asexual heteronormative'. Whilst an oxymoron, it is clear to see staff members are expecting Fred to 'perform' in ways associated with heteronormative masculinity such as having posters of women on his walls (Nielsen *et al* 2000), whilst simultaneously attempting to enforce a version of asexuality upon him.

It is evident in the case of Fred, and many of the other young men and boys who participated in the respective research projects, that the certainties that they experienced in schools were further reinforced by both families (in the case of Stuart) and services (in the case of Fred).

Whilst the findings of our research highlight that for a large number of participants the pressure to conform to the certainties imposed upon them was significant, it was interesting to note that many of the young men resisted the attempted imposition of these certainties and actively sought out the company of other gay men by attempting to spend time in a commercial gay space.

Discussing his experiences on the commercial gay 'scene', Fred explained how he was often confronted with negative attitudes to his presence in this space. Fred explained that out of the 30+ bars and clubs that exist within the space he was only able to access a small number of them. Fred explained that often 'door' staff would refuse to permit him to enter these venues. Whilst he often was given no reason or told that the venue was closed for a private function (however, Fred could see other people freely entering the venue) on other occasions he was confronted with extremely discriminatory remarks such as 'you should go back to your day-center'. Fred was by no means the only participant who reported these attitudinal barriers to accessing commercial gay space. Other participants revealed experiences including being ridiculed, being physically lead out of the space by non-disabled gay men who assumed that they must be lost and being told they could only enter the venue if a support worker was present etc.

Without exception, all of the men that participated in the research relating to commercial gay space stated that they felt that this space was unwelcoming and that they felt that they did not 'fit in'. Summing up his feelings, Fred stated that, 'It's like an exclusive club with them and us... it's like I'm not a member of that club and I never will be'.

CONCLUSION

The findings of both the research projects referred to in this paper indicate that disabled young men are presented with a range of 'certainties' regarding their sexuality throughout their lives. These certainties derive from and feed into a range of negative discourses that construct men with ID as 'asexual', 'undesirable', 'heterosexual', 'abnormal' and sexually 'confused'.

When undertaking the analysis of the young men's narratives both authors were struck at how many of the men appeared to have internalised many of these certainties. For example, phrases such as 'I just wanted to be normal' and 'What's the point nobody would want me' were common place throughout these men's narratives (Blyth and Carson 2007). The findings of these two projects would suggest that for many of the participants the certainties regarding their sexuality have resulted in what Thomas (2007) terms 'psycho-emotional disablism'. Exploring this concept, Thomas (2007) illustrates how the prevalence of negative discourses regarding individuals with impairments can lead to disabled people feeling '*worthless, useless, of lesser value, ugly, burdensome*'. The findings of our research would suggest that for men with ID, Thomas's social relational model of disability has specific relevance, in as much as they are confronted with a range of disablist heteronormative discourses on an almost daily basis. It is clear from these men's narratives that many of these discourses have lead to many participants feeling that expressing a gay identity within educational, social or home environments is an option that often leads to extremely negative reactions from others around them.

REFERENCES

Blyth, C. & Carson, I. (2007) 'Sexual Uncertainties and Disabled Young Men: Silencing Difference Within the Classroom' Pastoral Care in Education, Vol. 25, No. 3, pp 34-38.

Carson, I. (2002) 'An Inclusive Society? One young man with learning difficulties doesn't think so!' in Farrell, P. & Ainscow, M. [Eds] Making Special Education Inclusive, London, David Fulton Publishers Ltd.

Grieve, A., McLaren, S., Lindsay, W. & Culling, E. (2009) 'Staff attitudes towards the sexuality of people with learning disabilities: a comparison of different professional groups and residential facilities', *British Journal of Learning Disabilities*, Vol. 37, 1 pp 1-9.

Löfgren-Mårtenson, L. (2009) 'The Invisibility of Young Homosexual Women and Men with Intellectual Disabilities', Sexuality and Disability, Vol. 27, pp 21-26.

Nielsen, J., Walden, G. and Kunkel, C. (2000) Gendered Heteronormativity: Empirical Illustrations in Everyday life, *The Sociological Quarterly*, 41(2), pp283-296.

Thomas, C. (2007) Sociologies of Disability and Illness: Contested Ideas in Disability Studies and Medical Sociology, New York, Palgrave Macmillan.

Valentine, G. and Skelton, T. (2003) Finding oneself, losing oneself: The lesbian and gay 'scene' as a paradoxical space, *International Journal of Urban and Regional Research*, 27, 849 - 866.

Chapter 37

AN EXPLORATORY STUDY OF THE EXPERIENCES OF VICTIMS OF SEXUAL ABUSE WHO HAVE INTELLECTUAL DISABILITIES IN ACCESSING THE JUSTICE SYSTEM AND OTHER SUPPORT SERVICES

G. Koopman[1] and A. Roux[1]
[1]Cape Mental Health Society, Observatory 7935, South Africa

INTRODUCTION

In South Africa the rate of sexual assault in the general population is very high with 54 926 cases of rape and 9 805 cases of indecent assault reported between April 2005 and March 2006. According to the Medical Research Council only one in nine rapes in South Africa is reported, with approximately 460 000 rapes annually of which 52 000 to 55 000 will be reported. Despite statistics not being kept on complainants with intellectual disabilities (ID) in sexual assault cases in the justice system, there is considerable evidence both internationally and in South Africa that people with ID are at much greater risk of sexual abuse and assault than the general population. Research shows that the incidence of abuse among people with disabilities is as much as four times higher than it is among the non-disabled population (Dickman & Roux 2005).

Cape Mental Health's Sexual Abuse Victim Empowerment Programme (SAVE) attempts to offer complainants with ID the same access to justice as the general population. In the absence of such a programme complainants with ID may have the tendency to acquiesce and also not be able to take an oath. SAVE is a psycho-legal programme that involves psychological evaluation of the complainant's level of functioning, competence to act as a witness, capacity to consent to sexual intercourse as well as the emotional effect of the alleged sexual abuse.

The complainants level of intellectual functioning is assessed using the Individual Scale for General Scholastic Aptitude (Robinson 1994) and the Vineland Adaptive Behavior Scales

(Sparrow et al 1984). The level of understanding of sexuality and ability to consent to sexual intercourse as well as competence as a witness are assessed through interviews. In addition the psychologist acts as an expert witness to prepare the court for the complainant's testimony. Social workers provide ongoing support for the complainant and their family before, during and after the court case. This includes providing court preparation for the complainant. Training is also provided for police and prosecutors, when requested, so that they will be better equipped when working with a complainant with ID.

RATIONALE FOR THE STUDY

The aim of the study was to research the deficits in access to justice and service delivery to people with ID who have been sexually abused as well as highlight the prevalence and other factors surrounding sexual offence cases involving people with ID in the justice system.

RESEARCH METHODOLOGY

The study looked at approximately 300 complainants who had been supported through the judicial process by the SAVE programme. These complainants were referred to the programme by the justice system between 2000 and 2006. The outcome of the cases was established through police and justice department records. Interviews were undertaken with prosecutors and police to gauge attitudes, challenges and training needs when investigating and prosecuting these cases. Victim centered interviews were also undertaken to gain an understanding of the experience of the complainants in obtaining access to justice.

RESULTS

Characteristics of the Cohort

The majority of the complainants (79.5%) are resident in the urban areas of Cape Town with only 20.5% resident in areas outside Cape Town. The cohort consisted of 264 females (92.3%), of whom 15 were complainants in more than one case of sexual abuse, and 22 males.

The age of the complainants in the 303 cases at the time of the abuse ranged from 6 years old to 2 women of 60 and 62 years, with 132 complainants (43.6%) under the age of 16, which was legally the age of consent. Two hundred and fifty seven complainants (85%) were between the ages of 10 and 29 years.

The classification of ID as defined by the Diagnostic and Statistical Manual IV of the American Psychiatric Association, was used to categorise the level of ID of the complainants. This classification describes ID as follows: mild IQ 50-55 to approximately 70, moderate IQ 35-40 to 50-55, severe IQ 19 to 35-40 and profound IQ below 19. One hundred and eighty two of the complainants (63.6%) were functioning in the range of moderate ID or lower.

Charges Laid

Two hundred and forty eight of the cases, (81.8%) were rape charges; four of these involved an additional charge, such as indecent assault, abduction and attempted rape. There were 51 cases of indecent assault, which included the 22 cases of sodomy, in which the complainants were male and 29 cases involving females, which included 9 cases of sodomy. These cases were reported prior to the new sexual offences act being enacted and thus the charge was indecent assault. In terms of the new sexual offences act the cases of sodomy would have been classified as rape. The charge in the other 4 cases was attempted rape. There were more than one accused in a total of 32 cases, 26 rape cases, 5 indecent assault cases and a case of rape and attempted rape.

Ability to Consent to Sexual Intercourse and Competence to Testify

The level of understanding of sexuality and ability to consent to sexual activity as well as competence as a witness are assessed through interviews with the complainant. A very basic level of understanding is required of the mechanics of sexual intercourse and its implications in order for the complainant to be found able to consent. Assessment of competence as a witness depends on the supportive facilities and attitude of the court as well as on the abilities of the complainant. In the courts in Cape Town, there generally is an awareness of the particular needs of these complainants.

Of the 171 complainants who were 16 (the legal age of consent at the time of the assessment) and older, only 47 (27.5%) were found to be able to consent to sexual intercourse, 122 complainants, (71.3%) were found unable to consent and it was not clear about the ability of the other 2 complainants. Sixty nine percent (69%) of the complainants were found to be competent to testify in court with adequate court preparation and in some cases with extra support or an intermediary.

The Relationship between the Complainant and the Accused

Information was available on the relationship between the complainant and the accused in 282 of the cases. The accused was known to the complainant in 244 (86.5%) of these cases. Seventy two of the accused were neighbours, family friends or boarders. In 49 of the cases (17.4%), the accused was a family member; these included 17 cases of incest involving 13 fathers, 2 brothers and 2 grandfathers. In another case the mother was the co-accused. Five of the accused were the complainant's step father and 5 were their brother-in-laws. In addition 5 were the complainant's mother's boyfriend. Eight of the accused were staff members at the facility that the complainant attended, one of whose case had 4 complainants. In the remaining cases in which the accused was known, they were community members, acquaintances, members of the same church etc.

Outcome and Sentencing

The status of 293 of the cases was known. Fifty one cases were still ongoing, of which warrants of arrest had been issued in 5 of them. Of the 242 cases in which the outcome was known and that had been finalised, the accused was found guilty in 68 cases (28.1%) and was acquitted in 44 cases (18.2%). The matter was withdrawn in 130 cases (53.7%). The reason for withdrawal was not known in 107 cases. Thirteen cases were withdrawn as the suspect was undetected, in 3 cases the accused was deceased, in 1 the complainant was deceased, in 4 the accused were juveniles, and in another 2 the family did not wish to pursue the matter.

In 20 of the cases in which the accused was found guilty, the complainant had been found not competent as a witness. In 16 of these, there was a witness and in another we know there was DNA. One who was 28 years old at the time of the abuse had been found to be competent as a witness provided an intermediary was used. This is usually not done with adults. In this particular case the court allowed the use of an intermediary despite the complainant's age.

OBSERVATIONS

As would be expected in cases of sexual abuse most of the complainants (92.3%) were female. In a previous study (Dickman & Roux 2005) done on referrals to the SAVE programme 92.6% were female. The fact that 43.6% of the sample were under the age of 16 at the time of the abuse underlines the vulnerability of children with ID.

In this study only one of the perpetrators had an ID, which is reasonably surprising as other studies suggest that 40% of the abuse of people with an ID is perpetrated by another person with ID (Cooke & Sinason 1998; Furey 1994). This specific case was withdrawn before it went to court. In the Dickman & Roux 2005 study none of the perpetrators had an ID. This seems to suggest that there is underreporting of these cases. One interpretation may be that a perpetrator with ID cannot be held responsible for his actions or as discussed above, it might be seen as seduction rather than abuse. It is also possible that as this type of abuse would probably take place in facilities for people with ID, and the facility sees fit to deal with it internally rather than immediately seeking legal redress. Cape Mental Health has been consulted about some of these cases, although they have not been referred to the SAVE programme, and another issue that seems to arise is that if a person with ID is found guilty of such an offence, there are no specialised appropriate facilities for sentencing purposes, and the person would be very vulnerable in prison. Both this and the fact that these cases are not being prosecuted, is a cause for concern.

Research shows that the majority of perpetrators are known to the complainants (Brown et al 1995). In this study 86.5% of the perpetrators knew the complainants and one could therefore assume that they knew the complainant had an ID and was probably perceived as a 'soft target'. The large proportion of family members, 17.4%, and other trusted adults i.e. family friends, is also a disturbing statistic and this again illustrates the increased vulnerability of people with ID.

Sixty eight percent of the sample was functioning in the mild and moderate levels of ID. In terms of the prevalence of ID, this group is underestimated in the sample. A survey in Western Australia found 82.5% of people with ID were functioning in the mild and moderate levels of ID. South African figures estimate that 86% of people with ID have mild ID. This proportionate overrepresentation of the more severe levels of ID in this sample seems to be in line with other studies (Brown et al, 1995; Mansell et al 1992), which found a higher proportion of sexual abuse of people with more severe ID.

Only 27.5% of those complainants who were 16 and older at the time of the abuse were found able to consent to sexual intercourse. This is a considerably smaller percentage than the 46% in the previous study, (Dickman & Roux 2005) and is often the result of people with ID not being exposed to sex education, which in itself is both disempowering and another factor that could make them more vulnerable to sexual abuse.

The majority of the complainants (69%) were found able to testify in court, generally with adequate court preparation and in other cases with other extra support such as intermediaries. Although one presumes that this is a reasonably select sample as it is not possible to ascertain how many incidences are not referred to the SAVE programme, this reinforces the fact that cases in which the complainant has an ID can be prosecuted. In other cases where the complainant was not found competent to testify other evidence permitted the cases to proceed and as discussed above in 20 of these cases a guilty verdict was obtained.

The conviction rate of 28.1% of the finalised cases is slightly better than the best rates reported for the general population in the South African Law Commission research paper (2001), which reported a rate of 21%. The conviction rate in this study is the same as the one found in the previous study on cases that had gone through the SAVE programme, (Dickman & Roux 2005). Only 18.2% of the accused were acquitted in this study as opposed to 25% in the previous study, but the matter was withdrawn in 53.7% of cases as opposed to 47% previously. The figures in the Law Commission's paper show that in tried cases of adult rape almost twice the number of cases resulted in acquittals than convictions. In child rape cases the number of acquittals and convictions were equal. This sample has a better conviction rate possibly because of its selected nature.

This study confirms that the SAVE programme is the only way that people with an ID will have access to justice in cases of sexual abuse and the continuation and expansion of the programme is imperative.

Amanda Roux passed away in November 2008.

REFERENCES

Bailey A., Barr O. & Bunting B. (2001) Police attitudes toward people with intellectual disability: an evaluation of awareness training. *Journal of Intellectual Disability Research*, 45 (4): 344 – 350.

Brown H., Egan-Sage E., Barry G. & Mc Kay C. (1996) Towards better interviewing: A handbook for police officers and social workers on the sexual abuse of adults with learning disabilities. NAPSAC Series, Pavillion Publishing. Brighton.

Balogh R., Bretherton S., Whibley S., Berney T., Graham S., Richold P., Worsley S. & Firth H. (2001) Sexual Abuse in children and adolescents with intellectual disability. *Journal of Intellectual Disability Research*, 45 (3): 194 – 201.

Brown H., Stein J. & Turk V. (1995) The sexual abuse of adults with learning disabilities: report of a second two-year incidence survey. *Mental Handicap Research*, 8: 3-24.

Cooke L. B. & Sinason V. (1998) Abuse of people with learning disabilities and other vulnerable adults. *Advances in Psychiatric Treatment*, 4: 119-125.

Dickman B.J. & Roux A.J. (2005) Complainants with learning disabilities in sexual abuse cases: a 10 year review of a psycho-legal project in Cape Town, South Africa. *British Journal of Learning Disabilities*, 33: 138-144.

Furrey E.M. (1994) Sexual abuse of adults with mental retardation: who and where. *Mental Retardation*, 32: 173-180 .

Green G (2001) Vulnerability of witnesses with learning disabilities: preparing to give evidence against a perpetrator of sexual abuse. *British Journal of Learning Disabilities*, 29: 103-109.

Gunn M (1993). Competency and Consent The importance of decision making Ch 6 in Practice Issues in Sexuality and Learning Disabilities ed Craft A., Routledge, UK.

Joyce T.A. (2003) An audit of investigations into allegations of abuse involving adults with an intellectual disability. *Journal of Intellectual Disability Research*, 47 (8) : 606 – 616.

Kebbell M.R., Hatton C., Johnson S.D. & O'Kelly C.M.E. People with learning disabilities as witnesses in court. What questions should lawyers ask? *British Journal of Learning Disabilities*, 29: 98-102.

Keilty J. & Connelly G. (2001) Making a statement: An exploratory study of barriers facing women with an intellectual disability when making a statement about sexual assault to police. *Disability & Society*, 16 (2): 273 – 291.

Mansell S., Sobsey D. & Calder P. (1992) Sexual abuse treatment for persons with developmental disabilities. *Professional Psychology: Research and Practice*, 23: 404-9.

Milne R. & Bull R. (2001) Interviewing witnesses with learning disabilities for legal purposes. *British Journal of Learning Disabilities*, 29: 93-97.

Robinson M. (1994) Individual scale for general scholastic aptitude. Pretoria, Human Sciences Research Council.

South African Law Commission (2001) Conviction rates and other outcomes of crimes reported in eight South African police areas, *Research paper*, 18

Sparrow S., Balla D.A. & Cicchetti D. (1984) Vineland adaptive behavior scales, 4th ed. Interview version. Circle Pines, MN, American Guidance Service.

Chapter 38

SHARING STORIES OF EVERYDAY LIFE WITH ADULTS AND CHILDREN WHO HAVE SEVERE/PROFOUND INTELLECTUAL DISABILITIES

N. Grove[1], J. Harwood[1],V. Ross[1], L. Peacey[2], and M. Jones[3]

[1]Openstorytellers/ British Institute of Learning Disabilities,Campion House Green St Kidderminster Worcs, UK
[2]London Institute of Education, 20 Bedford Way London UK
[3]Talk4Meaning

INTRODUCTION

Narrative recall of personal experience is critical to the formation of personal identity, and is one of the main ways in which people make and sustain friendships over the lifespan. For people with severe and profound disabilities, this kind of anecdotal storytelling is extraordinarily difficult. Evidence (Grove, 2007; McHutchinson, 2006) suggests:-

Staff and families tell stories ABOUT people with high support needs, but not WITH them

Lives are dominated by routines, so there are few reportable experiences. This reduces the likelihood of recall, limits the potential for social learning and leads to a lack of motivation to tell

Experiences that could be made into stories pass unnoticed or are told only by staff

Social networks are restricted, so there are few people interested in hearing a story

Additional problems include the difficulties for families in recalling highlights from their children's lives and the prioritization of choice and control over issues of social inclusion.

STORYSHARING™ is a new approach to narrative for people with severe difficulties in language and communication, based on social constructionist models of narrative, and research into anecdotes told in conversational contexts (Labov & Waletzky, 1967; Peterson & McCabe, 1983; Norrick, 2000). The fundamental principles are as follows:-

Stories are created around unexpected – or at least, non-routine – events

Emotion and feeling lie at the heart of the story

We learn to tell stories by participating in the act of storymaking and storytelling

We tell stories collaboratively with others – and at first, adults "scaffold" storytelling with children, by accepting and extending their contributions.

Personal stories are repeated over and over again – we actively craft these little tales and roll them out at every social opportunity. This gives plenty of opportunity for practice.

The basic techniques include foregrounding of an experience at the time to establish a sensory representation; use of sensory cues in recall - smell, touch, sight, sound and voice. By emphasizing affect and intonation of what was said at the time we help people to tune into the meaning of the experience. In retelling the story, we look for what the person can contribute to the telling - vocalisation, gesture, facial expression or movement, and we tell it together, using sentence completion to prompt and minimizing the use of direct questions, which will create a pressurized interview, rather than a shared story. Finally, we repeat our good story again and again with new listeners,

STORYSHARING IN RESIDENTIAL HOMES

Five courses were run over two years with 21 people with severe and profound intellectual disablities and 13 staff, in 5 centers (four residential homes, one day center). Each course involved a two hour session once a week for 7 weeks, with two visiting storysharer tutors, one with intellectual disabilities acting as a peer tutor and role model. Staff completed diaries to record small key events of the week, which were shared collaboratively during the sessions. Families and keyworkers were interviewed to provide stories from the past. The final session was a celebratory "story café". Qualitative data were collected, including: observations of sessions and interviews with staff before and after the project.

The findings from this project highlighted some of the difficulties involved in using story in these contexts. Staff found it hard to move away from a directive, questioning interactive style. They perceived lack of time as a major barrier to telling stories on a regular basis. Family histories were often inaccessible or nonexistent, and families were often not in contact. Family members whom we did contact often failed to recall any events involving the individual. Finally the stories that did exist were often painful or difficult such as hospital treatments. However, there were very positive outcomes from the work. When staff changed to nondirective style of interaction, the balance of power shifted and the people with ID became much more involved as partners in the telling. Although family stories were in short supply, there were numerous small events of interest that happen during the week which people enjoyed recalling and sharing. Finally, individuals started to recall and engage with experience, and this increases with practice. A narrative culture began to develop in the service, for example by:-using shift changeover to share information with the whole community, and using tenants meetings as the context for recall. Everyday communication started to change, with more ongoing conversations about real events both observed and reported.

STORYSHARING IN SCHOOLS

In a second project, 4 schools participated in a storysharing project over one term. These were co-located special and mainstream schools for primary aged children, two based in a large city and two in a small rural town. The aims were to:

Develop empathy and friendship between children in mainstream and special schools
Show children how to share narratives in a collaborative and supportive way
Help the schools to work more closely together

In both sites, the work involved bringing in outside storytellers to work with small groups to develop and share personal narratives. The range in ages, abilities and school routines meant that implementation was somewhat different. Qualitative data were collected including interviews with children and staff, and observations of filmed sessions.

In the Country

8 mainstream children (5 F, 3M) aged 7-9 were paired with 8 special school children (6M 2F) aged 7-11 in groups of 4. All were white British with English as L1. The special needs of the children were predominantly emotional and behavioral + mild-moderate ID. All but one of the children were verbal. Sessions lasted up to 40 minutes for 5-6 weekly visits, and comprised a lot of collaborative narrative and reenactment, with artwork to illustrate the stories. There were 2 storytellers, 2 peer tutors with ID, and one volunteer.

In the City

6 mainstream children (3M 3F) aged 9-11, were paired with 7 special school children aged 8-11 (3M 4F). The origins of 10/13 were multi ethnic , and only 3 had English as L1. Special needs were moderate-severe ID, and communication impairments: only 2 children used short sentences, 3 used a few single words and 2 were nonverbal. There was 1 storyteller who rehearsed stories with the mainstream children and was then joined by the special school children and their classroom assistant for about 20 minutes- 4 sessions per group of 4 children

Our findings were that despite the relatively short space of time, the children did get to know each other, to strike up relationships and to learn how to share stories together. Some of the older mainstream children became particularly adept at sharing stories effectively. The children reported increased empathy and understanding. In both sites the project contributed to closer working between the schools at the level of pupil inclusion. Successful strategies used by MS children as tellers included: sign and gesture, pausing, checking, looking with attention at their partners and using anecdotal techniques such as repetition and exaggeration.

As listeners they echoed, elaborated, watched intently and checked. Even skilled children however were inclined to revert to direct questions when faced with nonverbal partners. Successful strategies in group narratives included: co-active movements and vocalisations; structured feedback responses, enactment, use of the big mac communication aid, props and artwork.

CONCLUSIONS FROM THE PROJECTS

Collaborative storysharing involves strategies that everyone uses, which can be successfully taught

Storysharing promotes real participation and engagement in everyday life

Services for both adults and chidlren need to prioritise friendship and the skills for establishing and maintaining relationships, as well as agendas of choice and control

ACKNOWLEDGMENTS

Storysharing projects with adults were funded by the Esmee Fairbairn Foundation

Storysharing in schools was funded by the Somerset Community Foundation, SENJIT & London Borough of Harrow

Thanks to all service users, children, families, staff, volunteers who took part and to peer tutors from Openstorytellers

Note: Openstorytellers is the new name of the project Unlimited Company of Storytellers with Learning Disabilities

openstorytellers, limited is registered in England and Wales. Registered company number 6829975 Registered office: 61 White Street, Horningsham, Warminster, Wiltshire, BA12 7LH; www.openstorytellers.org.uk

REFERENCES

Grove, N. (2007) Exploring the absence of high points in story reminiscence with carers of people with profound disabilities. *J Policy & Practice in Intellectual Disabilities*, 4, 252-259

Labov, W. & Waletzky, J. (1967) Narrative analysis: oral versions of experience. In J. Helm (Ed) *Essays on the verbal and visual arts: proceedings of the 1966 Annual Spring Meeting of the American Ethnological Society.* Seattle: University of Washington Press. (pp. 286-338).

McHutchinson, L. (2006) A comparison of communicative functions used by staff towards people with intellectual disabilities who are verbal or preverbal. *4th year BSc Dissertation, City University, London*

Norrick, N. (2000) *Conversational narrative: storytelling in everyday life.* Amsterdam/Philadelphia: John Benjamin.

Peterson, C. & McCabe, E. (1983) *Developmental psycholinguistics: three ways of looking at a child's narrative.* NY: Plenum.

You can find out more about storysharing on our website www.bild.org.uk/storytelling , www.storytracks.org.

The Unlimited Company is a project managed by the British Institute of Learning Disabilities, but is moving towards independent status as a social enterprise

PART VII. FAMILIES AND PARENTS

Living with a child or sibling with intellectual disabilities (ID) brings with it its own challengers. Such challengers can be quite demanding, but at other times can be very rewarding. *Steel and colleagues* investigated how siblings cope with a brother or sister with ID. They found that siblings have different experiences during childhood and adolescence. Supporting the wider context of family relationships is important rather than focusing narrowly on the individual with ID themselves. In terms of parental stress, a number of studies have demonstrated that parents of children with ID suffer from considerable stress and mental health problems, such as depression and anxiety. *Miodrag and Sladeczek* highlight the additional stresses experienced by parents of children with autism and Down syndrome The emotional stress often experienced by parents is not only to do with how things are now but is also related to the future. Parental hopes and worries about the future are ongoing concerns which are often not addressed. *Akerstrom and Nilsson* highlight the need for organizational support and forward planning to lessen such fears. Caring for a child or an adult with ID can at times be difficult but even more so when there are coexsistent mental health problems. *Gibbs and colleagues* highlight that often families accept mental health problems as being issues related to ID per se. Families are inadequately supported and often lack appropriate information about mental health issues in persons with ID.

Brown highlights the differences and similarities of family quality of life across a number of countries. Quality of life remains complex and may differ across countries, being affected by different subgroups of people with ID and the differences in family types. *Carr* as part of her ongoing longitudinal study highlights that parents of adults with Down syndrome aged 40 yrs generally function similarly to parents in the general population.Indeed some previous concerns appeared to be now less.

Chapter 39

HOW TO SUPPORT SIBLINGS OF CHILDREN WITH INTELLECTUAL DISABILITIES? A BRIEF OUTLINE OF A LONGITUDINAL, MULTI-PERSPECTIVE STUDY ON SIBLINGS OF CHILDREN WITH INTELLECTUAL DISABILITIES

R. Steel[1], S. Vandevelde[1], L. Poppe[2], and T. Moyson[3]

1Faculty of Social Work and Welfare Studies, University College Ghent - Ghent University, B-9000 Ghent, Belgium

[2]Faculty of Social Work and Welfare Studies, University College Ghent, B-9000 Ghent, Belgium

[3]Department of Experimental Clinical and Health Psychology, Ghent University, B-9000 Ghent, Belgium

INTRODUCTION

This short paper reports on an ongoing field study (2006-2009) into young and adolescent siblings of people with intellectual disabilities (ID). By developing support strategies for siblings, the project aims to improve the quality of life of the sibling and his/her family as a whole.Growing up in a family with a brother or sister with ID is something unique. The influence siblings with a disability have on their family members is difficult to describe and is characterized by its variable, dynamic and complex nature. Each family is unique, which also means that each typically evolving sibling in each family has a different story to tell.

By means of narrative as well as participative research methods, three different perspectives are being mapped: the perspectives of brothers and sisters, parents and professionals. The study aims at 1) recording narratives of siblings, parents and network members of children with ID, during different periods over a 3-year time span; 2) recording narratives of professionals working with (families of) children with disabilities, and map the actual services and provided family support; 3) exploring the family quality of life and the siblings' quality of life; 4) mapping the siblings' roles and positions in the provided family support and 5) developing, implementing and evaluating support strategies for siblings.

The objectives of this paper are twofold: (1) to sketch the research outline and methodology and (2) to present some exploratory results, confined, for the present, to an analysis of open – ended interviews with the siblings themselves.

RESEARCH OUTLINE AND METHODOLOGY

Participants

Twenty-five families living in the Province of East-Flanders (Belgium) participated in the study. In these 25 families, the researchers monitored one sibling and both parents, if possible.

Table 1. Family and family member characteristics

		(N)
Family size		
	2 children	8
	3 children	8
	4 or more children	9
Family structure		
	One parent	1
	Two parent	19
	Other (e.g. a stepfamily)	5
Gender of sibling		
	boy	13
	girl	12
Birth order sibling		
	Eldest child	12
	Middle child	8
	Youngest child	5
Number of siblings with ID		
	One child	23
	Two children	2
Type of disability		
	Down's syndrome	9
	Multiple disabilities	5
	Autism and ID	6
	Autism	1
	ID (unknown)	6

The siblings participating in the study were aged from 4 to 21 years old, at the start of the study. They were divided into four groups according to life stage. In each of the first three age groups (from 4 to 7 years, from 9 to 12 years and from 14 to 17 years) there are seven participating siblings (with more boys than girls). The last age group (18 to 21 years) is composed of four girls.

Families and individuals living in these families are differing on variables as family size, family structure, gender of sibling, birth order of sibling, number of siblings with ID and type of disability, resulting in a quite heterogeneous sample (Table 1). One family from each age group was selected as a case study.

Procedures and Instruments

Open-ended interviews and focus groups with siblings, parents and professionals were carried out. Several questionnaires and instruments were filled out by siblings and parents. In the case studies more participative and creative research methods were used, such as a photographic method.

The results presented in this paper are based on a content analysis of the interviews with siblings. They were interviewed individually three times, over a 2-year period, about different aspects of family life, especially about their relationships with their brother or sister, about their well-being at different domains (e.g school, leisure, friends, community), about social support and support from services.

ANALYSIS

The transcribed interviews were analysed by means of the qualitative software package MaxQDA2007 (Kuckartz, 2007). MaxQDA2007 is embedded in social interactionism and is based on the theory of Weber and Schütz. It considers reality as a social construction, which can be categorized (Vandevelde, Vandeplasschen & Broekaert, 2003). First, this process involved the identification of 'hermeneutic units'. Second, two independent researchers developed a separate coding tree structure. Third, after in-depth discussion, the two structures were integrated into a communal one. By comparing and discussing the coding process, the researchers gradually adjusted the definitions of categories and subcategories. During the next phase of the analysis, the researchers coded all hermeneutic units according to the refined tree structure, in order to maximize the reliability and validity of the coding process.

RESULTS

Three of the themes emerging from the comprehensive amount of data will be discussed.

Age Related Opportunities and Challenges

Siblings can have different experiences during childhood and adolescence. For instance, all young siblings in the study (aged 4 to 12 years) have many thoughts and experiences regarding *play and activities* with their brother or sister. Many siblings spoke of a moderate amount of playing together but little game playing. Some siblings often play alone which is tough on them. Many siblings have questions regarding the abilities of their brother or sister and have experiences with under- and overestimating them. They seek to join their brother or sister at play, and often use play situations to learn and teach the other sibling new skills. Playing is often accompanied by *quarrels and conflicts*. While some siblings report hardly any conflicts, others report plenty. Siblings report different ways of dealing with anger or aggression of the person with a disability: avoiding, understanding, getting angry and hitting back or getting an adult to intervene.

For many of the adolescent siblings (aged 13-21), *the future* is a very important topic, although there are various opinions on this. Some siblings have many worries and doubts about the future, others don't. What most have in common however, are different questions that are rising: "What will happen to my brother/sister?", "what will happen when my parents die?" and "what are my responsibilities?". In general, most adolescent siblings are willing to be involved in decisions on future planning. While some grope in the dark when it comes to the future, others are able to describe, in great detail, their future relationship and their role in the support of their sibling with ID.

Life-Changing Events

Many important transitions and major incidents were reported that may have a big impact on the life of the sibling, the child with ID and the family as a whole. These life-changing events are key markers in the family life of all families, but in families with a member with a disability, these events can have an additional weight or connotation. The following events may be illustrative: the birth of the child with ID; the medical diagnosis; discussion about guardianship; changes in school life for the sibling; changes in community services / schooling for the child with ID; hospitalization, intensive therapy or treatment.

Life Domains

Building on the framework of a 'Quality of Life' approach (Schalock & Siperstein, 1996; Poston, et al., 2003; Turnbull, et al., 2007; Kidscreen Group, 2006), the experiences of siblings on different life domains (leisure time, home, school, friends, neighbourhood and community, emotional well-being, future plans) were explored. Following experiences and thoughts of siblings are illustrative results.

For most siblings, having a place of their own is very important. This place is often defined as 'my own room', but can be placed in a larger perspective (space and/or time): e.g. separate leisure activities or their own friends.

Siblings expect their parents to search for fair (not equal) solutions in conflict situations and to divide their parental attention fairly (not equally) across the different children in the family.

The impact of the disability on family life is also apparent during holidays and leisure activities. Because collective activities have to be accessible and adapted to the child with a disability and because of the high organizational load, many families have to subdivide themselves to get most out of their leisure time.

Regarding school life, it is desirable for siblings to perceive openness among school staff and peers to talk about their sibling with ID, although it should not be imperative. In case of inclusive education, siblings report taking care of their sibling with ID, e.g. on the playground, and that teachers appeal to them in difficult situations.

CONCLUSION

When formulating support strategies for siblings, much has to be taken into account in order to do right to each sibling in each family situation, since each situation is characterized by its unique dynamics and complexity. The findings discussed above are exploratory but may lead to a better understanding of ways in which siblings could be better supported by their parents, other network members and professionals, although a more extended and in-depth analysis of the data is needed.

Nevertheless, some preliminary conclusions can be drawn. First, across the full lifespan, attention and support for siblings need to match the ever-changing opportunities and challenges of being a sibling of a person with ID. Second, the meaning of life-changing events for the sibling and his family needs to be investigated. Third, the importance of taking a 'widescreen' image of the life of siblings has been underlined, since having a brother or sister with ID affects many life domains.

REFERENCES

Kidscreen Group Europe (2006). *The Kidscreen questionnaires. Quality of life questionnaires for children and adolescents*. Pabst Science Publishers, Lengerich.

Kuckartz, A. (2007). *MaxQDA, The Art of Text Analysis*. VERBI Software, Consult, Research GmbH, Germany.

Poston, D., Turnbull A. et al. (2003). Family Quality of Life: A Qualitative Inquiry. *Mental Retardation, 41* (5), 313-328.

Schalock, R. & G. Siperstein (1996). Quality of Life. Volume I: Conceptualization and Measurement. American Association on Mental Retardation, Washington.

Turnbull, A. Poston, D. et al. (2007). Providing supports and services that enhance a family 's Quality of Life. In: Brown, I. & M. Percy (2007*). A Comprehensive Guide to Intellectual & Developmental Disabilities*. Paul H Brookes Publishing.

Vandevelde, S., Vandeplasschen, W. & Broekaert, E. (2003). Cultural responsiveness in substance-abuse treatment: a qualitative study using professionals' and clients' perspectives. *International Journal of Social Welfare, 12*, 221-228.

Chapter 40

PARENTAL WELL-BEING: COMPARING STRESS PROFILES IN MOTHERS AND FATHERS OF CHILDREN WITH AUTISM AND DOWN SYNDROME

N. Miodrag[1] and I. E. Sladeczek[1]
[1]Department of Educational and Counselling Psychology
McGill University, Montreal, Quebec, Canada

INTRODUCTION

Psychological stress can significantly jeopardize a person's physical health, social, interpersonal, and professional life (Singer, 2006), and is considered a major public health concern for families of children with ID (ID)(Perry, 2004). Parents of children with ID are a particularly vulnerable population that report significantly elevated levels of stress (Davis & Carter, 2008) as well as moderate and clinically significant mental health problems such as depression, anxiety, and somatization (Feldman et al., 2007; Olsson & Hwang, 2001; Weiss, 2002; Yirmiya & Shaked, 2005). There is evidence to suggest that parent stress varies as a function of the child's disability (Abbeduto et al., 2004), and emerging evidence to show that stress differs across parent gender (Ricci & Hodapp, 2003). Taken together, these findings reflect the need to explore further, the distinct stress profiles of not only mothers but fathers of children with particular ID. While families of children with autism and Down syndrome (DS) have gained ample attention on account of their unique and challenging experiences (Hutton & Caron, 2005), a call is made for further research in particular on the unique differences between mothers and fathers on children with DS (Hodapp, 2007).

Children with autism show marked impairments in reciprocal social interaction, communication, and restricted, repetitive, and stereotyped patterns of behavior (American Psychiatric Association, 2000; Perry et al, 2007); these behaviors can be especially taxing for parents (Tomanik et al, 2004; Pakenham et al, 2005). In contrast, children with DS tend to have gregarious personalities, are sociable, affectionate (Ricci & Hodapp, 2003), and easily accommodated (Holroyd & McArthur, 1976). They also display lower rates of maladaptive behavior and a lack of psychopathology relative to children in mixed etiological groups

(Dykens & Kasari, 1997; Hodapp et al, 2003; Ricci & Hodapp, 2003). Hodapp et al (2001) consider these etiology-related behaviors as a 'DS advantage', predisposing parents to less stress and more positive effects on well-being. However, a few researchers have found that parents of children with DS show comparable stress levels to children in mixed disability groups (Most et al, 2006; Stores et al, 1998), and no DS advantage in specific areas related to depression, stress, satisfaction with social support, and warm parenting beliefs and behaviors (Stoneman, 2007).

While generally, parents of children with autism report significantly elevated levels of stress when compared to other disability groups (Firat et al, 2002; Davis & Carter, 2008; Olsson & Hwang, 2001; Weiss, 2002), fewer studies have compared mothers of children with autism to mothers of children with DS (Holroyd and McArthur, 1976; Pisula, 2007), and no known studies have included fathers' perceptions of stress. The exclusive attention on mothers is a significant shortcoming in understanding the family as a whole because fathers are assuming greater responsibility in parenting and report stress as well. For example, McNeill (2004) found that fathers are significantly affected by their child's chronic health condition. They experience strong emotions of "...guilt, anger, pain, anxiety, and sadness" (p. 533), and worry and are uncertain about their child's future. Compared to mothers, little is known about the well-being of fathers of children with autism and DS. What is more, no known studies have compared a Canadian sample of mothers and fathers whose children are receiving early intervention or specialized services.

Given the increased prevalence rate of children identified with autism (Fombonne, 2005), the scarcity of research on fathers, the move towards an etiological approach in behavioral research (Hodapp, 2002), and the adverse effect of stress on families (Bishop et al 2007; Singer, 2006), the aim of this study was to examine perceptions of stress by comparing mothers to fathers in two prevalent disability groups to better understand the effects of disability and gender. Teasing apart who may be at risk for maladjustment can pinpoint where efforts are most needed to help alleviate stress. The research questions were: (a) How do the clinical stress profiles of mothers compare to fathers? (b) Does overall stress, child-related stress, and parent-related stress differ for mothers and fathers and if so, what specific dimensions vary? (c) Does overall stress, parent-related and child-related stress differ for four parent groups as a function of child disability? (d) Does a child's demandingness, inability to reinforce the parent and mood differ across the four parent groups? and (e) Do the four parent groups differ on depression and role restriction?

METHOD

Participants

Seventy-eight families of children with autism and DS participated in this study, with a total of 143 mothers and fathers (76 mothers, 67 fathers) completing the Parenting Stress Index. Participants comprised of 41 families of children with autism (28 males, 13 females) and 37 families of children with DS (19 males, 18 females). Children ranged in age from 8 months to 11.5 years (autism $M = 69.37$ months, $SD = 23.67$) and (DS $M = 61.89$ months, $SD = 35.22$). Children's diagnoses were garnered from a demographics questionnaire. Based on

DSM-IV criteria (American Psychiatric Association, 2000), 37 children had a diagnosis of Autistic Disorder and four had Pervasive Developmental Disorder Not Otherwise Specified (PDD-NOS). All but two children had DS because of Trisomy 21. The inclusion criteria for children were (a) between birth and 9 years of age, and (b) autism or DS diagnosis. All mothers were the biological mothers of the children. Mothers of children with autism were between the ages of 26 and 48 (M = 38.17, SD = 4.91) and fathers were between 29 and 55 (M = 40.54, SD = 6.43). Mothers of children with DS were between the ages of 27 and 48 (M = 40.14, SD = 4.94) and fathers were between 33 and 56 (M = 42.28, SD = 5.10). An independent samples t-tests showed a significant effect for parent age between mothers and fathers, F = .186, p = .015, which was then used as a covariate.

Measure and Procedure

The Parenting Stress Index (PSI, long version; Abidin, 1995) is a standardized 120-item self-report measure used to examine the level of perceived stress experienced by a parent in relation to their child in two domains: Child Domain, where sources of stress are attributed to child characteristics, (i.e., Distractibility/Hyperactivity, Adaptability, Reinforces Parent, Demandingness, Mood, and Acceptability), and Parent Domain, where sources of stress are related to parent characteristics (i.e., Competence, Relationship with Spouse, Isolation, Health, Role Restriction, Depression, and Attachment to Child). A Total Domain composite is generated by the Child and Parent subscales and yields scale scores for the Child and Parent Domain to locate sources of stress within the family (Abidin, 1995). Higher scores signify greater levels of perceived stress and a raw score at or above 260 identify individuals who should be considered for psychological services. This study was part of the larger National Early Intervention Research Initiative (NEIRI) tracking the developmental trajectories of families and children with DD. Data were collected from parents receiving early intervention services in Canada. Mothers and fathers completed the PSI independently.

RESULTS

Clinical Levels of Stress

Participants means were compared to PSI normative means (Abidin, 1995) to confirm previous findings that parents of children with ID show increased stress levels compared to the general population (e.g., Brehaut et al., 2004; Hodapp, 2002; Montes & Halterman, 2007; Singer, 2006; Sivberg, 2002; Smith et al, 2001). As confirmed, the current sample of mothers reported higher clinical total stress (M = 270.50 vs. M = 222.8), child-domain stress (M = 128.10 vs. M = 99.7), and parent-domain stress (M = 142.30 vs. M = 123.1) than the normative sample. This pattern was also confirmed for fathers showing higher total stress scores for the current sample (M = 250.96) compared to the normative sample (M = 201. 6), higher child-domain stress (M = 123.34 vs. M = 92.2), and higher parent-domain stress (M = 127.58 vs. M = 92.9), respectively. In Table 1, the mean stress scores and percentages of mothers and fathers that fall within the clinical range are reported. Fifty-seven percent of mothers reported overall clinical stress compared to 46% of fathers. As well, 49% of mothers experienced clinical levels of parent-related stress and 67% was child-related. Fathers showed the same pattern as mothers, albeit the percentage and clinical levels were not as high. Twenty-eight percent of fathers reported clinically significant parent-related stress and 60% was child-related.

Table 1. Parenting Stress Index Means and SD and Percentages at the Clinical Level

	M (SD)			% of clinical stress		
	Total Group (N = 143)	Mothers (n = 76)	Fathers (n = 67)	Total Group (N = 143)	Mothers (n = 76)	Fathers (n = 67)
Total Stress	261.34 (47.71)	270.50 (45.38)	250.96 (48.50)	52%	57%	46%
Parent Domain	135.38 (28.06)	142.30 (26.50)	127.58 (27.91)	39%	49%	28%
Child Domain	125.87 (25.30)	128.10 (25.47)	123.34 (25.06)	64%	67%	60%

Note. Appendix A in the Parenting Stress Index manual (Abidin, 1995) was used to calculate the percentage of critical stress for mothers, fathers, and the total group. Appendix A outlines means, standard deviations, and percentiles for the PSI total stress, parent-domain stress, and child-domains stress for children ages 1-3, 4-6, and 7-12.

Stress Differences Across Mothers and Fathers

To test whether the means of mothers and fathers differ significantly on stress, three separate one-way between subjects analysis of covariance (ANCOVA) were conducted using parent age as a covariate. The independent variable was parent group and included two levels: mothers (of children with autism and DS) and fathers (of children with autism and DS). The dependent variables were total, parent, and child-domain stress. Prior to conducting each ANCOVA, the homogeneity of slopes assumptions were tested and supported allowing for further analysis. Mothers had significantly greater total stress, $F(1, 140) = 5.03$, $MSE = 2197.53$, $p = .027$ and parent-domain stress $F(1, 140) = 9.44$, $MSE = 742.46$, $p = .003$ than fathers. However, there were no significant differences on child-domain stress, $F(1, 140) = .686$, $MSE = 635.24$, $p = .409$. As expected, mothers had significantly greater stress related to perceived depression, $F(1, 140) = 12.84$, $MSE = 35.06$, $p = .000$, role restriction, $F(1, 140) = 8.15$, $MSE = 38.35$, $p = .005$, and relationship with spouse, $F(1, 140) = 10.17$, $MSE = 26.95$, $p = .002$, than fathers.

Stress Differences across Parent Gender and Child Disability

Three separate 2 Child Diagnosis (Autism, DS) x 2 Parent Gender (Mother, Father) analysis of covariance (ANCOVA) were performed on total, parent- and child-domain stress, controlling for parent age and education. Independent samples *t*-tests identified significant differences between the groups for parent age, $F = .339$, $p = .026$ and years of education approached significance, $F = 5.04$, $p = .58$. Both were used as covariates.

The ANCOVA for total stress was significant, $F(3, 137) = 3.33$, $MSE = 2168.29$, $p = .022$. The strength of the relationship between the independent variable, parent group and total stress was small ($\eta p^2 = .068$) accounting for 7% of the variance. The means adjusted for initial differences were ordered as expected across the groups. Mothers of children with autism had the largest adjusted mean ($M = 277.17$), followed by mothers of children with DS ($M = 262.03$), fathers of children with autism ($M = 260.11$), and fathers of children with DS ($M = 239.73$).

The ANCOVA for parent-domain stress was significant, $F(3, 137) = 3.50$, $MSE = 749.70$, $p = .017$. As estimated by partial eta ($\eta p^2 = .071$), parent group accounted for 7% of the variance of stress. Mothers of children with autism had the largest adjusted mean ($M = 142.80$), followed by mothers of children with DS ($M = 141.70$), fathers of children with autism ($M = 130.29$), and fathers of children with DS ($M = 123.96$). As expected, depression differed significantly across the groups, $F(3, 137) = 4.22$, $MSE = 35.80$, $p = .007$. The effect size was small ($\eta p^2 = .085$) accounting for approximately 9% of the variance of depression. As predicted, mothers of children with autism followed by mothers of children with DS had the highest adjusted means; fathers of children with autism followed with the third highest adjusted mean, and fathers of children with DS had the smallest adjusted mean. Role restriction was also significant, $F(3, 137) = 3.87$, $MSE = 38.13$, $p = .011$. The effect size estimated was small ($\eta p^2 = .078$), at 8% of the variance. Mothers of children with autism had the highest adjusted mean followed by mothers of children with DS, fathers of children with autism, and fathers of children with DS.

The ANCOVA for child-domain stress was significant, $F(3, 137) = 3.90$, $MSE = 598.81$, $p = .010$. The effect size estimated by partial eta was $\eta p^2 = .079$ accounting for 8% of the variance. As supported in previous studies showing that child behavior problems are a significant predictor of parent stress (Plant & Sanders, 2007), the adjusted means were ordered as expected. Mothers of children with autism showed the largest adjusted mean ($M = 134.23$), followed by fathers of children with autism, ($M = 129.82$), mothers of children with DS ($M = 120.22$), and fathers of children with DS ($M = 115.69$). As predicted, subscales on child-related stress that differed significantly across the groups were demandingness, $F(3, 137) = 2.90$, $MSE = 39.53$, $p = .037$, reinforces parent, $F(3, 137) = 3.98$, $MSE = 14.83$, $p = .009$, and mood, $F(3, 137) = 5.60$, $MSE = 12.95$, $p = .001$. The strength of the relationship between parent group and demandingness, reinforces parent, and mood larger was expected to be larger than their respective 6, 8, and 11% of the variance.

DISCUSSION

The current study compared the perceptions of maternal and paternal stress in parents of children with autism and DS to understand differences by disability and gender, and to contribute to the dearth of literature examining fathers' perceptions of stress. Extending a consistent and large body of research, mothers of children with autism in this study experienced the most psychological stress when compared to other groups of parents (e.g., Abbeduto et al., 2004; Beck et al., 2004). Compared to fathers, they reported greater overall psychological stress and greater stress attributed to their own parent traits including depression, role restriction, and relationship with their spouse. This is consistent with Yamada et al. (2007) who found that emotional stress was higher for mothers than fathers in a sample of parents of children with pervasive developmental disorders. Typically, mothers are the primary caretakers involved in the daily hassles and demanding day-to-day caretaking tasks that can take a toll on their psychological well-being (Saloviita et al., 2003). They also show a greater propensity for psychological maladjustment related to depressive symptoms (Feldman et al., 2007; Singer, 2006). Mothers and fathers in general did not differ significantly on stress associated with children's characteristics as was the case found by Hastings et al (2005). However, parents reached clinical significance with respect to their child's characteristics, with 60% of fathers and 67% of mothers meeting the cut-off. Thus, it appears that fathers along with mothers perceive their children's difficult behaviors to be adverse, making it more challenging to fulfill the parenting role (Abidin, 1995) and playing a potential role in poorer well-being.

Further comparisons of stress across the four parenting groups confirmed the authors' hypotheses that mothers in both mother groups are affected more negatively than fathers. With the exception of child-related stress, mothers of children with autism, followed by mothers of children with DS showed greater stress than fathers of children with autism and fathers of children with DS, in that order. For child-related stress, mothers and fathers of children with autism showed greater stress than mothers and fathers of children with DS adding to previous research suggesting that adverse behavior problems in children with autism are highly predictive of parent stress (Davis & Carter, 2008; Tomanik et al., 2004). Specifically, parents of children with autism in our study perceived their children to be more demanding, less reinforcing, and moodier, which are consistent with the behavioral characteristics that many children with autism display (Pisula, 2007). More focused attention on interventions that help to alleviate clinical stress in mothers *and* fathers of children with autism should be made by professionals with every effort to decrease the behavioral problems that many parents of children with autism find so challenging.

REFERENCES

Abbeduto, L., Seltzer, M. M., Shattuck, P., Krauss, W. M., Orsmond, G., & Murphy, M. M. (2004). Psychological well-being and coping in mothers of youths with autism, Down syndrome, or fragile X syndrome. American *Journal on Mental Retardation*, 109, 237-254.

Abidin, R. (1995). Parenting stress index: Professional manual (3rd ed.). Odessa, FL: Psychological Assessment Resources.

American Psychiatric Association. (2000). Diagnostic and statistical manual of mental disorders, (4th ed., text revision). Washington, DC: Author.

Bishop, S. L., Richler, J., Cain, A. C., Lord, C. (2007). Predictors of perceived negative impact in mothers of children with autism spectrum disorder. *American Journal on Mental Retardation*, 6, 450-461.

Beck, A., Hastings, R. P., Daley, D. M., & Stevenson, J. (2004). Pro-social behavior and behavior problems independently predict maternal stress. *Journal of Intellectual and Developmental Disabilities*, 29, 339-349.

Brehaut, J. C., Kohen, D. E., Raina, P., Walter, S. D., Russell, D. J., Swinton, M., et al. (2004). The health of primary caregivers of children with cerebral palsy: How does it compare with that of other Canadian caregivers. *Pediatrics*, 114, e182-e191.

Davis, N. O., & Carter, A. S. (2008). Parenting stress in mothers and fathers of toddlers with autism spectrum disorders: Associations with child characteristics. *Journal of Autism and other Developmental Disorders*, 38, 1278-1291.

Dykens, E. M., & Kasari, C. (1997). Maladaptive behavior in children with Prader-Willi syndrome, Down syndrome, and non-specific mental retardation. *American Journal on Mental Retardation*, 102, 228-237.

Feldman, M. A., McDonald, L., Serbin, L., Stack, D., Secco, M. L., & Yu, C. T. (2007). Predictors of depressive symptoms in primary caregivers of young children with or at risk for developmental delay. *Journal of Intellectual Disability Research*, 51, 606-619.

Firat, S., Diler, R. S., Avci, A., & Seydaoglu, G. (2002). Comparison of psychopathology in the mothers of autistic and mentally retarded children. *Journal of Korean Medical Science*, 17,679-685.

Fombonne, E. (2005). Epidemiology of autistic disorder and other pervasive developmental disorder. *Journal of Clinical Psychiatry*, 66 (Suppl. 10), 3-8.

Gupta, A., & Singhal, N. (2004). Positive perceptions in parents of children with disabilities. AsiaPacific Disability Rehabilitation Journal, 15, 22-35.

Hodapp, R. M. (2002). Parenting children with mental retardation. In M. H. Bornstein (Ed.),Handbook of parenting (Vol 1. Children and Parenting) (pp. 355-380). Mahwah, NJ:Lawrence Erlbaum.

Hodapp, R. M. (2007). Families of persons with Down syndrome: New perspectives, findings, and research and service needs. *Mental Retardation and Developmental Disabilities Research Reviews*, 13, 279-287.

Hodapp, R. M., Ly, T. M., Fidler, D. J., & Ricci, L. A. (2001). Less stress, more rewarding: Parenting children with Down syndrome. *Parenting Science and Practice*, 1, 317-337.

Hodapp, R. M., Ricci, L. A., Ly, T. M., & Fidler, D. J. (2003). The effects of the child with Down syndrome on maternal stress. *British Journal of Developmental Psychology*, 21, 137-151.

Holroyd J., McArthur, D. (1976). Mental retardation and stress on the parents: a contrast between Down's syndrome and childhood autism. *Am J Ment Defic.* 80, 431-436.

Hutton, A. M., & Caron, S. L. (2005). Experiences of families with children with autism in rural New England. *Focus on Autism and Other Developmental Disabilities*, 20, 180-189.

McNeill, T. (2004). Fathers' experience of parenting a child with juvenile rheumatoid arthritis. *Qualitative Health Research*, 14, 526-545

Montes, G., & Halterman, J. S. (2007). Psychological functioning and coping among mothers of children with autism: A population-based study. *Pediatrics*, 119, e1040-1046.

Most, D. E., Fidler, D. J., Booth-Laforce, C., & Kelly, J. (2006). Stress trajectories in mothers of young children with Down syndrome. *Journal of Intellectual Disability Research*, 50, 501-514.

Olsson, M. B., & Hwang, C. P. (2001). Depression in mothers and fathers of children with intellectual disability. *Journal of Intellectual Disability Research*, 45, 535-543.

Pakenham, K. O., Samios, C., & Sofronoff, K. (2005). Adjustment in mothers of children with Asperger syndrome: An application of the Double ABCX model of family adjustment. *Autism*, 9, 191-212.

Perry, A. (2004). A model of stress in families of children with developmental disabilities: Clinical and research applications [Special Issue]. *Journal on Developmental Disabilities*, 11, 1-16.

Perry, A., Dunlap, G., & Black, A. (2007). Autism and related disabilities. In I. Brown & M. Percy (Eds.), A comprehensive guide to intellectual disabilities (pp. 189-203). Baltimore: Paul H.Brookes.

Pisula, E. (2007). A comparative study of stress profiles in mothers of children with autism and those of children with Down's syndrome. *Journal of Applied Research in Intellectual Disabilities*,20, 274-278.

Plant KM, Sanders MR.(2007). Predictors of care-giver stress *J Intellect Disabil Res.* 51 109-24.

Ricci, L. A., & Hodapp, R. M. (2003). Fathers of children with Down's syndrome versus other types of intellectual disability: Perceptions, stress and involvement. *Journal of Intellectual Disability Research*, 47, 273-284.

Saloviita, T., Itälinna, M., & Leinonen, E. (2003). Explaining the parental stress of fathers and mothers caring for a child with intellectual disability: a Double ABCX model. *Journal of Intellectual Disability Research*, 47, 300-312.

Singer, G. H. S. (2006). Meta-analysis of comparative studies of depression in mothers of children with and without developmental disabilities. *American Journal on Mental Retardation*, 111,155-169.

Sivberg, B. (2002). Family system and coping behavior: A comparison between parents of children with autistic spectrum disorders and parents with non-autistic children. *Autism*, 6, 397-409.

Smith, T., Oliver, M., & Innocenti, M. (2001). Parenting stress in families of children with disabilities. *American Journal of Orthopsychiatry*, 71, 257-261.

Stoneman z. (2007). Examining the Down syndrome advantage: mothers and fathers of young children with disabilities. *J Intellect Disabilt Res.* 51, 1006-1017.

Stores, R., Stores, G., Fellows, B., & Buckley, S. (1998). Daytime behavior problems and maternal stress in children with Down's syndrome, their siblings, and non-intellectually disabled and other intellectually disabled peers. *Journal of Intellectual Disability Research*, 42, 228–237.

Tomanik, S., Harris, G. E., & Hawkins, J. (2004). The relationship between behaviors exhibited by children with autism and maternal stress. *Journal of Intellectual & Developmental Disability*, 29, 16-26.

Weiss, M. J. (2002). Hardiness and social support as predictors of stress in mothers of typical children, children with autism, and children with mental retardation. *Autism*, 6, 115-130.

Yamada, A., Suzuki, M., Kato, M., Suzuki, M., Tanaka, S., Shindo, T., et al. (2007). Emotional distress and its correlates among parents of children with pervasive developmental disorders. *Psychiatry and Clinical Neuroscience*, 61, 651-657.

Yirmiya, N., & Shaked, M. (2005). Psychiatric disorders in parents of children with autism: A meta-analysis. *Journal of Child Psychology and Psychiatry*, 46, 69-83.

Chapter 41

Parent's Views on the Future for Their Disabled Child and the Family

B. Åkerström[1] and I. Nilsson[2]

[1]Mid Sweden University/Municipal R&D – Unit, County of Jämtland, Östersund, Sweden

[2] Swedish National Institute of Public Health, Östersund, Sweden

Introduction

The way society provides expert, educational and social support influences the parents possibilities to handle the strain of having a child with some form of disability. The present situation can also be decisive in forming opinions on how the future development for the child and the family will be formed. Swedish legislation gives children with a disability the right to habilitation as well as specialist care regarding child psychiatry, hearing impairment, visual impairment and diabetes through the Health Services Act, HSL, (SFS 1982: 763). Furthermore the Act Concerning Support and Services for Persons with Certain Functional Impairments, LSS, (SFS 1993: 387) gives children specified forms of support, respite care and right to special schooling through the Education Act (SFS 1985: 1100) if the child has an intellectual disability or an autism spectrum disorder. Children with other impairments who have profound and longstanding needs for support (e.g. children with cerebral palsy and normal IQ) can also get support and services from the LSS. Different forms of economical support are available through the social insurance system for example disability allowance and care allowance. Although the support system is well developed, has a longstanding tradition and is well-intended, studies show that parents to children with disabilities show more signs of stress (Olsson & Hvang, 2002) and rate their health lower (Åkerström & Nilsson, 2004) and have to develop coping strategies to manage. Similar results are also found in international studies (Llewellyn et al 2003; Kenny & Mc Gilloway, 2007). Factors that induce stress in the family situation could be characteristics of the child but also family characteristics and experiences of society's support system (economic compensation, satisfaction with schooling, habilitation and other support services). An interesting problem to investigate is how the parent's views of the future includes comments on these factors.

The aim of this paper was to describe and analyze parents written statements on the future for their disabled child and the family. Some related questions were:

- which words and expressions were used to describe the future
- were there different patterns of descriptions with regard to type of disability
- were there specific references to expected developments in economy, social care or education.

METHOD

Participants

The target population (after controlling for doubles, those who had moved and deaths) was 827 children registered in child and adolescent habilitation services, special schooling for children with ID and children with impairment in hearing or vision and children with diabetes. A total of 517 analyzable questionnaires were returned (63 % response rate). Of these, 358 (69 %) had also responded to the question of views on the future. Responses included 348 mothers (mean age 41.2 years) and 313 fathers (mean age 44.7 years). Children were 143 girls (mean age 12.2 years) and 215 boys (mean age 11.6 years).

Instrument

The complete questionnaire consisted of 90 pre coded and open ended questions. Parents were also asked to complete a Swedish version of the SF 36, a health survey (Sullivan et al., 1994; Ware et al. 2000). The questionnaire was constructed in cooperation with representatives from the local parent associations for children with disabilities. Main results from the survey are reported in Åkerström & Nilsson (2004).

The question analyzed in this study was:

"How do You think the future will be? Give your viewpoints, expectations and wishes regarding the development for the family and the child with disability."

Procedure

Answers from the pre coded questions were entered into a data analysis program (SPSS v 12.01) for analysis. Responses to open ended questions were written into a single file in a word processing program (MS Word) retaining the code for the questionnaire which gave information on what form of disability that was present in the child. Most statements regarding the future consisted of 1 – 4 sentences.

Data Analysis

All statements were read trough by the authors separately for finding important key expressions and themes. The authors then discussed together to find subthemes and more comprehensive themes comprising the material.

RESULTS

Table 1. Themes and subthemes with examples in parents statements about the future

	Hope	Worry
Economy	Things will be better and money will be invested in children with disabilities	Negative development due to financial cut-downs
Endurance	Hope to have the strength to go on	Can't manage to think about the future Taking it day by day
Independence - individual level	The child's individual development will give Possibilities for living an independent life	The child's severity of impairment will make it difficult to attain an independent life
- structural level	Hope that the habilitation and other services can give support also in the future	Support from habilitation, school and other resources will be cut down
Research	Research will give improvements	-
Schooling	Good support in schooling leading to a work in adult life	Worries about schooling, changing stages, entering gymnasium etc.
Struggle	Not to have to fight for services or rights	Fighting to get ones right
Parental role	Hope of relief from parental responsibilities	Continuing responsibility for the child/youth even in adulthood

Two themes were found to describe the parents views on a higher level characterized by the word pair "hope" and ""worry". Citations in the following text are translations from the Swedish original citation texts. A few statements expressed a general positive view on the future like *"bright and exciting"* or *"future will be good, the hard days are over"* and likewise there were general negative views like *"negative development"* or *"I don't have any expectations of any improvements within the nearest 5 – 10 years"*. For most other statements the hope – worry dichotomy could be expressed in several areas according to subgroups of statements.

Economy

Regarding economy the majority of statements belonged to the "worry" category. There were general worries about future developments

"Development looks gloomy due to all cutbacks everywhere. There is a lack of speech therapists and speech trainers."

There were also more individual or specific worries regarding the situation for the child and the family.

"Regrettably, I don't think that we will get support and help in the future. The resource person (in school) will be withdrawn. Our wish is of course that he (the child) can keep her."

Endurance

This theme concerns the energy and strength parents experience that they have in handling the situation with the child. Many statements includes formulations of not being able to think of the future.

"For the moment I don't have the strength to think on the future"
"To be honest I don't have the strength to think so far, as long as we function as a family it works for our daughter ----then?"
"HELP!! It's all about surviving the day and the moment"

Independence

Positive statements regarding individual level centered on hopes and wishes that development and support will result in that the child will become more and more independent growing into adulthood.

"Future looks good for the child. (We) have received support and help that made the child develop and (he) will perhaps not need so much help in the future"

Negative expressions also more openly considered the level of disability in the child estimating possible development in the future.

> "As he has a severe impairment I have small expectations that he will be able to function independently in society as it is now."
>
> "A lot of worries for the future. We can not se that she will be able to move out from our home in many years yet. She will need personal assistants but she will surely not receive that. We are wondering about what will happen in the future when we don't have the strength to take care of her."

Regarding the structural aspects of independence worries regarding possibilities for development into more independent life goes together with economic factors in society.

> "The child is registered in the child habilitation services which probably gives possibilities for coordination between all authorities so that he can get an education and a work that he can manage and like"
>
> "We wish that there will be more resources within the child habilitation services. Also when it comes to the integration of special schooling with (support from)traveling teachers, that there will be more resources."

RESEARCH

Statements about research leading to future improvements or cure of the child's disability were only mentioned by parents of children with hearing impairment and children with diabetes. The statements included formulations of hope (no explicit worries) on future research to lead to making it easier to live with diabetes, minimize need of taking injections and mentioning transplantation of insulin producing cells.

> "Our hopes and big expectations are that research within a near future will find a way to help persons with diabetes to manage without injections. A life without injections is our wish"

Schooling

Future schooling and resources needed in school was by far the area that was most often touched upon in the parents statements. Again the parents in the diabetes group did not mention schooling while all other groups commented needs in the school situation. Worries concerned, among other things, staff resources, needs of assistants, problem in going from one stage to another or changing from one school to another.

> "The child will begin school in the autumn and it will probably be a bit difficult. (We) hope that he will have his own assistant. It will probably take many years before he will speak."
>
> "Our worries are great facing his needs of support in upper secondary school and his needs of long-term preparation before he can move out from home."

Positive statements sometimes centered on a positive future goal picture perhaps based on good experiences from current schooling.

"In two years time he will attend a good upper secondary school with good dwelling arrangements, leisure time activities and a school that understands his disability, makes him interested and sees him as a whole person. Mother and father then find the time to rest and find new energy until he comes home again to his own dwelling."

Struggle

Parents often stated that they almost always have had to fight and struggle to get the support that they needed

"Wish = That children with disabilities and their families shall get the support they are entitled to according to legislation without always having to push/make war to get them."

Parental Role

Within many statements we could trace a hope regarding the child's development so that the parent can be relieved of responsibilities and do other things in life.
"That she continues to develop well and that I have the strength to be a good mother at the same time that I can go forward with my own working life."

The view of the parental role also includes the "struggle" dimension of having to struggle for services and so on and in the worries (or insights) are for some parents that they will have to continue to take a great deal of responsibility even when the child is growing into adulthood.

"Think that we always have to be parents giving support and being the link to other parts in the society. To never be able to let go and to always be a step ahead"
"As long as we are around and can support him he will manage, but how will things be after that?"

The last citation also illustrates worries about who will take responsibility for the son/daughter when the parents are gone. Can society be trusted to provide continuing support?

DISCUSSION

The analysis of parent's statements resulted in an higher order theme of hope and worries about the future. This word pair was exemplified in subthemes concerning economy, endurance, independence (individual and structural), research, schooling, struggle and parental role. Although there is a comprehensive system of legislation and support organized in Sweden, parents are clearly worried about stability of services in the future. The worries included cut downs on habilitation, schooling and other services and being forced to continue to struggle for services needed. Major concerns were expressed about life after school regarding dwelling arrangements and job opportunities. An opposite theme of hope and expected improvement and gradually more independence was also found. There was special mentioning of hope expressed in that future research would lead to improvements or cure for the child in parents of children with diabetes but not (perhaps surprisingly) in the other groups.

Comparing the different groups of parents (without building on any statistical analysis) our impression is that there were more of worries in the groups with children with multiple impairments like autism, intellectual disability and severe motor impairment registered in the habilitation services. Fewer worries were expressed in the groups with a more "singular" impairment like hearing impairment or diabetes. This would be an interesting area for future research as would be the relation between hope and other coping strategies used to manage a sometimes very difficult situation.

The concerns around the parental role expressed here have been discussed in earlier research especially regarding worries resulting in similar themes (Monsen, 1999; Koegel, 1992). A concluding impression of the hope – worry theme is that it also could be formulated in terms of "trust". If you could trust the societal legislation, organization and financial security regarding future support for child and family, worries would be diminished and risks for stress related problems in the parents would also probably be less prevalent. The conclusion is that organization of support needs to be provided in a comprehensive and "future – secure" way so that parents can rely on good services, if needed, during the whole life span.

REFERENCES

Åkerström B & Nilsson I. (2004) Samhällsstödet till barn och ungdomar med funktionshinder och deras föräldrar i Jämtlands län (Societal support to children and adolescents with disabilities and their parents in the County of Jämtland). Municipal R&D-Unit County of Jämtland (FoU-Jämt), report nr 2004:3, Östersund, Sweden.

Kenny, K., & Mc Gilloway, S. (2007). Caring for children with learning disabilities: an exploratory study of parental strain and coping. *British journal of Learning Disabilities*, Vol 35, 4, 221-228.

Koegel, R. L., Schreibman, L., et al., (1992). Consistent Stress Profiles in Mothers of Children with Autism. *Journal of Autism and Developmental Disorders*, 22, 2, 205-216.

Llewellyn, G., Thompson, K., Whybrow, S., McConnell, D., Bratel, J., Coles, D., & Wearing, C. (2003). *Supporting Families. Family well-being and children with disabilities.* University of Sydney: School of Occupation and Leisure Sciences.

Monsen, R. B. (1999). Mothers Experiences of Living worried When Parenting Children With Spina Bifida. *Journal of Pediatric Nursing*, 14, 3, 157 – 163.

Olsson, M. B., & Hwang, C. P. (2002). Sense of coherence in parents of children with different developmental disabilities. *Journal of Intellectual Disability Research*, 46, 7, 548 – 559.

SFS 1982: 763. Health Services Act.

SFS 1985: 1100. Education Act.

SFS 1993: 387. Act concerning Support and Services for Persons with Certain Functional Impairments, LSS,

Sullivan, M., Karlsson., & Ware, J. E. (1994). SF-*36 Hälsoenkät. Svensk manual och tolkningsguide (SF-36 Health Survey. Swedish Manual and Interpretation Guide).* Göteborg: Sahlgrenska universitetssjukhuset.

Ware, J.E. Jr., Kosinski, M. & Gandek, B. (2000). SF-36®, Health Survey: Manual and Interpretation Guide. Lincoln, RI: Quality Metric Incorporated (first printed in 1993).

Chapter 42

FAMILY QUALITY OF LIFE: A COMPARISON OF TRENDS IN EIGHT COUNTRIES

I. Brown[1]

[1]Factor-Inwentash Faculty of Social Work, University of Toronto. Canada

INTRODUCTION

Quality of life is a term that burst into popularity in the 1990s because it seemed to capture the life goals and interests of people in so many walks of life. The field of intellectual and developmental disabilities was no exception to the general enthusiasm shown for the term, and it was quick to adopt the overall philosophy that improving quality of life for people with disabilities was a *raison d'être* that made our work both important and relevant. As a result, academics and professionals in our field took the term quality of life and undertook strong efforts to develop its meaning, its measurement, and its application. Many families saw quality of life as a family challenge and adopted enhancing family quality of life as a personal goal. This work is continuing, and shows no sign of abating.

The field of ID has been one of the richest sources of developing the concept of quality of life (Brown, 1999; Brown, 2006). Numerous articles and texts have explored what quality of life means at a conceptual level (Brown & Brown, 2003; Schalock et al., 2002; Schalock & Verdugo, 2002), and large numbers of quality of life measures have been developed (see Australian Center on Quality of Life, 2005 for a current list of available QOL instruments). In recent years, the focus of quality of life work has been perhaps more on application, and on specific ways to put concepts into practice that result in observable improvement (e.g., Brown & Brown, 2003; Brown et al; Schalock et al, 2007).

FAMILY QUALITY OF LIFE

In the late 1990s, a new and dynamic focus emerged from within quality of life work – family quality of life. The focus on individual quality of life work for children and adults with disabilities was welcomed by parents and other family members, but they did ask periodically, "And what about *our* quality of life?" and "What about the rest of the family?" These questions built on accounts of family life that were widely read in our field (especially Turnbull & Turnbull, 1978, 1985), and on the less formal accounts that are heard in families and support organizations on a daily basis. Researchers quickly agreed that these were valid and important questions.

Families have always been a vital aspect in successful living for children and adults with intellectual and developmental disabilities, but, in recent years, families have become more important than ever. The enactment of laws that entitle all children to education in their local schools (in Ontario, Bill 82 provided this entitlement in 1980), meant that almost all children with disabilities could continue to live with their families and attend local elementary and secondary schools (in Ontario, young adults may attend secondary school until the end of the school year following their 21st birthday). In addition, government policy documents have increasingly called for a stronger role for families in providing support and making critical decisions. For example, Ontario's 2006 policy document *Opportunities and Action: Transforming supports in Ontario for people who have a developmental disability* (Ministry of Community and Social Services, 2006) clearly states policy changes that allow families to make more decisions about what kinds of supports are needed for their family member with disabilities, and about how to spend approved funding in the best ways to provide those supports.

The success of an increased role for families relies on assumptions by policy makers that most families are both able and willing to act as main caregivers and decision makers, and that family life will be enhanced as a result of their greater involvement. Research into family quality of life asks whether or not these assumptions are valid. More specifically, though, research into family quality of life aims to make these assumptions a reality by describing family life, determining aspects of family life that contribute to and detract from family quality of life, and suggesting how aspects of life can be improved to enhance overall family quality of life.

To address these questions, two important family quality of life initiatives sprang to life almost at the same time. In the United States, the Beach Center on Disability (2008) was a strong initiative that developed a conceptualization of family quality of life and a valid method for measuring it, which is being used to evaluate the success of supports to families. The second initiative included an international team of researchers from Australia, Canada and Israel who developed the *Family Quality of Life Survey 2000* (Brown et al, 2000), and collected data using volunteer parents from service organizations with which they were affiliated. Together, these initiatives resulted several academic articles being published (Brown et al, 2003; Isaacs et al., 2007; Park et al, 2003; Turnbull et al, 2007), and in the first-ever book the focused specifically on family quality of life (Turnbull et al, 2004).

The international team of researchers amended its survey and the resulting *Family Quality of Life Survey 2006* (Brown et al., 2006) is being used as a way to collect family quality of life data not only in the three originally participating countries, but also in several other countries as well. To date, the initial results from studies in eight countries have been put together. This report represents a first look at those results, using Attainment and Satisfaction as two measures of family quality of life.

METHOD

Participants

The participants in the eight studies reported here were the main caregivers in families that have at least one member with an intellectual or developmental disability. Each participant completed the *Family Quality of Life Survey 2006* (Brown et al., 2006), recording family quality of life from his or her own perspective. Although all eight studies used the same method, the participants did vary because the families were selected from available volunteers. For example, the average age for the family member with disabilities ranged from 9.7 to 32.7 (17.0 for Australia, 11.5 for Belgium, 21.7 for Canada, 10.4 for Israel, 32.7 for Japan, 12.3 for Nigeria, 11.6 for Slovenia, and 9.7 for the United States). Thus, families in some countries had younger children and families in other countries were more likely to have older children or young adult members with disabilities. The disabilities represented in the families varied widely in most countries, although the samples in Canada and the United States reported autism in about 30% of the families, and the sample in the United States was drawn fully from low income inner-city families. Level of support needed and level of communication ability also differed slightly for the samples in the eight countries.

Sample size differed among countries as well. The samples in the eight studies included 44 from Australia, 25 from Belgium, 64 from Canada, 69 from Israel, 140 from Japan, 80 from Nigeria, 20 from Slovenia, and 28 from the United States.

PROCEDURES

The main caregivers of families were identified independently by the research teams in the eight countries. Ethical approval, including informed consent, was obtained from the universities or other institutions with which the lead researcher was affiliated. Trained research assistants administered the *Family Quality of Life Survey 2006* in a one-on-one session, in small group sessions, or by mail following a telephone information session.

A datafile, developed for the international teams by researchers in Toronto, Canada, was used to enter the data gathered in all eight countries. Thus, the same data was available from all countries for comparison purposes. Descriptive statistics were generated for the purpose of the present report, using the statistical program SPSS.

Survey Used

The *Family Quality of Life Survey 2006* is a comprehensive instrument for assessing family quality of life. It collects information that is both quantitative (numbers) and qualitative (explanations, ideas, and comments) in nature. Quantitative information is essential for statistical analyses and facilitates comparisons, while qualitative information is usually very useful for providing explanations and a deeper understanding to the numbers.

The *Family Quality of Life Survey 2006* has an introductory section where information is gathered concerning the family makeup and the family member with disabilities. Nine sections follow, each one addressing what are considered to be important areas of family life:

Health of the family
Financial well-being
Family relationships
Support from other people
Support from disability-related services
Influence of values
Careers and preparing for careers (school)
Leisure & Recreation
Community interaction

In each of these sections, Part A gathers some factual information and Part B provides an opportunity to rate each area of life using 6 separate measures: Attainment, Satisfaction, Importance, Opportunities, Initiative, and Stability. Attainment and Satisfaction are considered to be the two outcome measures (direct measures of family quality of life), and Importance, Opportunities, Initiative, and Stability are explanatory measures (measures that help to explain Attainment and Satisfaction). A sample question for Attainment is, "To what degree do your family members enjoy good health?" and for Satisfaction, "All things considered, how satisfied are you with the relationships within your family?"

A final section of the survey asks participants to rate their overall family quality of life ("Overall, how would you describe your family's quality of life?"), and their overall satisfaction ("Overall, how satisfied are you with your family's quality of life?"). As well, there is a final opportunity for participants to make any additional comments and to identify other areas of family life that they consider also influence their family quality of life.

RESULTS

The analysis for this report included an eight-country comparison of the two main outcome measures of family quality of life, Attainment and Satisfaction. The relationship between these two measures was explored, and their relationships with global satisfaction with family quality of life and global family quality of life were also investigated.

ATTAINMENT

Attainment was measured on a 5-point scale: 5=A great deal, 4=Quite a bit, 3=Some, 2=A little, and 1=Hardly at all. The Attainment ratings by the main caregivers who participated in the projects in each of the eight countries are shown in Figure 1 for each of the nine family quality of life domains and overall (average rating of the nine domains).

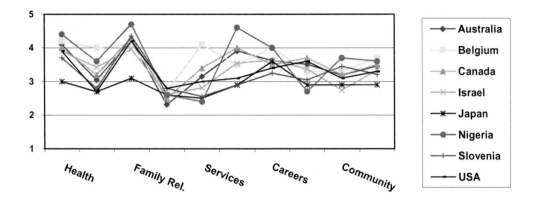

Figure 1. Attainment scores for nine domains of family quality of life for projects in eight countries.

The Attainment ratings showed a strong "W" effect for the first five domains, with Family Relationships consistently rating highest, and Support from Other People consistently rating lowest. The ratings for Support from Other People were very close among the eight country projects. There was more variation in the ratings for Support from Disability-Related Services, where ratings for Belgium were high and those for Japan, Nigeria, and Slovenia were considerably lower. The Influence of Values was rated high for Nigeria, where qualitative information suggested that religion was a very important aspect in the lives of the participants and their families. Nigeria showed considerable "up and down" in its pattern of Attainment ratings, compared with, for example, Japan where the pattern was flatter. The overall ratings were relatively close for most countries, and the country order for these ratings was not unlike that for a few of the domains (e.g., Health of the Family) but certainly not all. On the whole, the Attainment ratings showed that, for all country projects, there was variability across the nine domains, and that the pattern was similar among country projects for some domains and not for others.

SATISFACTION

Satisfaction was also measured on a 5-point scale: 5=Very satisfied, 4=Satisfied, 3=Neither satisfied nor dissatisfied, 2=Dissatisfied, and 1=Very dissatisfied. Figure 2 shows the Satisfaction ratings of the main caregivers for the projects in the eight countries and overall Satisfaction (average of the nine domains).

The "W" effect that was noted for Attainment was also evident in the Satisfaction ratings, except that satisfaction with disability-related services tended to be relatively low, flattening the final arm of the W. The exception was Belgium, where satisfaction with disability-related services was rated quite highly. It is clear that the patterns for Satisfaction ratings are somewhat flatter than those for Attainment, but Figure 2 also shows that participants did rate satisfaction differently across the nine domains and that the patterns across the nine domains were often quite similar among country projects. Again, the overall Satisfaction scores were relatively close and reflected the order of patterns in some, but not all, domains.

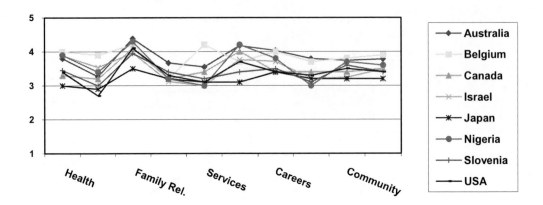

Figure 2. Satisfaction scores for nine domains of family quality of life for projects in eight countries.

Do Attainment and Satisfaction Measure the Same Thing?

One question that arises from looking at Figures 1 and 2 is whether or not participants were giving similar responses to both Attainment and Satisfaction. In other words, are Attainment and Satisfaction ratings almost the same thing? Certainly, the overall ratings seem to be quite similar. Figure 3 illustrates that for Canada and Nigeria the two overall ratings are the same, while Satisfaction ratings are higher than Attainment ratings for the other countries, especially for Australia and Japan.

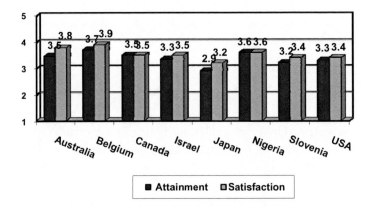

Figure 3. Overall Attainment and Satisfaction ratings for projects in eight countries.

Another way to look at the relationship between Attainment and Satisfaction scores is to calculate correlation coefficients. This measures the degree to which participants are likely to rate both measures in the same pattern. A correlation coefficient of 1.0 indicates a perfect correlation (all participants contributing to the patterns shown in Figure 3).

Pearson correlation coefficients for Attainment and Satisfaction ratings were computed using SPSS, and were as follows: Australia, .52; Belgium .75; Canada, .79; Israel, .82; Japan,

.63; Nigeria, .79; Slovenia, .63; and the United States, .82. All were significant at the .01 level of probability, meaning that we can feel confident that a positive relationship would occur more than 99% of the time. These results show that the pattern of ratings was relatively consistent for the projects in all eight countries, but that there was sufficient variation among individual participants in the way they rated Attainment and Satisfaction (especially Australia, Japan, and Slovenia) to indicate that both measures should probably be used.

Can We Just Ask One Overall Question on Satisfaction?

As indicated above, all participants completed a global satisfaction question, "Overall, how satisfied are you with your family's quality of life?" One reason for including this question was to ascertain whether the average of the ratings of satisfaction for the nine domains of life (overall Satisfaction) would be similar to the ratings for a global question on satisfaction with family quality of life. Figure 4 shows that the mean ratings for overall and global Satisfaction are similar for Belgium and Japan, but that they differ slightly for the other countries. For Australia, Nigeria, Slovenia and the USA, overall Satisfaction was rated lower than global Satisfaction, but the opposite is the case for Canada and Israel.

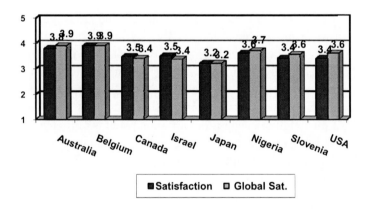

Figure 4. Overall Satisfaction and global Satisfaction ratings for projects in eight countries.

Again, Pearson Correlation coefficients for overall and global Satisfaction were computed as follows: Australia, .68; Belgium, .91; Canada, .76; Israel, .73; Japan, .58; Nigeria, .67; Slovenia, .59; and the United States, .76. All were significant at the .01 level. This analysis suggests that, for Belgium, overall and global Satisfaction measures are almost the same thing, but that it is less certain for the other countries' projects, and thus both measures should probably be used for the time being at least.

Can We Just Ask One Overall Question About Quality of Life?

A final question that was explored was whether or not the overall ratings of Attainment and Satisfaction might be reflected in just one global question on family quality of life: "Overall, how would you describe your family's quality of life?" Participants' ratings for this question are shown in Figure 5, and can be compared to overall Attainment and Satisfaction ratings in Figure 3 for the eight countries. Global Family Quality of Life ratings were lower than overall Attainment and Satisfaction ratings for all eight countries, with the exception of Attainment ratings in Slovenia which were marginally lower than global Family Quality of Life ratings. The specific reasons for global Family Quality of Life to be rated lower need to be explored further, but it seems clear that participants respond to this question differently than they respond to questions directly about attainment and satisfaction.

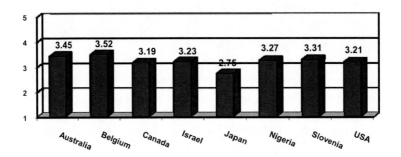

Figure 5. Global Family Quality of Life ratings for projects in eight countries.

Pearson correlation coefficients between overall Attainment and global Family Quality of Life ranged from .43 (Australia and Slovenia) to .70 (Nigeria), and were significant at the .01 level for all countries except Slovenia where the sample was small (20 families). Correlation between overall Satisfaction and global Family Quality of Life ranged from .32 (Japan) to .82 (Belgium), and again were significant at the .01 level for all countries except Slovenia. However, the two coefficients differed considerably for some countries (e.g., .43 and .67 for Australia, and .55 and .82 for Belgium), suggesting differing patterns of ratings. This analysis further supports the view that participants were responding differently to questions about Attainment, Satisfaction, and their global impression of family quality of life, and thus that all three measures should be used in future studies for the time being.

FUTURE ANALYSES

The information shared in this paper represents a first look at Attainment and Satisfaction as measures of family quality of life in projects in eight countries, looking at nine areas of family life. It showed that the two measures are related, but somewhat different, and thus it is important to use both measures. It also showed that there is a striking similarity in the way the main caregivers of families rate Attainment and Satisfaction in some domains of family life, and that there is more variation in other domains. Finally, it showed that, although we can ask one simple global question about Satisfaction and a similar global question about Family Quality of Life, the ratings resulting from these questions differ somewhat from the Satisfaction and Attainment scores derived from each of the nine domains of family life.

This initial analysis, interesting as it may be, needs to be followed up with additional analyses to clarify the meaning of the scores obtained, and to develop ideas about what they mean for support to families who have a member with a disability. First, the relationship between the two outcome measures – Attainment and Satisfaction – and four explanatory measures – Importance, Opportunities, Initiative, and Stability – needs to be explored in detail. Second, family quality of life as measured by Attainment and Satisfaction may differ for some subgroups of people with disabilities, or some family types. Third, we need to determine what lessons emerge from our family quality of life data that might help us to make changes to practice to enhance individual and family life. Putting such knowledge together in a more general way also enables us to generate useful advice to policy makers, so that methods of funding and methods of carrying out support services can be closely related to the overall objective of improving family quality of life.

AKNOWLEDGMENTS

The author is very grateful to the researchers and their teams in seven countries for sharing their data and completing data analysis: Fiona Rillotta, Australia; Riet Steel and Stijn Vandevelde, Belgium; Dana Roth and Shimshon Neikrug, Israel; Ryo Takahashi, Japan; Majda Schmidt and Branka Čagran, Slovenia; Paul Ajuwon, USA and Nigeria; and Preethy Samuel, USA. The author also recognizes the considerable efforts of the research team in Toronto Canada for their work in collecting and analyzing data: Nehama Baum, Roy Brown, Meaghan Edwards, Barry Isaacs, and Nicole Petrowski, and Jonathan Schmidt.

REFERENCES

Australian Center on Quality of Life. (2005). *Instruments*. Retrieved June 15, 2008 from http://acqol.deakin.edu.au/instruments/instrument.php

Beach Center on Disability. (2008). *Beach Center on Disability*. Retreived September12,2008from, http://www.beachcenter.org/Default.aspx?JScript=1

Brown, I. (1999). Embracing quality of life in times of spending restraint. Journal of *Intellectual & Developmental Disability, 24*(4), 299-308.

Brown, I., Anand, S., Fung, W. L. A., Isaacs, B., & Baum, N. (2003). "Family quality of life: Canadian results from an international study": Erratum. *Journal of Developmental and Physical Disabilities, 15*(4), 377.

Brown, I., & Brown, R. (2003). *Quality of life and disability: An approach for community practitioners*. London: Jessica Kingsley Publishers.

Brown, I., Brown, R., Baum, N. T., Isaacs, B. J., Myerscough, T., Neikrug, S., et al. (2006). *Family Quality of Life Survey: Main caregivers of people with intellectual or developmental disabilities*. Toronto, ON: Surrey Place Center.

Brown, I., Brown, R. I., & Neikrug, S. (2000). *Family Quality of Life Survey: Main caregivers of people with intellectual disabilities*. Toronto, ON: Surrey Place Center.

Brown, R. I. (2006). Editorial. *Journal of Policy and Practice in Intellectual Disabilities, 3*(4), 209-210.

Brown, R. I., Schalock, R. L., & Brown, I. (in press). Special issue on quality of life application. *Journal of Policy and Practice in Intellectual Disability, 6*(1).

Isaacs, B. J., Brown, I., Brown, R. I., Baum, N., Myerscough, T., Neikrug, S., Roth, D., Shearer, J., & Wang, M. (2007). The international family quality of life project: Goals and description of a survey tool. *Journal of Policy and Practice in Intellectual Disabilities, 4*(3), 177-185.

Ministry of Community and Social Services. (2006). *Opportunities and action: Transforming supports in Ontario for people who have a developmental disability.* Retrieved September 12, 2008 from, http://www.oasisonline.ca/mcss-policy/government-documents

Park, J., Hoffman, L., Marquis, J., Turnbull, L., Poston, D. J., Marquis, J., et al. (2003). Toward assessing family outcomes of service delivery: Validation of a family quality of life survey. *Journal of Intellectual Disability Research, 47*, 367-384.

Schalock, R. L., Brown, I., Brown, R. I., Cummins, R. A., Felce, D., Matikka, L., et al. (2002). Conceptualization, measurement, and application of quality of life for persons with intellectual disabilities: Report of an international panel of experts. *Mental Retardation, 40*, 457-470.

Schalock, R. L., Gardner, J. F., & Bradley, V. J. (2007). *Quality of life for people with intellectual and other developmental disabilities.* Washington, DC: American Association on Intellectual and Developmental Disabilities.

Schalock, R. L., & Verdugo, M. A. (2002). *Handbook on quality of life for human service practitioners.* Washington, DC: American Association on Mental Retardation.

Turnbull, A., Brown, I., & Turnbull, R. (2004). *Families and persons with mental retardation and quality of life: International perspectives.* Washington, DC: American Association on Mental Retardation.

Turnbull, A. P., Summers, J. A., Lee, S., & Kyzar, K. (2007). Conceptualization and measurement of family outcomes associated with families of individuals with intellectual disabilities. *Mental Retardation and Developmental Disabilities Research Reviews, 13*(4), 346-356.

Turnbull, A. P., & Turnbull III, H. R. (1978). *Parents speak out: Growing with a handicapped child.* Columbus, OH: C. E. Merrill.

Turnbull III, H. R., & Turnbull, A. P. (1985). *Parents speak out: Then and now.* Columbus, OH: C. E. Merrill.

Chapter 43

EXPERIENCES OF FAMILY CARERS OF PEOPLE WITH INTELLECTUAL DISABILITIES AND A DIAGNOSED MENTAL HEALTH CONDITION

M. Gibbs[1], H. Priest[2] and S. Read[1]

[1]KeeleUniversitySchoolofNursingandMidwifery,UniversityHospitalofNorthStaffordshire, Stoke-on-Trent UK
[2]Shropshire and Staffordshire Clinical Psychology Training Programme, Staffordshire University, Stoke-on-Trent, UK

INTRODUCTION

It is widely acknowledged that people with intellectual disabilities (ID) at all levels of severity are at greater risk of experiencing mental health problems than the general population (Department of Health [DH], 2009). It follows, therefore, that family members who assume the role of carer for a person with an intellectual disability may, in addition to the long recognised burden of care in this context, have to face an additional burden in identifying and responding to mental health needs.

Little is known about the impact of the duality of ID and mental health problems within the family context. This chapter explores the experiences, skills and knowledge of family carers for people with ID (and in particular, adult children) who also have a diagnosed mental health condition. It aims to add to the current limited evidence base, while also giving voice to members of a marginalised group.

WHO ARE THE CARERS?

The people who are the focus of this chapter are those who care for and support relatives with intellectual disability. The concept of caring as a 'role' or identity is relatively new and has only been used formally since the 1970s (Finch, 1993); prior to this time, care was often viewed as part of the everyday role of a wife or female family member. Caring can be understood as a distinct way of being, thinking, believing and acting that calls for commitment, knowledge and skill (Cheung & Hocking 2004). Barton (2000, p.42) pointed out that such care is 'informal in that it does not form part of a paid contract; instead, it relies on a sense of responsibility for, and commitment to the other, driven by feelings of love, duty or concern'.

It is estimated that in the UK, around 60% of adults with ID live at home with their families (Emerson et al., 2001). Today the family is recognised as 'the main source of love, care and support for children and adults with learning disabilities', especially for those with complex needs (DH, 2009, p.44-5).

PEOPLE WITH ID AND MENTAL HEALTH PROBLEMS

This group of people share a set of characteristics. Firstly, they have an intellectual disability. While terminology and definitions vary internationally, within the UK this implies difficulties in both intellectual and social functioning and an intelligence quotient (IQ) below 70, with the level of disability ranging from borderline to severe/profound.

Secondly, they are experiencing a difficulty with their mental health, which has resulted in a referral to a specialist psychiatrist and a formal diagnosis. Broadly speaking, a mental health problem exists when there is a significant change in a person's mood, behavior and thought processes that singly or in combination adversely affects their everyday life. While ID are present from birth or acquired in childhood and are enduring, mental health problems can develop at any age and may be either temporary or enduring. There is a tendency, however, for them to recur and lead eventually to progressive deterioration in cognitive, social and behavioral functioning.

The third shared characteristic is the coexistence of the intellectual disability and mental health condition, sometimes unhelpfully referred to as 'dual diagnosis', and finally, the nature of the combined disability and condition often results in the person's need for care from a family member.

THE BURDEN OF CARE

The concept of mental illness in people with ID has only gained prominence in recent years and there is limited literature available in relation to the families of people with this dual disability (Maes et al., 2003; Priest & Gibbs, 2004). However, a good deal is known about the burden of care for informal carers where there is a family member with ID alone. Much of this literature points to the negative effects (see Table 1).

In bringing together the two elements of ID and mental health conditions, there may be a factorial affect, whereby the addition of 'labels' increases the disabling effect and distances the person from appropriate services. It could thus be predicted that the negative effects on family carers and family stress will be considerable (Maes at al., 2003; McIntyre et al., 2002), and that specific support will be needed to help family carers understand the nature and cause of mental illness, to acquire relevant skills, and to access appropriate services (Maes et al., 2003). While there are many organisations, training programmes and support systems for professional carers working with people with ID and mental health problems, little is available for or aimed at the needs of informal family carers (Gratsa et al., 2006; Spiller & Hardy, 2004).

Table 1. Examples of the literature of carers of people with ID

	Negative effects		Positive effects
Bayley 1973	'A daily grind'	Mulroy et al. 2008	Good sibling relationships
Barr 1996	Social isolation Perceived lower social acceptance Fear for the future	Dykens 2005	Greater tolerance, understanding and viewing life as more valuable
Beck et al. 2004	Mothers more negative towards child with ID than		
McConkey et al. 2008	sibling. Adverse effects on family mental health		
Barr & Millar 2003	Breakdown in family relationships Negative definitions		
Saloviita et al. 2003	of the child (e.g. behavioral problems and social acceptance) predict parental stress.		

Similarly, there are numerous studies identifying the effects of caring for a person with a mental health problem (see Table 2).

Table 2. Examples of the literature on carers of people with mental ill health

	Negative effects		Positive effects
Pejlert 2001	Sorrow, anguish, constant worry, guilt, shame, stigma.	Marriot 2000 Whelton 1997	Achievement Family involvement can improve mental health of the carer
Jeon & Madjar, 1998	Being unable to make long term plans.		

The Family Carers Study

We set out to explore the impact of the duality of ID and mental health problems in the family context within one county in England. Approval was obtained from the local NHS Research Ethics Committee and Research Governance office. Participants were four families: 2 biological mothers, I adoptive mother, 1 grandmother, 1 grandfather; 3 sons, and 1 daughter. The average age of the cared-for person was 32 and the most frequent mental health condition was depression, with anxiety, obsessive-compulsive disorder, bipolar disorder, psychosis, and self-harm being experienced by some.

Semi-structured interviews were conducted with the family carers who were asked to talk about experiences of caring, knowledge about mental health issues, coping strategies and skills, family relationships, aspirations, concerns, and support. Interpretive Phenomenological Analysis (IPA; Smith and Osborn, 2003) was used to facilitate participants' describing and making sense of their experiences. Analysis and interpretation involved reading and reflecting on interview transcripts; identifying and labelling themes; developing theme clusters; and producing a summary table.

Four main themes emerged from the analysis: support; family relationships; information and knowledge; the caring role and its impact on the self. Here we illustrate themes with the participants' own words (names and details have been changed to protect anonymity).

Support

Andrea (mother of Russell, suffering from Depression:

"Somebody came to see me and said we could do two things. Put him on medication to keep him drowsy the whole time, or send him away to residential and you just have him back for holidays.

I says no! To both!. I said, I'm not having him on medication, you don't know what's wrong with him so how do you know what medication to put him on?... and I says, I'm not having him like a zombie its not fair and I'm not having him put away, ..."

This illustration points to an incomplete or inaccurate understanding of Russell's problems, together with a lack of consideration of the carer's perspective in offering what was seen as inappropriate and unacceptable support.

Family Relationships

Elizabeth (mother of Kate, suffering from depression and auditory hallucinations, and who self-harms):

"She'd been hearing voices telling her she was bad, she'd got to cut herself, she scraped her arms with broken glass and she'd taken an overdose ...I did get very upset about the fact that she hadn't felt she could tell me, but the social worker [said] ... it's all part of the illness, they do try to hide it. ... How could I have missed her going into depression ...? I still don't know how I missed it. I do communicate [now] in a different way ... I'm always questioning when she says something ... I'm thinking, 'is she telling the truth?'"

In this illustration. Kate's mental health problems have adversely affected her relationship with her mother, who no longer trusts her to be honest about her experiences and symptoms.

Information and Knowledge

Celia (mother of David, suffering from depression, in response to the interviewer asking if she had enough information about David's condition):

'Definitely not! What I do get doesn't come from the right quarters, it is not detailed enough. He ... gets depression and anxiety, but it is difficult to get information to support people who have a mixture of Down's syndrome, autism and mental health problems!'

Celia explains that because professionals do not always have the necessary knowledge, the information that she does get comes from informal sources.

The Caring Role and Impact on the Self

Celia: "I am pleased that I can be there for David, my caring role for so long now means that I recognise when he is uncomfortable or has problems, which is most of the time, although I often misunderstand the situation at my expense"

Celia "I've learned what to say and what not to say, trying to avoid so many things that are stressful to him".

Celia's comments make it clear that carers are constantly developing new skills and strategies when attempting to deliver care. For Celia, her caring role has begun to shape and to some extent control her own behavior.

DISCUSSION AND CONCLUSION

Despite a small sample, this study enabled a meaningful and powerful insight into the unique challenges and opportunities experienced by these carers. Key findings indicate that the development of mental health conditions is accepted by families as just another problem to deal with; a part of the person they care for. However, family dynamics are affected, and carer strain is evident; families do not have adequate information about mental health conditions and may not access appropriate services. When services are involved, their response is not always appropriate or acceptable, and there is some suggestion that health care professionals, too, lack appropriate knowledge and skill.

The study had the additional benefits of empowering and giving a voice to a marginalised or invisible group. The project is ongoing and intends more involvement with families; and joint interviews with carers and cared-for persons to create informative case studies of these unique caring relationships.

REFERENCES

Barr O (1996) Developing services for people with intellectual disabilities which actively involve family members. A review of recent literature. *Health and Social Care in the Community*, 4(2), 103-112.

Barr O, Millar R (2003) Parents of children with intellectual disabilities: Their expectations and experience of genetic counselling, *Journal of Applied Research in Intellectual Disabilities*, 16(3),177-188,

Barton R (2000) In: M Davis (Ed) The Blackwell Encyclopaedia of Social Work. Wiley-Blackwell, Oxford, p.42.

Bayley M (1973) Mental handicap and community care. London: Routledge & Kegan Paul

Beck A, Daley D, Hastings R P, Stevenson J (2004). Mothers' expressed emotion towards children with and without intellectual disabilities. *Journal of Intellectual Disability Research,* 48(7), 628-638.

Cheung J, Hocking P (2004) Caring as worrying: the experience of spousal carers. *Journal of Advanced Nursing*, 47(5), 475-482.

Dykens E.M. (2005) Happiness, well-being, and character strengths: Outcomes for families and siblings of persons with mental retardation. *Mental Retardation*, 43, 360-364.

Department of Health (2009) Valuing people now: a new three-year strategy for people with learning disabilities. London: Department of Health.

Emerson E, Hatton C, Felce D et al. (2001) Intellectual disabilities: the fundamental facts. London: The Mental Health Foundation.

Finch J (1993) The concept of caring: Feminist and other perspectives. In: J Twigg (ed), Informal care in Europe. 5-21. York: Social Policy Research Unit.

Gratsa A, Spiller MJ, Holt G et al (2006) Developing a mental health guide for families and carers of people with intellectual disabilities. *Journal of Applied Research in Intellectual Disabilities,* pp1-10.

Jeon Y, Madjar I (1998) Caring for a family member with chronic mental illness. *Qualitative Health Research*, 8(5), 694-707

Maes B, Broekman TG, Došen A et al 2003 Caregiving burden of families looking after persons with intellectual disability and behavioral or psychiatric problems. *Journal of Intellectual Disability Research*, 47(6) 447-455.

Marriott A, Donaldson C, Tarrier N et al. (2000) Effectiveness of cognitive-behavioral family intervention in reducing the burden of care in carers of patients with Alzheimer's disease. *British Journal of Psychiatry*, 176:557-562

McConkey R, Truesdale-Kennedy M, Chang M, Jarrah S, Shukri R (2008) The impact on mothers of bringing up a child with intellectual disabilities: a cross-cultural study. *International Journal of Nursing Studies*; 45 (1): 65-74

McIntyre LL, Blacher J, Baker BL 2002 Behavioral/mental health problems in young adults with intellectual disability: the impact on families. *Journal of Intellectual Disability Research*, 46(3):239-249

Mulroy, S.; Robertson, L.; Aiberti, K.; Leonard, H.; Bower, C (2008) The impact of having a sibling with an intellectual disability: Parental perspectives in two disorders. *Journal of Intellectual Disability Research*, 52(3),216-229,

Pejlert A (2001) Being a parent of an adult son or daughter with severe mental illness receiving professional care: parents narratives. *Health and Social Care in the Community*, 9, 194–204.

Priest HM, Gibbs M (2004) Mental health care for people with intellectual disabilities. Churchill Livingstone, Oxford.

Saloviita T, Italinna M, Leinonen E (2003) Explaining the parental stress of fathers and mothers caring for a child with intellectual disability: a double ABCX model. *Journal of Intellectual Disability Research*, 47(5) 300-312

Smith JA & Osborn M (2003) Interpretative Phenomenological Analysis: In JA Smith (Ed). Qualitative Psychology: A practical guide to research methods. Sage, London, pp. 51-80.

Spiller M and Hardy S. (2004) Developing a guide to mental health for families and carers of people with intellectual disability. *Learning Disability Practice*, 7(8) 28-31.

Whelton C, Pawlick J (1997) Involving families in psychological rehabilitation. *Psychiatric Rehabilitation Journal*, 20(3), 57-60.

Chapter 44

FAMILIES OF 40-YEAR OLDS WITH DOWN SYNDROME AND OF A COMPARISON GROUP

J. Carr

Formerly of St George's Hospital, London, UK

INTRODUCTION

This paper presents the findings from the latest phase of a long-term study of people with Down syndrome (DS) and their parents, and of a comparison group of parents of people without disabilities, both groups having been followed since the 40-year-olds were infants. The data are derived from Rutter's Malaise Inventory (see Carr 2005) and semi-structured interviews with the survivors of each group. Health, social life and friendships of both groups will be considered, and, for the families of people with DS, their experience of services.

PARTICIPANTS

At the outset there were 45 families of people with DS, each matched for sex, age and social class with a non-disabled child and his/her family. Numbers declined over the years, due to deaths of both people with DS and of their parents. At age 40 there were 21 people with DS with at least one parent, seven fathers and 18 mothers, still alive. In three cases both parents, including one step-father, were alive. In the comparison group, 16 families were still in the study, 12 with both parents alive. Average age for mothers of people with DS was 75.9 and for fathers 75, these being some six and four years older respectively than for mothers and fathers of the comparison group.

RESULTS

Mothers' Health

As in previous phases of the study, mothers rated their own health (Table 1). Proportionately rather more mothers of people with DS, two-thirds, compared with half of comparison mothers, said their health was good, while more comparison mothers said it was poor. In contrast to the findings at all previous stages of the study, fewer mothers of people with DS than of those in the comparison group said they currently felt run-down or depressed. Mothers' health was not related to a wide range of factors connected with themselves (age, marital status, loneliness etc) nor to any connected with the people with DS except for independence: poorer health was reported by mothers whose family member with DS was thought not capable of going out alone beyond the garden.

Mean scores on the Malaise Scale were lower for both groups than at age 35, down by 0.72 points for the mothers of people with DS and by 0.25 points for the comparison group mothers. Factors which had previously been significantly related to Malaise scores (poor health, loneliness, feeling run-down or depressed) were not now significant, although trends were the same. Older mothers now had a higher mean score ($p=<.05$), as did mothers with fewer friends ($p=<.05$), as was found also at age 30 (Carr 2005). Of factors connected with the people with DS, again, only independence featured, with higher Malaise scores in those whose offspring could be left alone in the house for not more than half an hour, and this too has been found at previous stages of the study (Carr 1995, 2005).

Table 1. Mothers' self-perceived health

	DS group %	Comparison group %
Overall health		
Good	60	50
Fair	28	28
Poor	12	21
Felt run-down &/or Depressed		
Run-down	6	7
Depressed	11	7
Both	11	29
Neither	72	57
Malaise Scale		
Mean	2.56	2.25
Range	0-7	0-5
Score 6+	11	11

Looking at Malaise scores over the years, the mean for mothers of people with DS was highest, at 3.33, and that for the comparison group lowest, at 1.5, at 11 years. At age 40 the difference between the two was lower than at any other time.

Social Life

Mothers were asked about going out, alone or with a partner, attendance at social and leisure events, friendships and holidays. Mothers of people with DS went out somewhat less, and more would have liked to go out more often, compared with the comparison group (Table 2). As at ages 21, 30 and 35, fewer were able to have a holiday without the adult person but the difference is not now significant.

A composite social life factor was arrived at by combining scores for going out, club and leisure attendance, and holidays. The mean score for mothers of people with DS was lower, indicating a more restricted social life, but not significantly so. Analyses of all the above factors, to take into account, first, mother's age, and second, whether the person lived at or away from home, showed that younger mothers tended to have a more active social life, as did mothers whose person with DS lived away from home, significantly more having holidays independently (p=.011).

Where friendships and family relationships were concerned, there was little difference between the groups in contact with friends (Table 2). Mothers of people with DS had rather fewer contacts with other family members than did the comparison group, but said they had a good deal of help from them.

Table 2. Mothers' social life and friendships

	Down's Syndrome %	Control %
Went out 1pm+		
-accompanied	23	58
-alone	50	50
-to clubs etc	60	55
Would like to go out more	35	20
Had a holiday last year		
-no, or only with N	60	33
Has no or few friends	42	53
Has many friends	26	40
Sees family 1pm+	74	93
Family gave much help	71	-

Fathers and Siblings

Data on fathers and siblings were gained from reports by mothers, and, in the case of fathers of people with DS, from a very small number. Over 70% of fathers in both groups were said to be in good health; two-fifths of fathers of people with DS were said to be run-down and two-fifths of comparison fathers to be depressed. The remainder were neither run-down nor depressed. Asked about worries about their other children (mainly health problems), 17% of mothers of people with DS and 54% of the comparison group said they had, a difference that just fails to reach significance. At least it may be concluded that mothers of people with DS were not dealing with a greater number of serious problems than did other mothers.

SERVICES

Mothers of people with DS rated their satisfaction with a range of services on a scale from 1 (very dissatisfied) to 5 (very satisfied). Table 3 shows the number who had had contact with each service and the percentage dissatisfied (1 and 2) and satisfied (4 and 5).

Table 3 Satisfaction with services (percentages)

Service	n	Dissatisfied %	Satisfied %
GP	30	3	93
Hospital Doctor	12	-	100
Dentist	23	4	91
Optician	18	11	89
Social Worker	18	39	50
Speech Therapist	2	-	50
Chiropodist	17	6	88
Day Center	23	13	83

Figures exclude those neither satisfied nor dissatisfied with a service.

Over 80% were at least satisfied with each service apart from that given by social workers and speech therapists (only two having had contact with speech therapists). No mother was dissatisfied with all services, and 56% were satisfied with all. As before (Carr 2005) there was a (non-significant) trend towards more mothers in manual workers' families to be satisfied with all – 64% compared with 31% of mothers in non-manual workers' families.

DISCUSSION

As was found at previous stages of the study, these, now very elderly, parents were functioning similarly to parents in the general population. Higher stress scores were found in older mothers and those with few friends, but where the people with DS were concerned, only dependency was related to mother's stress, as it was also to her health ratings. Both dependency factors were significantly related to IQ (with going out alone, $z=-2.35$, $p=.018$:

with staying home alone, z=2.42, p=.015) so the mothers' decisions may have been quite realistic.

The data on other family members, despite being derived from the mother's reports, are in broad agreement with other research (Krauss & Seltzer 1993, Cuskelly & Gunn 2006) showing fathers and siblings of older people with DS to be well adjusted. Among this group of parents there is no evidence that their lives have become more stressful over the years. If they had known this when their babies were first diagnosed, when apprehensions about the future loom large (Kingston 2007), they would I believe have been greatly comforted.

REFERENCES

Carr, J (1995) Down's Syndrome: Children Growing Up. Cambridge: Cambridge University Press.

Carr, J. (2005). Families of 30-35 year olds with Down's Syndrome. *Journal of Applied Research in Intellectual Disabilities*, 18, 75-84.

Cuskelly M, Gunn P. (2006). Adjustment of children *J Intellect Disabil Res*. 50:917-25.

Kingston, A.K. 2007. Mothering special needs. Jessica Kingsley Publishers. London.

Krauss, M.W., & Seltzer, M.M. (1993). Current well-being and future plans of older caregiving others. *Irish Journal of Psychology*, 14, 48-63.

PART VIII. QUALITY OF LIFE AND SPIRITUALITY

Individuals with intellectual disabilities (ID) are on a daily basis confronted with a number of barriers preventing them from accessing fully their community and thereby having a better quality of life. Such barriers may be those experienced by individuals with physical disability. *Monninger and Tsakarestos* and *Tillmann and Haveman* highlight a number of issues related to public transport for children with ID. Being freely mobile is an essential part of self-independence, which in turn is the basis of a good quality of life. This is further highlighted by *Farrell* and *Verdonschot and de Witte* who demonstate that identifying priorities by individuals themselves and focussing on specific environmental factors can lead to an improvement quality of life.

For the general population spiritualty remains a crucial part of human experience. The role of spirituality in ID is not understood and very little research has been undertaken on this matter. *Meininger* highlights a number of issues for persons with ID accessing protestant churches. *Bernhard* discusses the benefits of improved pastoral care for people with ID in religious congregations. *McNair* comments on the issues of Christian social constructs of disabilities. *Gaventa* in a number of papers remarks on the wider aspects of spirituality and its role in the life of individuals with ID, particularly related to end of life issues.

Chapter 45

PHYSICAL AND PSYCHOLOGICAL BARRIERS IN PUBLIC TRANSPORTATION FOR SCHOOL CHILDREN WITH INTELLECTUAL DISABILITIES

D. Monninger[1] and A. Tsakarestos[1]

[1]Technische Universität München, Chair of Traffic Engineering and Control,Germany

AIM

When people with intellectual disabilities (ID) wish to use public transport independently they are confronted with a wide scope of barriers. While people with physical disabilities already benefit from a lot of measures allowing barrier free access to public transport, the same cannot be said for people with ID. However, as most of them are not able to acquire a driving license, the issue of independent use of public transport is even more important. This is particularly essential in rural areas, where most everyday activities can not be carried out within walking distance.

An important basis for improving this situation is profound knowledge about which elements within the transportation chain actually constitute a barrier for people with ID. The aim of this text contribution is to bring this knowledge together, to analyse and systemize it, and to discuss possible measures to eliminate these barriers.

The presented work is part of the German research project MOGLI[8], where children and young adults with ID (between ages 9 to 19) will be equipped to use public transport independently to achieve their own mobility as far as possible. These skills will be learned on their daily way to school. The participants receive support from two sides: mobility training, designed by specialised pedagogues, and enhancement of the public transport system, carried out by transportation engineers. A pilot application of this project is taking place in the County of *Grafschaft Bentheim* (Lower Saxony, Germany) in close cooperation with the *Vechtetal Schule*, the local school for children with ID. Through this project a process will be initiated and promoted, which intends to address the backlog in scientific understanding regarding barrier-free accessibility, mobility and behavior of this sensitive target group.

Initially participants learn to manage independently their daily way to school and back. As soon as they have gained enough experience and self confidence, they are encouraged to use public transport also for other trip purposes like leisure or shopping. This anticipates a lifelong dependency on special individual transport services. After the participants have successfully completed a remedial education to learn all necessary specific transport skills, they are ready to manage their daily trip to school independently. Starting in April 2009, the first group 40 pupils from the *Vechtetal Schule* will have achieved this stage. In autumn 2009 a further 50 pupils will follow.

METHOD

Until now there have been no studies that bring together and analyse the mobility behavior of people with ID in detail. Prior knowledge is distributed in single scientific studies regarding specific skills or is part of teachers' experiences from different special schools. To bring together all of this knowledge and to acquire the necessary additional information was a big challenge in this project. The chosen method included literature research of existing scientific studies, an experimental investigation of all pupils participating in the project and subsequently a systematic analysis within an interdisciplinary workshop.

To find out which barriers actually exist in public transport for people with ID, a pilot investigation was carried out with several participants from the *Vechtetal Schule*. The pupils' challenge was to handle a complete door-to-door trip by public transport. Each pupil was accompanied by a teacher and a member of the project team, allowing all potential barriers along the complete trip to be collected. Afterwards a workshop was carried out dealing with the issue of barriers in public transport. This interdisciplinary workshop was attended by transport engineers and pedagogues as well as representatives from the local municipal administration and the local transport company.

The objective of this workshop was firstly to define the term "barrier" in this context to assure a joint understanding of the subject. In a second step all potential barriers (noted in the pilot investigation or resulting from the participants' experiences) were collected and classified. Finally possible solutions for their elimination were developed.

BARRIER DEFINITION

To establish common terms, the following definition was agreed:

> "Barriers in public transportation for people with intellectual disability are obstacles, which impede or even prohibit a self-dependent usage of public transportation. Barriers can be constructional, technical and/or organisational and can result from operational and communicative situations and activities."

It becomes apparent, that the term "barrier" covers in this context a wide area; it is not restricted to physical and tangible barriers, but also to specific situations and social interaction.

Table 1. Overview about the categories and their description and some examples of barriers identified

Category	Description	Barriers identified (examples)
Information about the transport system	Preparation for the trip before leaving the door; study of the public transport system; geographical orientation; distinction of the different means of transportation in public transport; searching for a suitable connection using the passenger information available (time table book, network map, connection information via internet)	Missing local understanding, no orientation; reading the timetable-book; buying the right ticket; understanding the passenger information on the internet; having a sense of time, being able to read the clock; difficulties in reading and understanding characters
Bus stops and vehicles	Orientation at bus stops and in vehicles, comprehensibility of passenger information at bus stops and in vehicles, willingness of the driver to give information if required, friendliness of the driver	Signage at bus stops is not consistent; timetable at the bus stop is incomprehensible (structure and content); information is not up-to-date; announcements are not comprehensible; passenger information concept is not consistent; bus driver doesn't provide adequate information
Boarding, deboarding, transfer and waiting	Problems which can arise during boarding, deboarding, transfer and waiting, such as problems with disembarking correctly, no orientation at changing points, etc…	No ability to assert oneself; problems with waiting alone; assaults; limited or blocked waiting space; too short or too long changing times; too long or unsafe footways at changing points; no orientation at changing points; bad weather conditions
Bus riding	Availability of enough seats, behavior of pupil with ID, behavior of the other passengers, general fears and uncertainties	Not enough seats, not enough grab handholds; improper behavior from pupils with ID as well as from other passengers or the bus driver; rough driving manoeuvres; precariousness, fears
Footways	All barriers alongside footways	Footway not recognisable; no illumination; no footway at all; bumpy surface; unsafe street crossing (streets with 3 or more lanes, short green period); wrong role models

Incidents	Every occurrences, which describe a disturbance according to the daily routine of the door-to-door trip for people with ID	To miss the bus; to board the wrong bus; to get off at the wrong bus stop; bus ride is delayed or even cancelled; no connection on a changing point (because of delay)
Other barriers	Everything that doesn't fit into any other category	Blind confidence towards other passengers; way to school is too long with public transportation

BARRIER CATEGORISATION

Barriers can occur in every sub area of a door-to-door trip. The variety reaches from physical objects and constructions to cognitive difficulties and psychological processes, social interaction with one's own environment as well as with other passengers. Due to the plurality and complexity of the barriers a categorisation was made by dividing the chain of transportation into different parts. Table 1 gives an overview about the categories and their description and some examples of barriers identified.

GENERAL MEASURES TO ELIMINATE BARRIERS

The elimination of barriers for people with ID is a challenge that has to be handled on different levels. These levels, reaching from constructive changes and improvements in organisation up to technical assistance and pedagogical support cover a multitude of institutions and responsibilities, which usually have to cooperate with each other.

Constructional measures do make sense, where physical barriers can be easily eliminated structurally. A bus stop, for example, located on a street with high traffic load with difficult access for pedestrians and undersized waiting space, is a problem which should be solved structurally. This barrier can be removed by building a safe footpath to the bus stop and sufficient waiting space. Is this not possible – in case of too high costs or not enough space – a reasonable measure would also be to displace the whole bus stop to a more suitable location.

Some barriers can be eliminated by improvements in the organisation of the public transport system. For example, an important essential is good passenger information that is clearly structured and easy to comprehend. Completely different passenger information styles can often be found at the same bus stop, if there are several transport companies operating in the same district. A consistent and understandable system, completely independent from the transport company, would improve significantly the convenience of passenger information. Lots of people with ID have difficulties with reading. Thus it is very important to use colours and pictograms for passenger information.

In addition, technical measures can be effective to disarm some barriers. A system that automatically announces the next bus stop, for example, helps to avoid disembarking at the wrong stop. Technical support is particularly important in the case of an incident. The development of an incident management system is also part of the MogLi project. This system will be based on a public transport control system, which can recognize incidents and delays in real time. This information will be personalised, individually edited and finally transmitted to special mobile end devices especially adapted for the pupils participating in the project. By equipping the pupils with these devices it is also possible to call for help, if individual problems occur.

In addition to transport related measures, pedagogical support is also a major issue. This implies practicing an independent use of public transport and learning how to cope with existing barriers; either by overcoming or by avoiding them. This is of utmost important because, due to the high investment cost, not all barriers can be eliminated by transport related measures. Moreover, there are barriers that appear in an individual manner and concern only single persons – so a collective measure is not appropriate here. Finally, for some barriers the only solution available is learning to deal with them, which relies solely on pedagogical support and training. One problem for example, is the imitation of wrong role models, like ignoring red traffic lights at pedestrian crossings. A large percentage of young people copy the behavior of others. This applies particularly to people with ID. Irregular behavior of other traffic participants, which sometimes implies high risks, can spontaneously be taken over, although the imitators might not have the same possibilities to act and react in the same way as their role model. Thus it is important to learn how to distinguish between correct and irregular behavior and to act according to the traffic rules. Correct behavior in traffic has to be exemplified and exercised in the respective personal milieu also.

CONCLUSION

A plurality of barriers can be eliminated by constructional, technical or organisational measures. Lots of the barriers discovered impede not only people with ID, but also other groups of passengers (e.g. elderly people) or the entire population. An elimination of these barriers will help to make the whole system of public transportation more attractive. Removing these barriers provides a basic supply of barrier free accessibility. However, some barriers can occur in an individual manner and are also very much dependent on the type and level of the intellectual disability. This is a major difference to people with physical disabilities, where barriers can usually be identified clearly. Thereby it is necessary to examine precisely which measures are suitable to eliminate these barriers in the specific case. A mixture of different measures might be an appropriate solution.

It also became apparent that many barriers which have a psychological or social basis can not be eliminated physically. Therefore pedagogical support in terms of transport training and behavior practice is essential.

Chapter 46

PUBLIC TRANSPORTATION AS A MEANS OF SOCIAL INTEGRATION FOR SCHOOL CHILDREN WITH INTELLECTUAL DISABILITIES

V. Tillmann[1] and M. Haveman[2]

[1]Faculty Rehabilitation Sciences,Baroper Str. 279,
44227 Dortmund, Germany
[2]Faculty Rehabilitation Sciences, Emil- Figge Str. 50,
44221 Dortmund, Germany

INTRODUCTION

Mobility is a basic need and a precondition for a self determined life and participation in community living. People with an intellectual disability (ID) are often restricted in their mobility and they depend on other people for being mobile (Stöppler, 2002). In Germany school children have to get to school independently. It's of their parents' and of their owns' responsibility to get there. Individual transportation like school busses or taxis are only provided for children with special needs. This puts them in an even more special situation and leads to social exclusion.

In addition to the way to school the public transportation system is also an adequate way of being mobile independently, in leisure time. For people with ID the access to it isn't as easy as it should be out of two main reasons. First of all the public transportation system is not completely barrier- free. A hard or even impossible to read bus schedule or a confusingly signed bus station are just two examples. The second reason is the lack of adequate knowledge in terms of using the public bus system. They were hardly ever taught in a sufficient and structured way how to take part in traffic or how to use the bus safely and efficiently.

In consideration of these aspects the main goal of the three year intervention and research project "MogLi" (2007- 2010) in a rather rural are in Germany, is to enable children and young adults with ID to use the regular public transportation system to get to school independently. To achieve this goal it is necessary to reduce and eliminate the mentioned problems as far as possible and to ensure long term effects.

The research project started with different interviews to get a baseline for further steps. The children of the participating school, the teachers and the parents were questioned in adequate ways and for different purposes, which are described in the following. The school children (N=124) were interviewed in the beginning of the project with a structured list of items about their roles in traffic, traffic routes and their desire for mobility. These interviews were a first guideline to match the children's needs. The questionnaire was modified to match the participants' strengths and qualities e.g. by using pictures and easy language.

The results show that most of the children do have experiences in travelling with public busses in company of their parents or teachers (82%), but only a few have been on a bus before on their own (14%) and only 2% use it to get to school and not even 1% use it in leisure time. In contrast to this is the childrens' desire of using public buses independently. More than half of the children say they would like to use it on their own.

The parents are a very important part in the project. They were questioned as well to get information about their concerns, which need to be considered for following actions. As expected the main concern is their children's safety. To get more specific information about theses safety issues, the parents were asked to review certain situations.

75% think that a crowded bus, where people get pushed, is at least "partly dangerous" on a scale from "not dangerous" to "very dangerous". 76% classify hostility on the bus as at least "partly dangerous" and 76% also see difficulties in changing busses. Despite of these concerns more than 85% want their children to take part in traffic more independently during leisure time and only a little less do want their children to take the bus to school.

The teachers were mainly interviewed about their motivation of participating in the project and about their knowledge of mobility education. The most relevant reason for the teachers to take part in the project is the expected increase of their students' independency (93%). In addition to this 90% say that personal interest in the subject of mobility education is another reason and 76% expect to gain more knowledge of the subject.

In addition to this, they point out that they haven't really learned how to teach mobility education in a professional way during their study and their whole apprenticeship. This might be an explanation for the rather sparely done traffic education during their lessons. The topic of using the bus is even less taught. Since they do see the importance of this subject the whole staff is motivated to take part in the project and has a focus on mobility education during the next school year.

Considering the childrens', parents' and teachers' wishes of more independency and participation for the children and young adults with ID, the need of better traffic skills and less barriers, condensed the capability of the independent use of the public transportation system, is obvious. In terms of a better mobility education at school, a comprehensive curriculum for mobility was developed and established at the participating school. All previous tests, studies and analysis like the different interviews, a children's test of competences and an evaluation of the different barriers were considered. This lead to a collection of 167 learning targets including the needed materials.

The Curriculum has been split into the different areas of mobility education, safety-, environment-, health- and social- education. Further on the learning targets have been attached to the subjects taught at school. In addition to this the areas of "basic training", "traffic specific basic training", "training for pedestrians" and finally "training for using the public transportation system" were marked and can easily be separated to match the children's individual competences.

At the end of the research project "MogLi" in 2010 about 100 school children are going to use the public transportation system to get to and back from school. In addition to this they can use the public transportation system in leisure time as well. The interdisciplinary mobility concept gives these children and young adults the chance of being more mobile in all aspects of life and taking a huge step to a more independent life and participation.

REFERENCE

Stoppler, R. (2002). Mobilitäts- und Verkehrserziehung für Menschen mit geistiger Behinderung. Bad Heilbrunn. Klinkhardt.

Chapter 47

THE QUALITY OF LIFE OF PEOPLE WITH DISABILITIES IN IRELAND IN 2007

M. Farrell

Delivering Outcomes to People Project & St. Michael's House, Dublin

INTRODUCTION

The purpose of this study was to establish a national baseline on the quality of life of adults with a disability in Ireland in 2007. Such a baseline would provide a reliable measure by which to examine future progress in enhancing quality of life for people with disabilities, and to compare this data with others internationally; also, for the person with a disability, the information gathered is a valuable starting point for building a person-centerd plan. The extract above from 'John's Story' indicates the reality and bleakness of life for some people with disabilities in Ireland today. The study 'The Quality of Life of People with Disabilities in Ireland 2007', was conducted during 2007 by Dr. Bob Mc Cormack & Margaret Farrell, as part of the Delivering Outcomes to People Project, funded by the Irish Government initiative Enhancing Disability Services, under the Dept. of Justice, Equality and Law Reform.

METHODOLOGY

The Survey Instrument

The Study used The 23 Personal Outcome Measures (POMS), (Gardner & Carran 2005; Schalock et al, 2007). Personal Outcome Measures cover all major aspects of a person's life and were developed by Dr. Jim Gardner and his colleagues at The Council for Quality and Leadership (CQL www.thecouncil.org). Twenty-three discreet dimensions, The 23 Personal Outcome Measures, were identified by people in answer to the question: 'Can you tell me what's important in your life?' These dimensions include relationships, work, living arrangements, community involvement, personal choices, health, safety, rights and personal goals. (Appendix 1. for full list)

The Personal Outcome Measures approach is a radically different approach to Quality of Service work, it focuses on customer – driven service, with key concepts being 'The Whole Person' as reference point, flexibility in service design, and agency responsiveness to the individual's priorities, and the information gathered is valuable in the development of person-centerd plans. Currently, 9 Irish agencies are accredited by The Council on Quality and Leadership (CQL), with some 30 agencies using their Quality Measures 2005 as an ongoing external quality enhancement and evaluation system; and are also used widely throughout the English-speaking world (US, Canada, Australia).

The POMS Instrument allows measurement of participants' answers to 3 main questions:

Which of the 23 POMS are present for this person at this time?
Are there sufficient agency supports in place to achieve/maintain these 23 POMS?
Which three POMS are the person's own unmet priorities which they wish to realise?

Sample - Who Did we Meet?

The Project used stratified random sampling to ensure samples were representative of the agency's population in respect of age, gender and level/type of disability. A total of 300 adults were selected, representing c.5,000 adults with disabilities, across 27 different disability service providers in the Republic of Ireland. These service providers volunteered to participate, they were all members of the Outcomes Network of Ireland (an umbrella group of Irish disability providers interested in this approach), and were among 28 member agencies invited to participate. The sample comprised 85% people with intellectual disabilities/learning (75% mild/moderate, 25% severe/profound), 5% severe autism, and 10% physical/sensory disabilities, based on their primary disability. All participants availed of specialised disability service provision at least twice per week. Services received included day and / or residential service and/or respite and/or clinical provision. The sample grouped people into 2 age-bands: 18-35 years and 35 years and older. These 300 individuals were approached to participate, and were given accessible information on the study and its purpose. Where a person declined to participate, a replacement person was randomly selected fitting the same criteria.

Interview Process, Reliability and Scoring

The information was gathered from participants, and people who know them well, by teams of POMs - trained interviewers, working together using a fixed set of information-gathering and information-scoring questions. In each agency, a certified POMS trainer reviewed the information gathered and scoring, and where necessary, the evidence for particular scores were reviewed and re-scored. Following completion of the data collection process, the anonymised scoring sheets were forwarded by the local study Co-ordinator to the Project office for data inputting, checking and analysis. Analysis was undertaken by the Project team using the statistical software programme SPSS V.14.

(For example, in scoring for the Personal Outcome 'I have Friends', friends are defined as people apart from family members and staff. *We Explore:* 1. Does this person have friends? 2. Do they have enough friends? 3. Do they have enough contact with their friends? If the answers are *Yes*, the Outcome is considered fully present. If not, is this due their personal choice and *not* through lack of experience or having no clear choice? Friendships have to be reciprocal and cannot include paid staff. People do not have to have friends, if that is their choice and not through lack of opportunity.

We also explore the effectiveness of the supports for the Personal Outcome 'I have Friends' as provided by the agency. Agencies cannot manufacture friendships for people, but they can be nurtured and the agency must support opportunities where friendships may develop. 1. Does the agency know the person's preference and need for friends? 2. Are supports provided to assist the person with developing, maintaining and enhancing friendships if needed? If the answers are *Yes*, the Support is considered present. For example, supports might include transport, help with phone calls, text-messaging, facilitating social gatherings, support with learning about social skills.)

Priority Outcomes.

In terms of improving a person's quality of life, the starting point is the person's own priorities. These emerge clearly from the discussion about their current quality of life. What aspects of life does the person want addressed without delay? What are their priorities? Knowing the person's priorities creates an excellent starting point for person-centerd planning. Information gatherers were asked to elicit each person's top 3 priorities for the purpose of this study.

THE FINDINGS OF THE SURVEY

Our research findings showed that, on average, 10 out of the 23 Personal Outcomes were present for people in the study, with a range 0-23. There was no difference on basis of age or gender, but the arrangements in which people lived made a difference, and the type & severity of disability also made a difference. Overall, we found that the level of disability and living arrangements mutually interacted. People with severe /profound level of Intellectual Disability were more likely to live on campus settings (that is, with 10 or more residents) and this group had the lowest number of Outcomes present, that is, seven out of a total of twenty-three.

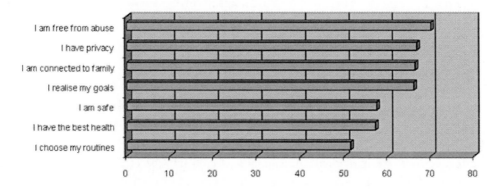

Figure 1. Personal outcomes most often present (%).

The Personal Outcomes which were most frequently present are shown in Figure 1 below. Most participants reported that they were free from abuse, neglect, mistreatment and exploitation (70%), that they had adequate privacy (67%), had enough contact with their families (66%), felt safe (58%) and had the best possible health (62%), while just 51% choose their daily routine.

The Personal Outcomes least often present are shown in Fig 2, these include: people choosing their living arrangements (17%) and work (22%) options, living including working and spending leisure time in an integrated environment (25%), choose personal services such as hairdresser, dentist or doctor (25%), understanding and exercising their human rights (18%). These are also probably challenging areas for most service providers in many other parts of the developed world.

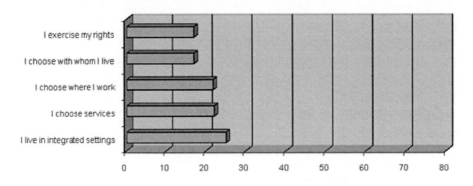

Figure 2. Personal outcomes least often present (%).

Effective Supports

An effective support means supports that the assessor was confident would result in the desired outcome being achieved in the next 6-12 months, depending on the particular outcome in question. Finding a new job or place to live might take much longer than joining a club or arranging a health check-up. The participants in the survey had effective agency supports in place for 10 of the 23 POMS, on average.

Are Outcomes and Organisational Supports Linked?

We found a strong association between Outcomes and Supports, (N=288, SRh = 0.744, sig +0.000). Where the Outcome was present, the support was also likely to be in place. Blanket supports are often not effective, one size does not fit all – individualised supports are more effective. For one individual, the supports offered may be effective, and for another person living in the same house, that level of support may be restrictive.

Priorities

The most frequently identified Priorities by people in the study are:
I choose my own goals – 'I do not want others choosing my goals for me!'

I choose where I work – 'I want to have some options to choose from, just like others'.

I choose where and with whom I live – and find out about what options are available.

I participate in my community – my own community, not just the community of people with disability and their staff.

I have the best possible health.

I want to be treated fairly & learn about exercising my rights, 'rights that are important to me'.

REFLECTIONS ON THE FINDINGS

While no-one's quality of life is perfect or fully to their satisfaction, these findings show that there is much to be desired – we have plenty of work to do to enhance the quality of the lives of people with disabilities in Ireland today. After a period of unprecedented economic growth in the country, 25% of the people in this study had 5 or less of the 23 Personal Outcomes fully present at the time of the study.

What influenced Quality of Life?

People who lived in campus settings and had severe or profound ID generally achieved fewer personal outcomes. In other words, people with more severe disabilities living in larger congregate settings are likely to have a poorer quality of life. This is hardly surprising. They will require more individualised support than others to achieve their personal outcomes. While we cannot change their disability, changing the setting would offer more opportunities for community integration, participation and interaction.

In this study, there was no significant difference based on the size of agency. Smaller agencies were as effective as larger agencies in achieving outcomes and providing effective supports for people. There is probably a trade-off here between the better-resourced larger agencies and more flexible local service. This finding differs from CQL's much larger scale research with 3,630 people from 552 agencies in the United States, which found that people supported by small-to-medium sized agencies (26-200 people) had more outcomes present. (Gardner et al 2005).

Accredited or Not?

At the time of the survey, there were 6 agencies fully accredited with CQL, and the survey showed that these achieved almost twice as many outcomes and supports present as non-accredited agencies. It is likely that the decision to seek accreditation gave a focus to efforts that motivated management and staff, with improved individual planning and responsiveness to addressing people' own priorities. At the end of the day, it is more important that we work consistently to improve people's quality of life, than that agencies get the kudos of accreditation. But, it is clear that seeking accreditation focuses and motivates agencies to support people achieve more personal outcomes.

What if the Person Communicates Differently?

The 22% of people in the survey with severe or profound ID were supported to some degree at the interview by a proxy. The study set out to limit the influence of proxies by having participants always present for at least part of the interview, and encouraged to respond directly using their preferred means of communication, and by using interviewers who were familiar with the person. An Accessible POMS Boardmaker Symbol Pack developed (Accessible POMS Pack 2006) to support POMS, was also available for use by information-gatherers.

How Do We Explain 'I Am Free From Abuse, Neglect, Mistreatment and Exploitation' at 70%?

No outcome was fully present for everyone in the survey. Outcomes are strictly assessed and any doubt regarding the presence of any aspect, will result in the outcome being considered 'not present'. An example might be where the outcome is present in the service setting, but not in the home or community. Also, possibly in the case of abuse, neglect, past events which have not been fully resolved to the person's satisfaction, may result in the person considering the outcome not present. These are possible factors which may account for the fact that 30% of respondents indicated that they were not fully free from abuse, neglect etc; an additional factor is that this outcome includes mistreatment and exploitation, and physical/verbal abuse by people other than staff, other people using the service, the public.

What is the Value of Measuring Outcomes and Supports?

By creating valid and reliable data, this survey allows agencies to measure progress in a number of ways: mapping individual change, monitoring organisational progress over time, comparisons with national and international data to identify relative strengths and challenges, as a check on internal organisational systems and checking of effectiveness of person-centerd planning systems. In this way, POMS data can fulfil a range of mapping, monitoring and verifying functions within an agency, giving the management team continuous data to evaluate organisational systems and agency effectiveness.

What Are Some of the Challenges for Organisations in Supporting the Person?

Low expectations of the person with disabilities, and devalued social roles;
Duty of care overriding 'dignity of risk' (O'Brien 2007) and the rights of the person;
Family wishes taking precedence over person's wishes;
Medical / Expert model - Professionals knowing best;
Person and staff wanting to please - acquiescence, the 'culture' of agency;
Opinions not being heard, and the person's communication not valued;

Tokenistic opinion-seeking.

What Helps in the Enhancement of Quality of Life of People with Disabilities?

Use the information gathered from the person to drive individualised actions on their priorities.

Use data given by people to plan changes in service delivery, and in re-allocation of scarce resources.

Adopt human-rights based approaches in the agency.

Involve people supported by services in decision-making structures, eg. Case Conferences about the person, and in Rights Review Committee, Workers' Comm, Board of Directors.

Support internal and external Advocacy, including self-advocacy and citizen-advocacy.

Implement supported decision-making assisted by a trusted individual, and ensure support for diverse communication systems.

Make all key information, for example, agency policies accessible to the people whose lives they affect.

Involve people in agency work to influence positive change in community perceptions.

CONCLUSION

Given half a chance, the people in the study were keen and able to talk about their quality of life, and say what was important and a priority for them. Many of their priorities are written into the UN Convention (2006), (Quinn 2006), for example, Article 19 says: 'Parties to this Convention recognise the equal right of all persons with disabilities *to live in the community* **with choices equal to others.** 'Persons with disabilities have the opportunity *to choose their place of residence and where and with whom they live* **on an equal basis to others***, and are not obliged to live in a particular living arrangement'*.

When POMS is used in individualised, person-directed planning approach and used in organisational development, it can impact strongly on the responsiveness of the agency and hence, enhance the quality of life of individuals with disabilities.

'As parents and family members, we expect our son to have a good life; when he wants to do wilder things, supported to do them as safely as possible; we need your support and expertise to help us let go and let him really live'.

Jim, the parent of a man with severe ID and autism.

And some final words from John's story:

The way I look at it ...
There's a guy I live with that shouts at me a lot.
He bangs on my door.
I don't like that but I try not to pay any heed.
He's being at that for many years.

I don't like it
I want to tell my story.
The way I look at it....
They said I will be moving out soon to a place with no stairs.
I'll do what I want to do then - I'd like that...
Sometimes I'm afraid when I think about leaving. When I'm in my own place I could catch the bus - to go to work.
I want to tell my story.

These findings are presented very briefly here, for further information and discussion, the full report, including an Easy-Read version, is available on www.outcomestopeople.ie and in a forthcoming article in the British Journal of Learning Disabilities issue late 2009.

REFERENCES

The Council on Quality and Leadership (CQL), www.thecouncil.org . Gardner, J.F. & Carran, D.T. (2005), Attainment of Personal Outcomes by People with Developmental Disabilities'. J. of Mental Retardation, 43, 157-174 www.thecouncil.org

Kendrick, M. (2000) 'When People Matter More than Systems' www.kendrickconsult.net

Mc Cormack, B. & Farrell, M. (2007) The Quality of Life of People with Disabilities in Ireland in 2007'. www.outcomestopeople.ie

O'Brien, P. (2007) 'Supporting Families to support Self-determination'. Paper delivered at Delivering Outcomes to People Conference, Ireland.

Quinn, G. (2007). 'The UN Convention on the Human Rights of Persons with Disabilities'. Paper delivered at Delivering Outcomes to People Conference, Ireland.

Speech and Language Therapy Accessible Information Working Group (2006). Accessible POMS Pack. Email: sltaccessibleinfo@gmail.com

Schalock, R. L., Gardner, J. F. & Bradley, V. J. (2007) Quality of Life for People with Intellectual and other Developmental Disabilities. Pg. 162. American Association on Intellectual and Developmental Disabilities.

United Nations (2006). Convention on the Rights of Persons with Disabilities.

APPENDIX 1. PERSONAL OUTCOME MEASURES 2005

MY SELF

I am connected to natural support networks.
I have intimate relationships.

I am safe.

I have the best possible health.
I exercise my rights

I am treated fairly.

I am free from abuse and neglect.

I experience continuity and security.
I decide when to share personal information.

MY WORLD

I choose where and with whom I live.
I choose where I work.

I choose my daily routines.*

I have time, space and opportunity for privacy.*
I use my environment.

I live in integrated environment

I interact with other members of the community.

I perform different social roles.

I choose services.

MY DREAMS

I choose personal goals.
I realise personal goals.
I participate in the life of the community.
I have friends.
I am respected.

Chapter 48

Getting by Better with Help From My Friends -Social Capital and its Contribution to Lives of Irish People with Intellectual Disabilities

M. Farrell

Delivering Outcomes to People Project & St. Michael's House, Dublin

Introduction

What is Social Capital? - 'Social Capital refers to ….The connections among individuals – their social networks and the norms of reciprocity and trustworthiness that arise from them', The core idea of social capital theory is that 'social networks have value', 'It is the glue that binds communities together', according to Putnam (2000) in his seminal work on the topic - Bowling Alone: The Collapse and Revival of American Community. It refers to 'The networks together with shared norms, values and understandings that facilitate co-operation within or among groups'. (OECD, 2000). As stated in the Irish Health Strategy, Quality and Fairness - A Health System for You 'Strong social support contributes to health by providing people with emotional and practical resources.' (Irish Health Strategy, 2001). The National Economic & Social Forum (NESF)(2003) in Ireland, describes key aspects of Social Capital, as:

Having regular contact with other people,
Feelings of mutual obligation,
A willingness to reciprocate,
Engagement in your community,
Volunteering,
A shared sense that you can effect change in your community, and
Having trust in institutions.

The NESF Report (2003) that some groups of people in modern society are 'at risk' from being disadvantaged from accessing social capital, including the aging population, people living in rural and large urban centers, lower socio-economic groups, those who are disabled and those engaged in home duties.

The Synergy view of social capital attempts to connect the network and institutional approaches by recognising …'the potential complementarity of state institutions to social networks, and the impact of institutional performance on networks embedded in those institutions'. Woolcock and Narayan (2000). 'Social Capital can help mitigate the insidious effects of socio-economic disadvantage'. The work environment is a very positive venue for building social capital and creating opportunity for establishing better social networks. Putnam (2000).

Braddock and Parish (2001) state that 'The disability rights struggle of the first half of the 21st century will fundamentally be a struggle to delink the enduring and oppressive relationship between poverty and disability', with both factors driving inequality and, the relevance in this paper, is in the resulting negative effect on the stores of Social Capital that the person with Intellectual Disabilities (ID) can access. The person with ID, generally has limited access to other sources of 'capital', such as intellectual capital through education or financial capital other than through inheritance.

So, Do People with ID Have Good Stores of Social Capital? Or Can They Be Supported to Increase Their Stores of Social Capital?

Types of Social Capital

Bonding Social Capital

Bonding Social Capital is what we have with people who are similar to us and already are part of our social circle, family of origin, life-long friends and neighbours.

Bridging Social Capital

Bridging Social Capital is the type we have from our relationships with others, who are less like us, and who exist outside our typical social circle, often accessed through the workplace.

Linking Social Capital

Linking Social Capital.refers to ' vertical dimension' of bridging social capital, referring to ties between different social strata of wealth and status and key to leveraging resources, ideas and information from formal institutions beyond the immediate community.

People with ID have little access to 'Bridging Social Capital (CQL 2005), but they often have strong Bonding Social Capital, through their families of origin, where the person with ID sometimes is as dependent recipient, and frequently is not a reciprocal partner. The person can _treated_ as the 'eternal child'.

Baron and colleagues (2001) state that: 'People with ID have access to mainly special forms of Social Capital with little access to the forms, which enable the transition to full adult status' including: Employment, Independent living, Intimate personal relationships, Self-selected reference groups. These strong, asymmetrical, non-reciprocal forms of bridging social capital, do not enable the negotiation of 'risk' – which these authors term 'the key to current social life'.

Gardner (2003) states 'Promoting choice and connections to the community and relationships, help to promote and sustain the basic protections of health, safety and wellness, finding that there was 'No negative relationship between the personal outcomes related to quality of life and social capital and those of the basic assurances of health, safety and wellness'.

Informally, people with ID often tell us in their planning / review meetings that they would like more friends and more contact with existing friends, more contact with people outside of the service circle, that they experience loneliness and isolation, they want to get out more often to places of their choice. People often want more involvement in their wider community, for example, through work, social contact, and less isolation. Many people with ID have limited valued social roles in their communities, have limited social networks and many people are separated from their natural support networks, i.e. family members and other close ties. Services, while providing generally safe environments, can sometimes erode or block opportunities for people to really engage with their community, in our efforts to protect people and occupy their time.

THE PURPOSE OF THIS STUDY

The purpose of this preliminary small-scale study was:

- To explore the contribution of Social Capital for people with ID using a personal outcomes approach in an Irish context.
- To see how people with ID, apparently at the forefront of opportunity in their communities, fare on the Social Capital front as measured on various tools.
- To provide direction for service providers in 'how-to' maximise benefits and highlight the contribution of Social Capital to people with ID in an Irish context.
- To look 'through the Social Capital lens'.

METHODOLOGY

Survey Instruments

The study used two instruments to gather data:

(i) Personal Outcome Measures (POMs)
Personal Outcome Measures (POMs) were developed by the U.S.-based Council on Quality & Leadership (CQL, 1997) and validity and reliability were reported on in two U.S. surveys (Gardner et al, 1997; Gardner & Carran, 2005). The survey instrument has 25

indicators or 'Personal Outcome Measures'; the present survey used a subset of 9, which specifically addressed the social capital area. (Table 1).

Table 1. POMS: A subset of the 25 POMS used in this study

I choose where and with whom I live
I choose where I work
I am connected to my natural support network
I live in an integrated environment
I participate in the life of my community
I interact with my community
I perform social roles
I have friends
I am respected

The survey elicited information on:

Which of these 9 personal outcomes are fully present for this person at this time?

The scoring of each POM is based on information gathered from the person and from whoever knows them best, as well as from observations and (if necessary) from existing documentation. The information gathering process for the subset of 9 POMS used in this study normally takes about 90 minutes, but may take longer where follow-up calls or visits are deemed necessary. The data collector then reviews the information gathered and determines whether a particular outcome is fully present or not, based on a set of model questions. Determinations regarding outcomes are based on stepwise decision questions (e.g. 1.Does this person have friends? 2. If not, is this through personal choice? 3. Does the person have enough friends? 4. Does the person have enough contact with their friends? If the answer to Q.3 & 4 is yes, the Outcome is present.)

(ii) National Economic and Social Forum's Social Capital Survey (NESF 2003)

This Survey consists of a 20-Item Questionnaire, devised originally by the project group on Social Capital of the National Economic and Social Forum, (NESF 2003) as a national household consumer survey in Ireland in 2002, as referenced in The Policy Implications of Social Capital (NESF 2003). The purpose was to take a quick picture of some key dimensions of the concept of Social Capital, using the following:

1. Community engagement and volunteering;
2. Community efficacy;
3. Political and civic participation;
4. Informal social support networks/sociability; and
5. Norms of trust and reciprocity.

The survey instrument was used in this preliminary study, with permission of the NESF, to obtain further information on Social Capital using a nationally recognised tool, which had already been used with an Irish population and could therefore be used comparatively. This instrument was conducted by the researcher verbally, immediately after the POMS information was gathered, and scored using the weighting variable supplied.

Subjects

The subjects consisted of a group of 14 people with ID supported by a large ID services provider in Dublin city, who were at the forefront in terms of opportunity and level of independence in accessing community involvement. All were selected on basis of being relatively independent, communicative, and keen to talk about their experiences.

A total of 9 adults were in the 30-50 years, who were living at home or community houses (maximum 6 residents) owned by the agency, and in supported employment 5 hours+ per week. The other 5 were young adults aged 18-20 yrs, who were attending or had attended mainstream primary and secondary school, at college or working independently, and were all still living at home with parents.

All 14 subjects were competent communicators and there was no involvement of proxies. Consent was sought from all to participate through supported decision making, with no significant communication issues. All consented to participate.

Findings

This section contains a summary of the main findings of this small-scale, preliminary study, with the more details in the full report available on request from the author.

(i) Data Set 1 - Personal Outcomes Measures

In the sample, shown in Figure 1, just one person had all 9 POMS fully present, with one having 8 POMS present, spread across the younger group still in education and those having supported employment. The most frequently present POM was People are Connected to their Natural Support Network, usually considered family and extended family at 93%, (85% of the sample had lived in their current home all their lives, which *may* account in part for this outcome being present for many). People Choose where they Work (85%), and People Choose where and with whom they Live (78%) were also most often present. The POMS least often present were People Live (*and* Work and spend Leisure Time) in Integrated Environments (43%), People have Friends, (including number, type and frequency of contact) 43%, and People are Respected (50%).

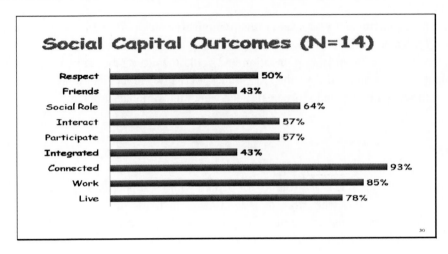

Figure 1.

(ii) Data Set 2 - National Economic and Social Forum's Social Capital Survey (NESF 2003)

The following is a short overview of the results of the NESF Survey:

When asked, 64% said they felt isolated, for reasons including not having enough friends in the first place, others being too busy to meet them or 'pretending' to be too busy, transportation difficulties, not being allowed/or being afraid to go out at night.

ACTIVE COMMUNITY INVOLVEMENT AND VOLUNTEERING

Figure 2 shows the levels of Active Community Involvement and Volunteering defined as follows:

(A) Take Part = Take a regular part in any type of unpaid voluntary activity or service outside the home or workplace in the past 12 months, as participant.

(B) Actively involved in any type of voluntary or community group in the past 12 months, taking on a specific role or function.

Much of the Volunteering activity reported by people, was with disability-related groups, eg. Special Olympics and ARCH Social Clubs.

Civic Engagement included the % of people, who in the last year engaged in the following:

Attended a public meeting;

Joined an action group of any kind;

Contacted an appropriate organisation to deal with a particular problem (Co. Council, residents association);

Contacted a local politician, public official, or local representative; or

Made a voluntary donation of money e.g. to charities, school, church.

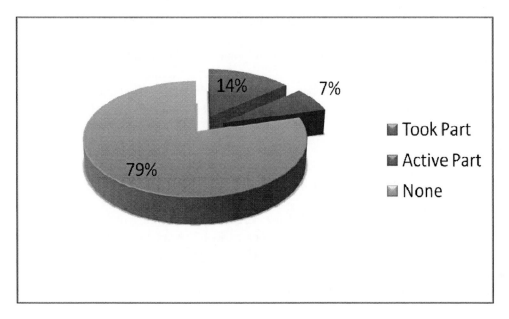

Figure 2.

Figure 3 showed that the sample in this study did not differ greatly, other than making a donation, from the National Consumer Sample reported by the NESF Survey (2003).

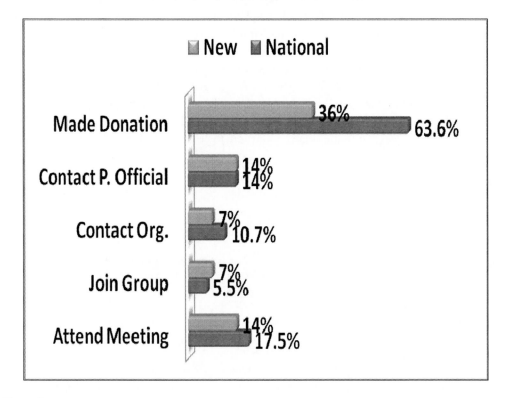

Figure 3.

Informal Social Contact over the previous 4 weeks period, was reported as follows:

(a) Made a social visit to someone in their home other than family member or relative = 36%
(b) Received a visit from someone at home other than family member or relative = 43%
(c) 57% reported have neither made or received a social visit, from other than family/relative, over the period.

SOCIAL SUPPORT NETWORKS

Social Support Networks identified the percentage of people with 3+ Close Friends - defined as people you feel at ease with, can talk to about personal matters, share confidence, seek advice or call on for practical help, including Neighbours, Work Associates, Relatives, others. In the sample, 36% reported less than 3 close friends in any of the categories, with 14% or 2 individuals reporting no Informal Social Contact or Social Support Network of 3 or more close friends.

Combined Sets of Data

The 9 POMS and the NESF Social Capital Survey, were examined together, and, while caution is necessary given the very small numbers and the exploratory nature of the study, there are some points of note. The 3 people with the lowest number of POMS present, were also those who reported no Active Community involvement, minimal Civic Engagement and no Informal Social Contact in the previous 4 weeks. All indicated in their POMS that they would like more frequent social contact and a greater degree of social/community engagement. 'I'd like to have more contact with people who don't have a disability', 'I'd like to be able to meet up with friends from the centre or work after work and at weekends', I don't go out at the weekend, I don' t have anywhere to go and I get into town anyway'.

Comments From Participants and Families

'She's built in(to this community) like bricks in the wall'.
'I have so many friends, I don't know what to do!'
'They treat me ordinary here (in work), just like anyone else, not 'special'.'
One person's perceptions of the value of Volunteering: 'I wouldn't Volunteer, my Mam says: 'If you work for nothing, you'll never be idle!'
'Special Olympics is my life!'
'I don't do things with friends from work after work'.
'If we weren't there at Mass or the pub, people would say: 'Where are they?' and they'd ask us the next week.'
'Friends are important to have, be nice, no fighting, no bad names'.
'Some people talk down to me, like I'm invisible. Once my dad's friend gave me a balloon – I was 18 years old!'.

Some Reflections on Findings

This small-scale exploratory study yielded useful information about the lives of these 14 people with ID considered to be at the forefront of this population, relatively speaking, in terms of their level of independence, community opportunities and inclusive experiences. Information included aspects of personal outcomes about choice, affiliation to and engagement in their community, and the social networks and supports people have or accrued in their lives thus far. A key concept of this approach is, that the information is firmly based on what people themselves had to say. The low level of active engagement in communities, in which many people lived a long time, and the fact that people said they would like more engagement, gives cause for concern. Also, the fact that much of the engagement was within 'special' groups with membership largely restricted to people with ID, is of concern. This concurs in with the literature on the 'strong, asymmetrical, non-reciprocal bonding social capital', referenced by Baron and colleagues (2001), which does not facilitate the 'negotiation of risk' and the transition to real adulthood.

Even where agencies have a strong community base, efforts still are largely to provide services 'within walls', with special activities, special buses, special places, and 'groups' of people with disabilities. Services have to strive to ensure that opportunities are deliberately nurtured and individualised to maintain old or weak networks and create new social networks and non-traditional connections for the person in a range of immediate and wider environments. The Social Capital literature suggests the need for 'generalised reciprocity' (Putnam 2000); for agencies in the disability sector, this may mean greater reciprocity between the provider and local communities, greater use of generic services, as well as nurturing more individualised opportunities for people to contribute to their communities, for example, volunteering in local Tidy Towns Committee or residents associations.

People with ID, who are more independent, well-supported by their families, and at the forefront of opportunity, through mainstream education and having ordinary paid work, are often not priority for providers over people with higher support needs, and the view may be that, given resource demands and competing priorities, these people 'can do it for themselves' with family. But a small, individualised budget can a long way....

The organisation needs to reformulate its role from 'services provider' to being a 'bridge' for people into their community. O'Brien in the 90's states: 'Services choosing to act like a ***bridge*** supporting people to access communities instead of walls that divide communities'. Gardner et al (2007).

Social capital contributes to our efforts on reformulating organisational roles. Disability organisations, like other bridging organisations in the community, can enhance networks and social capital for people. The Synergy Model – proposed by Woolcock & Narayan (2000), suggests the need for agencies to engage in increased reciprocity with community resources and service networks in their external environment, with agencies needing to adopt a 'Facilitator Role' seeking to *compliment* community supports and the person and their families' own resources.

CONCLUDING COMMENT

There are strong indicators that, not only is the concept of Social Capital very relevant to people with ID, there are strengths and also gaps in the social networking and variety of opportunities people have, for making a contribution, and engaging in and building reciprocal social supports in their local communities. According to the literature, those with high stores of Social Capital, there is a net benefit over time on their physical and emotional health and well-being, leading to positive outcomes on their quality of life. Therefore, service providers need to be aware of the 'social capital lens', and be cognisant of these net benefits to the people they support, and that the services we develop, and strive to promote opportunities for people to cash-in on these benefits, while helping them to stay healthy..

SOME WAYS TO BUILD YOUR SOCIAL CAPITAL[*]:

Draw up a diagram of your own social network, and help people supported to draw diagrams of their own social networks. Who do you have strong ties with? Are these reciprocal? Look at weak ties? How do these link you in with new networks and different experiences? Help people identify people they have lost contact with, and with whom they would like to try to re-connect. Help people find out names and addresses of people they have weak ties with and identify new opportunities.

Many people with disabilities are time rich. What about talking to a local Community Forum about setting up a Time - Bank? (Figure 4).

Go out and explore the local community for new, untapped resources.

Appreciate the Value of Volunteering in a Consumerist world – talk to Volunteering Ireland

Look at policies and procedures in your agency through the 'social capital lens'. Does the policy/procedure help to build social networks? Or is it, inadvertently, blocking or even damaging opportunities for building social ties?

Get involved in Neighbourhood Watch, Tidy Towns schemes / Residents Associations – many people supported are very observant and could have a lot to offer their community in this role.

Take in the garbage bins off the road for your neighbours, who are out all day, if you live in a residential area.

Offer your services as a volunteer at a local nursing home.

Offer your day unit to the local resident's committee to meet in at night.

Go to the local shops regularly. And visit local (farmer's) markets.

Offer your unit bus to a local community group during your quiet times.

Tell Luas Ltd. how this new local train service helps you to get around now.

Say 'Hello' to people, staff and customers in the local shops, get to know the staff by name.

Be aware (and supportive) of opportunities for staff to build social capital in the local community & workplace.

---

[*] Abridged from an Information Leaflet 'What is Social Capital? And Where can I get some?', produced by the Delivering Outcomes Project 2008 and available from www.outcomestopeople.ie

Use local, generic services where possible, local GP, dentist, pharmacy, local hairdresser.
If you're invited into someone's house, GO!
If you like animals, offer to walk the neighbours' dog, or feed their cat or goldfish, while
    they're away.
Go to local community meetings.

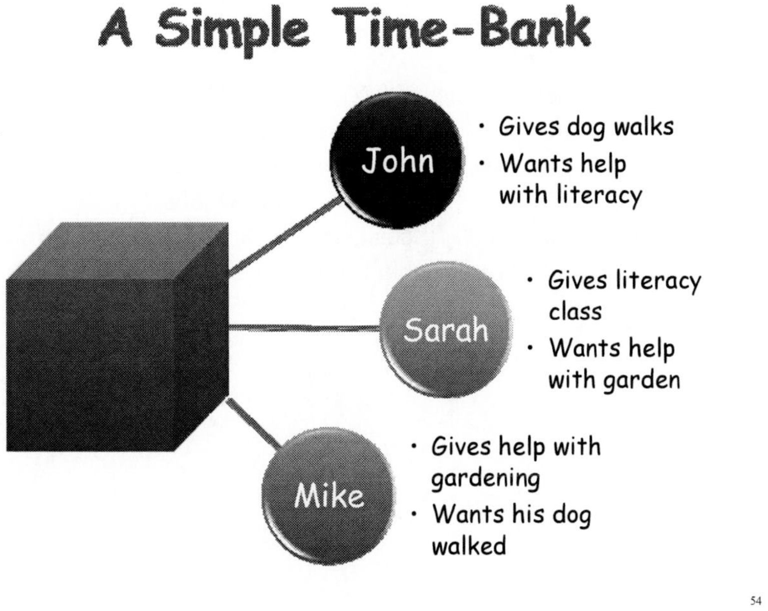

A Simple Time-Bank

Figure 4.

If you have other ideas, please forward them to the author!

REFERENCES

Baron, S., Field, J. , Schuller, T. (2001) in Social Capital: Critical Perspectives. P 252-253.
    Oxford University Press.

Braddock, D.L., and Parish, S.L. (2001). 'An Institutional History of Disability' pgs 45-50 in
    Albrecht, G., Seelman, K., Bury, M. Editors. Handbook of disability Studies. Sage
    Publications.

CQL (2005) Social Capital Index on www.thecouncil.org

Gardner, JF., Nudler, S. & Chapman, M. (1997) 'Personal Outcome Measures of Quality'.
    Mental Retardation, 35, p. 295-305.

Gardner, J. (2003) Capstone. www.thecouncil.org

Gardner, J. F. & Carran, D. (2005) Attainment of personal outcomes by people with
    developmental disabilities. *J. AAMR*, 43, 157-174.

Gardner, J (2007) in Schalock, R., Gardner, J. & Bradley, V. (2007) Quality of Life for
    People with Intellectual and other Developmental Disabilities. AAIDD.

National Economic & Social Forum's Social Capital Survey Instrument. Healy, T.(2003) Social Capital: Challenges for its Measurement at International Level. NESF. Government Publications.

O'Brien, John, (1991) http://soeweb.syr.edu/thechp/sgbcontr.htm

OECD (2000a) Report on The Well-Being of Nations, The role of Human and Social Capital, Centre for Educational Research and Innovation. Paris. OECD.

Personal Outcome Measures (2000). The Council on Quality and Leadership in Supports for People with Disabilities. Maryland.USA. www.thecouncil.org

Putnam, R. D. (2000) Bowling Alone – The collapse and Revival of American Community. Simon & Shuster. New York.

Quality and Fairness – A Health System for You (2001) The Health Strategy. Dept of Health and Children. Government Publications Office. Dublin.

The Policy Implications of Social Capital: Forum Report No. 26 (2003). National Economic and Social Forum. Government Publications Office. Dublin.

Woolcock, M. & Narayan, M. (2000) 'Social Capital: Implications for Development Theory, Research and Policy'. The World Bank: Research Observer: 15, 225-229.

www.outcomestopeople.ie

Chapter 49

COMMUNITY PARTICIPATION AND THE INFLUENCE OF ENVIRONMENTAL FACTORS

M.M. Verdonschot[1] and L.P. de Witte[1]

[1] Vilans, Center of expertise for long-term care. Utrecht, The Netherlands

INTRODUCTION

Community participation is a major goal for all disabled persons, but one which can be particularly difficult to achieve for adults with an intellectual disability. Over the last thirty years persons with intellectual disability (ID) have increasingly been living in community settings rather than in segregated facilities. Past studies have found that community presence' and enhanced opportunities are more readily attained than actual participation (Myers et al., 1998; Verdonschot et al., 2009).

Participation can be defined as the performance of persons in actual activities in social life domains through interaction with others in the context in which they live, and includes four social life domains: 1) domestic life; 2) interpersonal life; 3) major life areas consisting of education and employment; 4) community, civic and social life (WHO, 2001; Dalemans et al., 2008; van der Mei et al., 2006; Verdonschot et al., 2009). To be able to support people with ID in participating in community as much as possible and desirable, knowledge about factors that enhance participation is important.

THE ROLE OF THE ENVIRONMENT

Present models of disability emphasize the environment as an important determinant of disability. This is true for the World Health Organization (WHO) model (WHO, 2001), the Quebec model (Fougeyrollas et al, 1991) and the model of the American Association of Intellectual and Developmental Disabilities (AAIDD) (Luckasson et a., 2002). The models state that disability cannot be fully understood without consideration of the environmental context. The Quebec model, published by Fougeyrollas and colleagues (1991), was the first to articulate unreservedly how environmental factors influence social participation of persons with disabilities. The AAIDD model explicitly describes functioning in persons with an intellectual disability in five dimensions. One of these dimensions is the context (Buntinx, 2006). WHO's International Classification of Functioning, Disability and Health (ICF) is the most prominent international model advancing the importance of environmental factors. In ICF, environmental factors are considered external to the individual but interact with health conditions to produce disability outcomes at all levels (body structure and function, activities of daily life, participation in society). In the ICF environmental factors are assigned to five chapters: 1) products and technology; 2) natural environments and human-made changes; 3) support and relationships; 4) attitudes; and 5) services, systems and policies.

An important support question, for persons with ID, is how contextual conditions could be improved to achieve a productive, fulfilling and participative life in community.

By now little is known about the impact of environmental factors on participation of people with ID. Verdonschot and colleagues (2009) conducted the first systematic review concerning the influence of environmental factors, as defined in the ICF (WHO, 2001), on the community participation by persons with ID. By conducting a wide search strategy in several databases they could identify a number of environmental factors positively affecting participation, like: opportunities to make choices; variety and stimulation of the environment of facilities; opportunities for resident involvement in policy-making; small residential facilities; opportunities for autonomy; vocational services; social support; family involvement; assistive technology; and positive staff attitudes. Also a number of environmental factors negatively affecting participation were identified: lack of transport and not feeling accepted. Besides those factors, other factors will play an important role in community participation, for example legislation and policies, as part of the domain 'services, systems and policies'. Those environmental factors are mainly described in policy reports, which weren't included in this review (Verdonschot et al, 2009).

According to Verdonschot and colleagues (2009) the identification of the environmental factors, as defined by ICF, was difficult, because the included studies hardly refer to valid conceptual frameworks as a result of which a clear definition of participation and environmental factors was lacking and the studies used different measurement methods. Therefore, the researchers recommended that in future research researchers should try to identify and reach agreement on the range of environmental factors, relevant for community participation by persons with ID, and define a general and valid theoretical framework for identifying environmental factors of influence on community participation by persons with ID. The ICF can be the basis for the framework development, as ICF (WHO, 2002) is the only framework which classifies environmental factors. Furthermore Verdonschot and colleagues (2009) recommended to focus in future research on valid and suitable instruments to assess the influence of environmental factors on community participation by people with ID. The ICF can be recommended as a theoretical backdrop for the development of such instruments. The relevance of the ICF for the field of ID is even more obvious since it has been demonstrated that this framework is compatible with the AAIDD functional model of intellectual disability (Luckasson et al, 2002; Buntinx, 2006).

MEASURING THE IMPACT OF ENVIRONMENTAL FACTORS ON PARTICIPATION

An example of an existing measure of the interaction of person and environment is the Measure of the Quality of the Environment (MQE) – version 2.0 (Fougeyrollas, 1999). Although the MQE provides guidance for features of the environment that apply to participation restrictions for many individuals with disabilities, the specificity often important for homogeneous groups' (e.g. persons with ID) interaction in different environments is not addressed by this measure.

Also Whiteneck (2001) developed a measure; the Craig Hospital Inventory of Environmental Factors (CHIEF). The CHIEF items are scored for the frequency of encountering environmental barriers and the impact of the barriers on participation. The specificity of environmental features that may influence participation in major life activities for persons with one disabling condition is limited, since the item development was based on a heterogeneous group of disabling conditions. In addition, specific environmental facilitators of participation for persons with different impairments are not included in the CHIEF. Thus, the use of CHIEF for studying within-group variability and planning relevant interventions may face some limitations.

Because of the limitations of existing instruments, Vilans, center of expertise for long-term care in the Netherlands, started to develop an instrument for assessing environmental factors of influence on community participation. The objective of the instrument to develop is to assess the level of community participation of persons with ID and the impact of environmental factors. The outcome should help to assess support needs in the area of community participation. These needs can be the basis for organizing individual support with respect to community participation.

The draft instruments exist of a proxy version and a client version. Both versions exists of seventeen items covering all ICF participation domains. Those items assess the level of participation. Each participation item consists of two sub-items: 'Does the person perform the activity?' and 'Would he/ she like to change the current level of engagement?'. In all participation items the answering categories are similar. The first sub-item can be answered by: (1) no; (2) yes, with help from other persons and/ or assistive technology;(3) yes, independently. Per item examples are given. The second sub-items can be answered by 'No' or 'Yes'.

Each restriction in participation can be caused by several specific environmental factors. Therefore nine modules with a series of environmental factors of influence on a particular participation domain are developed. Each module is linked to one of the seventeen participation items.

Each module contains a number of specific environmental items. Items are based on ICF environmental factors (WHO, 2001), other instruments with similar objectives such as: MQE (Fougerollas et al., 1999); CHIEF (Whiteneck, 2001); LIFE-habits (Fougerollas et al., 1998); IMPACT© (Post et al., 2008), and contributions of persons with ID and experts in the field. Per item examples are given. For all items scores are similar. Each item can be answered in three steps.

When a person responds to a participation item that he or she wants improvement on that specific participation domain, the modules linked to this item should be completed to evaluate the role of the present environment in this process.

A small pilot was organized to evaluate the draft instrument. Twenty adult persons with a mild or moderate ID ($35 < IQ < 70$) administered the client version and for each client two support assistants administered the proxy version. Additionally both client and support assistant administered a feasibility questionnaire. For both proxy and client version the feasibility and score distribution were analyzed. Based on the results the participation items of the instrument seem promising. The modules with environmental items need further improvement.

In the light of these results the authors suggest further development of the instrument. An important step in this process is to develop a digital version of the instrument. This will offer several opportunities for further improving feasibility, such as the possibility of personalizing items, eliminating items that are not applicable, giving additional information when needed and summarizing results. Furthermore, a digital version offers opportunities to save results.

The development of the above mentioned instrument can be seen as an important step in the process of improving community participation in persons with ID.

ACKNOWLEDGMENT

Information on the instrument and the further improvements is available at Vilans, center of expertise for long-term care: Manon Verdonschot, m.verdonschot@vilans.nl.

REFERENCES

Buntinx W.H.E. (2006). The relationship between the WHO-ICF and the AAMR-2002 system. In Switzky H. & Greenspan S. What is Mental Retardation? Ideas for an Evolving Disability in the 21st Century (p.303-323). Washington: AAIDD

Dalemans R. J. P., de Witte L., Wade D.T. & Van den Heuvel W. (2008). A description of social participation in working-age persons with aphasia: a review of the literature. *Aphasiology*, 22, 1071–91

Fougeyrollas, P. (1991). The handicap creation process. *ICIDH International Network* (4) 1-2.

Fougeyrollas, P., Noreau L., Bergeron H., Cloutier R., Dion S.A., St-Michel G. (1998). Social consequences of long term impairments and disabilities: conceptual approach and assessment of handicap. *International Journal of Rehabilitation Research*, 21, 127-41

Fougeyrollas, P., Noreau, L., St Michel, G., & Boschen, K. (1999). *Measurement of the quality of the environment. V2.0.* Lac St. Charles, Canada: INDCP

Luckasson, R., Brotwick-Duffy, S., Buntinx, W., Coulter, D., Craig, P., Reeve, A., Schalock, R., Snell, M., Spitalnik, D., Spreat, S. & Tassé, M. (2002). *Mental retardation: Definition, classification, and systems of support.* Washington: American Association on Mental Retardation.

Myers F., Ager, A, Kerr, P., Myles, S. (1998). Outside looking in? studies of the community integration of people with learning disabilities. Disability & Society 13, 389-413.

Post, M.W.M., Witte, de L.P., Reichrath, E., Verdonschot, M.M.L., Wijlhuizen, G.J., & Perenboom, R.J.M. (2008). Development and validation of IMPACT-S, an ICF-based questionnaire to measure activities and participation. *Journal of Rehabilitation Medicine*, 40.

Van der Mei , S.F., Krol, B., Van Son W.J., De Jong, P.E., Groothoff, J.W., Van den Heuel, W.J.A. (2006). Social participation and employment status after kidney transplantation: a systematic review. *Quality of Life Research*, 15, 979-994.

Verdonschot, M.M.L., de Witte, L.P., Reichrath, E., Buntinx, W.H.E., Curfs, L.M.G. (2009). Community participation of persons with an intellectual disability. A review of empirical findings. *Journal of Intellectual Disability Research*, 53, 303-318.

Verdonschot, M.M.L., de Witte, L.P., Reichrath, E., Buntinx, W.H.E., Curfs, L.M.G. (2009). Impact of environmental factors on community participation of persons with an intellectual disability: a systematic review. *Journal of Intellectual Disability Research*, 53, 54-64.

Whiteneck, G.G. (2001). Validated measures of participation and the environment from the Craig Hospital: CHART and CHIEF. Paper presented at UN International Seminar on the Measurement of Disability, New York, June.

World Health Organization (WHO) (2001). International Classification of Functioning, Disability and Health (ICF). Geneva: WHO.

Chapter 50

PERSONS WITH INTELLECTUAL DISABILITIES AS SUBJECTS IN THEORY AND PRACTICE OF DIACONAL WORK

H.P. Meininger

Faculty of Theology, VU Unverist Amsterdam, The Netherlands

INTRODUCTION

Protestant churches in European welfare states have almost entirely lost sight of persons with intellectual disabilities (ID) as a target group of their diaconal work. Most governments have completely taken over care and support formerly in hands of churches and church affiliated organizations. Yet, the view of persons with ID as mere objects of diaconal care is still very much part of church thinking and the activities of local diaconal work. That kind of thinking easily returns in full force if political or economic circumstances change. The question then is what role persons with ID could play if they are viewed and approached as subjects in diaconal work and not merely as objects. In answering this question I will first make some remarks about views on church diaconal activity. Then I will discuss what 'being a subject' means in this context. Finally, I will summarize some implications of these reflections.

DIACONAL PARADIGM

The German practical theologian Herbert Haslinger (1996) has explored prevailing views in Protestant diaconal theory and practice from three points of view: from the "outside" point of view of society, from the "inside" point of view of church and theology and finally from the point of view of those at whom diaconal activities are directed. Attention to the last group seems in particular to be lacking almost entirely in existing diaconal theory and practice. This leads him to the conclusion that the usual diaconal practice is grafted on to a model in which those helping are subjects and those in need of help objects.

Both diaconal theory and practice are thus permeated by the interests of those helping. This helping plays a confirming role with respect to both society and the church. From the viewpoint of society, it is a stopgap that perpetuates unjust structures. From viewpoint of the church, it sometimes had the function of 'winning souls' and is nowadays increasingly acquiring the function of legitimating the church's existence vis-à-vis secular society. But at the same time, in the perspective of most churches diaconal work is viewed as a marginal phenomenon to which generally less significance is attributed than to the proclamation of the Gospel and to worship. The marginality of diaconal work leads to people in need being seen increasingly as deviant and infirm beings. In this way, the social stigmatization to which they are subject in society reproduces itself within the churches.

However, Haslinger also gives examples – often taken from personal contacts with persons with ID - of actual respect for the other in need and of a solidarity that does not remain detached. In the analysis of these examples he finds that the subject status of people in need can only be restored if diaconal work is oriented to the stories of the people in need themselves. On that basis he formulates a number of fundamental criteria regarding diaconal activity.

BEING A SUBJECT IN DIACONAL ACTIVITY

'Being a subject' in diaconal activity is not the same as being a subject in the current sense of full citizenship: mature, vigorous, self-determining, bearing rights, independent. Being subject in the diaconal-theological sense rests on a different concept of humanity, where being human is viewed as the existence of an individual before the face of God. Being human is thus always an existence in relationship with the other, with God and with human beings. Diaconal activity must therefore also be intersubjective activity, not a relationship in which the one party always stands on the receiving end and the other on the giving, not a relationship in which one sets the norm and the other can be said to have been "helped" if he also meets the norm. In short, it is not to be structured as a subject-object relationship. Such diaconal activity is not directed at an 'object' but at a goal, namely that the good news of God's Kingdom becomes continually more visible and tangible in the social lives of people.

Based on this principle of diaconal work as an intersubjective process focused at the subject status of human beings, Haslinger's criteria for diaconal action can be elaborated more specifically in three closely associated aspects of a diaconal relationship with persons with ID: coping, listening and acknowledgement.

DEALING WITH RESISTANCE

Persons with ID do not only have to deal with the functional impediments that their disability entails. They mainly suffer from the way others react to those impediments. Diaconal activities therefore have to display an awareness of the stigmatization and discrimination fostered by existing prejudices. Moreover awareness is needed of the roots these prejudices have in the theologies, the social conventions and the dominant opinions within many churches.

That requires, among other things, that church members have to deal with resistance and ambiguous feelings. Much has been written about coping and acceptance by parents of children with ID. But never has something similar been written about all those others who encounter these children – and later adults. However, for each of these others – whether they be family members, careworkers, volunteers or neighbours – coping and acceptance is also involved. It is vitally important to see this. Many parents have learned to live with their disabled child after a great deal of wrestling but in the process encountered a more or less silent lack of understanding among their fellow church members and pastors.

It would be an important diaconal task to request that attention be paid to the necessity of processes of dealing with ambiguous feelings and learning acceptance in encounters with persons with ID. Persons with ID themselves and their parents can fulfill a counseling role in guiding these processes. Such coping processes can lead to a habit of receptivity and to ways of dealing with the inner resistance in which the ambiguous feelings are not denied but are handled in a way that justice is done to the other.

LISTENING TO THE STORIES

The perspective of those directly involved remains underexposed in many diaconal practices and actually plays no meaningful role in diaconal theory. Haslinger therefore asks that attention be paid to stories of those directly involved, in this case the stories of those with ID and their family members. Diaconal activity is often informed by quite abstract and therefore not very motivational details on the concrete needs of people. A great deal of value is attached to the academic reliability of such details. What is indicated as a problem must also, according to academic standards, be a problem of a nature and extent that legitimizes diaconal activity. However, in such presentations of a situation the lived reality and the own insights of those directly involved is often lost.

Their stories must be told and heard. That requires the willingness to tell and listen and thus certain skills on the part of both narrator and listener. The context of social prejudice and personal resistance is a complicating factor here, because they compel the listeners to force unique stories into existing stereotypes. Persons with ID and their parents then eventually lose the desire to tell their stories. Sometimes, persons with ID need help to express their story. Often, they even are not invited to tell something about themselves and their attempts to tell their own stories are may be cut short or shouted down. They need support in the form of specific – but open – questions. Listeners must also learn to receive subtle nonverbal signals because they often lack the patience and the skills to understand and interpret these signals in the right way.

Helping to tell and to listen could be a task for a diaconate that is directed at being subject and at people living together before the face of God in view. In that case the diaconate would direct itself primarily to the stories of those who can hardly speak or whose voices can scarcely be heard.

ACKNOWLEDGING THE GIFT

The growth towards subject status is entirely dependent on the acknowledgement of this subject status by others. We receive who and what we are, our personal and our social identity, from one another. This interdependence is underestimated or even ignored in the notion of civil subject or citizenship, but it is essential for the subject that lives before the face of God. Acknowledging the other is grounded in the belief that people owe their existence to a God who acknowledges them, takes them seriously and is solidary with them.

The intersubjectivity and the liberating authenticity of diaconal activity should lead to the acknowledgement of the unique contribution that persons with ID make to the celebrating, learning and serving community. It must therefore be acknowledged that persons with ID have something to give – in addition to receiving something. This giving by persons with ID could particularly consist in the continuous invitation their mere presence implies for a transformation in thinking, feeling, willing and acting. Such a transformation can liberate us from our individualism, our rationalism, our one-sided appreciation of the cognitive and our limited interpretations of what passes for faith, usefulness or achievement. Wherever diaconal activity really is intersubjective, it reveals this giving by persons with ID. This, however, can only emerge in personal encounters in daily life: by spending time together, playing together, chatting, going out, celebrating and grieving.

Coping, listening and acknowledging are probably not immediately the first words to occur to us when we think of diaconal work. But they do reflect the idea that the most important thing diaconal work can do for persons with ID consists in being the kind of community and the kind of people that churches and Christians are supposed to be based on their calling. We truly serve the other when we work incessantly on those changes in our being church and in ourselves that can liberate persons with and without ID to live together before the face of God.

REFERENCES

Haslinger, Herbert (1996). Diakonie zwischen Mensch, Kirche und Gesellschaft. Eine praktisch-theologische Untersuchung der diakonischen Praxis unter dem Kriterium des Subjektseins des Menschen. Würzburg: Seelsorge Echter.

Chapter 51

RELATIONSHIPS BETWEEN PEOPLE WITH AND WITHOUT INTELLECTUAL DISABILITIES IN CONGREGATIONS: A MATTER OF TRANSFERRING SPECIAL KNOWLEDGE?

A. Bernhard

University for Humanistics, Utrecht, The Netherlands

INTRODUCTION

In this chapter I wish to discuss the question to what degree volunteers who are committed to people with intellectual disabilities (ID) in congregations could be provided with special knowledge. My presentation is based on the observations in a workshop developed to experience a kind of inclusive pastoral care.

THE WORKSHOP: EXPLORING LIFE STORY WITH A "BASIC PUZZLE"

In the context of social integration, the Dutch ecumenical platform 'SGGD' started to organize conferences for people engaged in transforming congregations into communities where people with ID can feel at home. To accommodate different professional interests, several taskforces/groups were offered, each concentrating on one feature of congregational life. The workshop mentioned above was developed in the context of the taskforce 'pastoral care'.

This taskforce found significant deficiencies in pastoral care given to people with ID in congregations: they often were not seen as persons seeking some kind of pastoral support, their stories were not heard or understood as stories with unique importance to their own spiritual life of that of their congregations. In order to address this problem, we first conceptualized what inclusive pastoral care should entail: focusing attention on the unique features of a person's individual life story and creating a relationship wherein the person seeking pastoral care feels valued and appreciated. We thought that a workshop would offer useful experimental space to put this concept of inclusive pastoral care into practice.

Knowing that spoken language is not always a useful tool for intellectual disabled people to communicate their experiences, we developed a tool which could help intellectual disabled people and volunteers alike to explore their life stories. We found a theoretical framework in the theory of spiritual guidance by T. v. Knippenberg[1]. This theory contains three elements:

a basic model featuring tensions with time, relationships and transcendence human beings are dealing with in their daily life,

a hermeneutical frame describing several levels how something that is told could be understood,

a methodical framework to initiate and sustain the process of telling and understanding.

Drawing on the basic model, we translated the structures of life into a "basic puzzle" representing the lifecycle. The methodological choice to use big puzzle pieces utilized insights of total communication. The "basic puzzle" could be filled up by pictograms or objects representing the storyteller's main activities. During the workshop we provided the participants with the "basic puzzle", a set of pictograms and various objects. We asked them first to compose their puzzle in small groups and to share their stories with all participants later on, so that in the end one large picture might emerge.

OBSERVATIONS

We presented the workshop on four conferences in different places. In total 64 participants took part, among them 10 people with ID. We had no problems to get people interested for the topic of inclusive pastoral care. All felt comfortable with exploring a life story and came up with very different ways of filling up the puzzle and sharing their stories.

During the process of sorting out pictograms and objects we saw interesting interactions: people with as well without disability started sorting out objects spontaneously. While negotiating the place where objects could be set they showed some kind of mutuality: 'We could do it like this…'. This changed when they used pictograms. People with disabilities quickly recognized pictograms as tools to get things said or done without words. Some of them started immediately to sort out which ones they would like to set in the puzzle. People without disabilities showed more difficulties to understand pictograms. Some of them discussed the meaning of a pictogram in the group, ending up with choosing a place for the pictogram together. Others encouraged people with disabilities to tell them more about it but corrected the place first chosen – even when the man or woman with a disability was protesting. When presenting the findings of the small groups only one out of the twelve small groups let a woman with disability do the job.

When we offered the workshop outside the conferences to a group of volunteers committed to people with disabilities in congregations we found that just a few people were interested in. These people were interested in exploring an unique life story, but rejected to

---

[1] Knippenberg, T. van (2000) Towards Religious Identity. An exercise in Spiritual Guidance. Assen: Van Gorcum.

use the 'language' of pictograms. They asked why they had to learn a new language and why they had to abandon their own symbols or rituals. Although they were committed to welcome people with disabilities in their parishes, they obviously resisted changes associated with it.

INSTITUTION AND CONGREGATION: TRANSFER OR TRANSLATION?

This observation raises the question to what degree we really could transfer special knowledge useful in an institutional setting to the context of a congregation. Both settings have in common that they need a kind of narrativity to value an individual person as an entity, with an unique story of life. Without valuing individual differences a system could become inflexible and inhuman, thereby risking to lose its right to exist.

Otherwise there are some differences: The purpose of an institution is to enhance a client's quality of life by addressing special problems and needs, using a professional (mostly client centered) relationship. The purpose of a congregation or parish is to gather as human beings around the story of God . These communities can be supported by a professional pastor, but most of the work is done by people with very different education, experience and expectations. These regular members can't be expected to act like professional spiritual caregivers in an institution. Accordingly, the concept of relationships with intellectual disabled people will differ: it may not be a client centered relationship, but might very well be a mutual one, where the voices of volunteer and disabled person receive equal weight.

This has consequences for the use of communication tools in relationships. While pictograms have proven useful in answering the communicational needs of intellectual disabled persons in an institutional setting, these are less useful in a congregational setting, as members of the congregation may not understand their meaning and are not necessarily ready to learn something new. They prefer forms of communication that correspond to their own spiritual needs. Accordingly, the effort of sharing each other's life stories requires a kind of double translation: for the parishioners a translation of the pictogram into signs which are useful to them and for disabled persons a translation of the spiritual language into forms they can understand. This translation could provide the participants with a language that enables booth partners to share their individual experiences and to link this with the shared spiritual experience of the community.

CONCLUSION

We started our supportive program with a workshop focusing on exploring the individual life story, intending to follow up with a workshop dealing with the features of a mutual relationship. Reflecting on the observations, we found that it might be more useful to start our program the other way around: first starting with an exploration of communicational and relational tools that volunteers and disabled people could share alike, and then, if necessary, translating these to get the individual life stories heard within the context of a community.

Chapter 52

CHRISTIANS' SOCIAL CONSTRUCTIONS OF DISABILITY

J. McNair
California Baptist University, Riverside, CA, USA

INTRODUCTION

The following is a synopsis of three research projects examining Christian's social constructions of disabilities. The first looks at perspectives of individuals who are church attenders (Cas) and the second church leaders (CLs). These two studies have been published in the Journal of Religion, Disability and Health (JRDH) (McNair, 2007, McNair & Sanchez, 2007). The third study is of adults with intellectual disabilities (ID)(McNair, Soper & McNair, 2008), however, the data provided here is preliminary. The completed study will be submitted to JRDH.

SOCIAL CONSTRUCTIONS

Bogdan and Biklen (1977) stated, "The social construction of disability is based on the theory of social construction, which asserts that meaning is created, learned and shared by people. Created meaning is then reflected in the behaviors, objects and language used by people."

Other aspects of social constructions include notions of "constructed obstacles leading to a lack of inclusion" (Devine, 1997, p 1), "severe economic and social deprivations encountered by disabled people (that) cannot be explained simply with reference to individually based functional limitations" (Barnes, 1995, p 9), disability as a actually a social disadvantage imposed on physiological impairment, resulting in people who "see themselves as pitiful because they are socialized into accpeting disability as a tragedy personal to themselves" (Oliver, 1990, p 82), and disability then, "becomes the primary basis of identification, one which mutes other characteristics (Fritsch, 2004, p 2).

Thus, using the example of Down's syndrome, we might accept the prescriptive nature of society's social construction, that it is a family tragedy, a genetic disorder, it results in severe intellectual disability, people "suffer" from the syndrome, it ruins families, and that the only option is therefore "prevention" through prenatal diagnosis and abortion. In contrast, we might embrace a cultural replacement narrative about Down's syndrome that, 90% of those affected have mild/moderate ID, if they suffer it is largely due to discrimination by society, they tend to be friendly and loving people, and that as a group they are caring and gentle people.

METHODOLOGY

Our interest in completing these three studies was to determine whether people involved in the Christian church might reflect various social constructions. To this end, the three surveys were undertaken. The first used opportunity sampling of attendees (89) of seven local churches in Southern California. The second, contacted a random sample of leaders in churches self-identified as accessible congregations and listed on the National Organization on Disability's website (42 responses, 19% response rate). In the third study, adults with ID attending a church were interviewed (preliminary data is reported based upon 30 respondents from two churches).

RESULTS

Data will be reported in three general categories: "Who are people with disabilities?", "Why do people have disabilities?" and "Issues related to church programs for persons with disabilities." For the purposes of this report, results will be integrated across the three studies.

WHO ARE PEOPLE WITH DISABILITIES?

CAs (33% agree, 37% unsure, 30% disagree) and CLs (36% agree, 31% unsure, 33% disagree) were mixed in their ideas of whether persons with intellectual disability suffer from their disability. CAs were also mixed about whether they should have children of their own (36% agree, 28% unsure, 36% disagree) ,whether AIDs were heroes because of the challenges their disability presents (CAs 57% agree, 22% unsure, 21% disagree and CLs 47% agree, 18% unsure, 35% disagree) or whether adults with ID were angels unaware (CA 54% agree, 22% unsure, 24% disagree and CLs 22% agree, 29% unsure and 49% disagree).

CAs (75%) and CLs (77%) disagreed that persons with ID have a poor quality of life. Those with disabilities also disagreed (57%) although 52% responded yes to the question of whether their disability "makes you sad." CAs (46%) and CLs (64%) thought adults with AID were aware of their disability, that they were created in the image of God (CAs 74%, CLs 100%) and CLs (98%) that those with or without disability are equal in God's sight.

WHY DO PEOPLE HAVE DISABILITIES?

Although church leaders (CLs) felt that families of adults with ID were not selected by God to have a child with ID (62%) Church attenders (CAs) were divided (38% agree, 48% disagree). When asked if God gives someone a disability because there is something special for that person to do, CLs disagreed (63%) while CAs were again divided (45% agree, 38% disagree). Adults with ID also felt there was something special for them to do (80%). Both CAs (89%) and CLs (95%) indicated that a person's disability was not a result of parent's sin. Responses were mixed to the question of whether people have a disability to teach those around them lessons about life (CAs 35% agree, 25% unsure, 40% disagree and CLs 27% agree, 20% unsure, 53% disagree).

Both CAs (73%) and CLs (95%) disagreed that with sufficient faith a person could be healed of their disability. Relatedly, 73% of adults with ID had prayed to be healed of their disability.

Of CAs, 78% did not feel a fetus with ID should be aborted which was supported by 83% of adults with ID who, however, had mixed feelings about having a baby with a disability like their own (41% yes, 55% no and 4 % I don't know). CAs (81%) disagreed with the statement that care of persons with disabilities is the government's responsibility. CAs (80%) also indicated that if a child with disability were born to them, it would not cause them to question their faith.

CHURCH PROGRAMS AND PERSONS WITH DISABILITIES

CLs (36% agree 59% disagree) were mixed about whether lots of training is needed for church ministry. They (90%) also felt congregational members are building relationships, and they (62%) are recruiting persons with disabilities for church membership. CLs (69%) also felt persons with disabilities are given opportunities for leadership in church settings.

Finally, CLs indicated that persons with disabilities, are not expensive to the church (85%), do not drive other members away (95%), do not take excessive time away from other areas of service (100%), are not already saved by virtue of their disability (90%) and that persons with cognitive disabilities have the ability to make a commitment to Christ (100%). Adults with ID (97%) felt they are a part of their church.

SOME GENERAL CONCLUSIONS

There appears to be some confusion in the Christian community about who persons with ID are. One would think, for example, questions of suffering from disability would be understood if churches were working to include adults with ID. The mixed responses to this and other questions may indicate a disconnectedness socially and intellectually with people who have disabilities.

Social constructions (that people with disabilities are heroes, angels, have something special to do, or utilitarian reasons for their disability among others) were evident to some degree in the responses from each of the three groups. The answers from adults with ID must be considered carefully. It is suspected that they may have been told many of the social constructions regarding who they are (heroes, angels, etc.), however, they also may just enjoy the notion of considering themselves such.

Significant lessons might be learned from responses about church programs and persons with ID. Specifically, ministries are largely characterized as not requiring a lot of training, resulting in relationships with congregational members, leading to some level of integration via recruitment, and offer the potential for positions of responsibility. Religious leaders should reflect on the fact that adults with ID are not deemed detrimental to the church, and have the ability to respond in typical ways to Christian church involvement, as well as evidences of spiritual commitment.

REFERENCES

Barnes, C. (1995). *"Cabbage Syndrome": The social construction of dependency*. London, UK: The Falmer Press.

Bogdan, R. & Biklen, D. (1977). Handicapism. *Social Policy, 7(3),* 14-19.

Devine, M. (1997). Inclusive leisure services and research: A consideration of the use of social construction theory. *Journal of Leisurability, 24(2).* RetrievedOctober1,2005,from http://www.lin.ca/resource/html/Vol24/v24n2a2.htm

Fritsch, K. (2004). SuperCrip strikes again: Or mine-body dualism. Conference proceedings, Disability   Studies   Association.   Retrieved,   October1,2005,from http://www.disabilitystudies.net/dsacont2004/fullpapers/fritsch.pdf

McNair, (2007). Christian social constructions of disability: Church attenders. *Journal of Religion, Disability and Health, 11(3),* 51-64.

McNair & Sanchez, (2007). Christian social constructions of disability: Church leaders. *Journal of Religion, Disability and Health, 11(4),* 1-4.

McNair, Soper & McNair, (2008). Christian social constructions of disability: Adults with intellectual disability. Article submitted for publication.

Oliver, M. (1990). *The Politics of Disablement*. NY: Macmillan.

Chapter 53

Enhancing Spiritual Supports and Faith Community Leadership: Unique Opportunities for University Centers on Intellectual Disabilities

W.C. Gaventa

The Elizabeth M. Boggs Center on Developmental Disabilites, UMDNJ, New Brunswick, NJ USA

Introduction

At first glance, the title of this paper and presentation may seem like an oxymoron. Most university based centers devoted to research and training in the field of intellectual disabilities (ID) have rightly been committed to scientific excellence and funded by public or "secular" sources. Their mission is usually defined as strengthening the quality of human services and supports for people with disabilities and their families, a mission that does not relate directly to religious organizations, faith communities, or places that train leaders in those communities. "Scientific" and "religious" perspectives and services have clashed just as often as they have collaborated. Understandings of "professional" practice have assumed that one should separate "professional" roles from spiritual beliefs, or that values and beliefs should be separated from public roles. Those concerns arose from an understandable fear of proselytizing and seeing the ways in which religious perspectives have sometimes oppressed people with disabilities.

There are, however, many compelling rationales for university centers of research and training to include spirituality and spiritual supports. In the west, the values of independence, productivity, integration, and self determination are often cited as central to the mission of research and services. Those values are affirmative answers to core spiritual/philosophical questions of identity (Who am I?), purpose (Why am I?), community (Whose am I?) and power (choice/control.).

Spiritual traditions and faith communities also provide ways in which many people find answers for those fundamental human questions. If professional research and practice is committed to understanding and strengthening the kinds of supports available to people coping with the experience of disability, then university programs have an obligation to help professionals and service providers understand the ways in which spirituality and faith can be utilized to support individuals and their families.

Rationales for including research and training related to spirituality include understanding the ways that beliefs about what is sacred impact people and their decisions, understanding ways that people use faith to find meaning and to cope, understanding ways that religious beliefs and practices shape cultural understandings of disability and responses to disability, understanding ways that spiritual supports impact quality of life, and understanding the ways that spirituality and faith relate to the commitment and motivation of human service professionals and faith communities as they respond to individuals with disabilities and their families.

Viewed from a life span perspective in the lives of people with disabilities and their families, spirituality and faith can also play crucial roles. How do families respond to a birth or diagnosis of a child with a disability? Do religious education programs for all children include children with disabilities? Do the children have the opportunity to included in the rites of passage into adulthood and community membership (e.g., baptism, bar mitzvah, etc.)? How might faith communities assist in helping young adults find jobs or valued roles in community life. How does faith and religion impact the many ethical questions that arise in human and scientific services and supports?

The "public," "secular," or "scientific" core of a university center's mission is, paradoxically, one of its greatest assets in relating to spirituality and faith issues. That can enable it to be a neutral point where different faith perspectives can come together. Leading researchers and educators can also have a great impact on leaders in faith communities by recognizing and affirming the importance of their roles in the lives of people with disabilities and their families. Most university centers also define themselves as "interdisciplinary," a definition that could and should include research and training in spirituality and faith. The impact of spirituality on health and quality of life is receiving great attention in many countries, but little of that has extended into the realm of intellectual disability.

In the United States, a number of University Centers of Excellence in Developmental Disabilities are beginning to develop significant initiatives that recognize and enhance the powerful supports that spirituality, faith communities, and faith community leadership can have in the lives of individuals with disabilities and their families. Some examples include:

1. The Elizabeth M. Boggs Center on Developmental Disabilities, where my role there began with a statewide New Jersey survey of ways that congregations were providing supports and ministries to people with disabilities. That survey led to the formation of a statewide interfaith Coalition for Inclusive Ministries, in which The Boggs Center has served as that very neutral base described above. The Boggs Center has also been accredited as a site for Clinical Pastoral Education, so that seminarians and clergy can join other traineeship programs in learning professional skills in the field of disability. Our Center is working with seminaries in New Jersey and Pennsylvania on ways to include issues related to disability in seminary curriculum. In response to requests and initiatives from two different disability advocacy and support networks, collaborative task forces worked with us to develop resource guides for

congregations in the area of brain injury and autism. (Both resources available on The Boggs Center website:

2. In Arkansas, the University Center there has worked with congregations to develop respite care programs for families and to organize parent support groups. They have hosted meetings and conferences, as other centers have done, that attract congregational leaders (clergy, religious educators, misson coordinators, childhood and youth program leaders) to share ideas, resources, and best practices that can be adopted by faith communities. They discovered that holding training events for parents and families on positive behavior supports in churches attracted and drew more parents than in other settings because families trusted information and training offered in their faith community. (For information, contact David Deere, Director. deereglen@uams.edu).

3. In Kentucky, the Center on Human Development has collaborated with Lexington Theological Seminary on conferences, and, most recently, expanded its Family Mentorship program to include seminary students along the same model used with medical students. (Director: Harold Kleinert, Ed.D., hklein@uky.edu)

4. In Tennessee, the Kennedy Center in Nashville is developing a Religion and Disability program, and finding that there is great interest in faith communities and families in a place where they can come together in an interdisciplinary, interfaith location to share ideas and receive training. (Courtney.taylor@vanderbilt.edu)

As university centers think from a systematic perspective about inclusion of spirituality and faith in its services, areas to consider are:

Links to seminaries and other pre-service training programs in their area, e.g., religious educators.

Inviting faith community leadership to community training initiatives

Including faith communities and its leadership in dissemination.

Providing training and technical assistance to faith communities and leadership as they seek to develop supports for individuals and families.

Including bibliographic and video resources in libraries for use by trainees and community members. There are growing numbers of excellent resources in this area of service, including the 2007 book by Erik Carter from Brookes Publishing Company entitled *Including People with Disabilities in Faith Communities: A Guide for Service Providers, Families, and Congregations.* Video resources could include the excellent documentary, *Praying with Lior* (www.prayingwithlior.com), a documentary about the spiritual gifts of a young man with Down syndrome and the gift of an inclusive faith community.

Developing strategies for assessing the role of spirituality in interdisciplinary, clinical services.

Encouraging research and writing in the area of spiritual supports. One example is project, "*A Space to Listen*," a collaborative research and training project between the University of Aberdeen in Scotland and the nation-wide Foundation for Learning Disabilities.

As university centers in the field of intellectual and developmental disabilities begin to address issues related to spirituality and enhancing community based spiritual supports, there is a growing number of international networks and resources which they can utilize. A number of them are connected through the Taylor and Francis *Journal of Religion, Disability, and Health*. The power of spirituality, faith and spiritual communities in the lives of people with disabilities and their families cannot be ignored as nations seek to enhance rights and community inclusion. The challenge and opportunity for University Centers is for them to help that power be developed and utilized in ways that are helpful to individuals and families, rather than avoiding an important area that can contribute, both positively and negatively, to quality of life.

Chapter 54

FAITH, BIOTECHNOLOGY AND DISABILITY

W.C. Gaventa

The Elizabeth M. Boggs Center on Developmental Disabilites, UMDNJ, New Brunswick, NJ USA

BACKGROUND

In 2000, the National Council of Churches of Christ in the United States voted to convene an ecumenical task force from its member faith organizations to write a new policy statement that would address the growing number of ethical and theological issues arising from new scientific and medical developments in biotechnology. The National Council of Churches had issued an earlier statement in 1986 entitled "Genetic Science for Human Benefit." This 2002 Task Force worked over a three year period. It included representatives from a number of Protestant and Orthodox faith communities. I was invited to be on the Task Force as a clergyperson working in the field of disability, with part of my role to ensure that the policy statement addressed the issues related to disability and the concerns of people with disabilities.

The decision to do a new position statement to guide its member denominations came from an awareness of a wide variety of challenges:

The huge new array of biotechnologies arising from work related to the genome project.

The ways in which traditional understandings of creation are being questioned by experiments that lead to cloning of animals of many kinds.

The tendency towards polarities in which the scientific and religious communities end up not talking to one another, much less collaborating, because of scientific reductionism on the one hand and religious fundamentalism on the other. (One could exchange those adjectives and nouns and still have the same meaning).

New understandings of disability as "diversity" rather than "illness" or "defect," expanding the range of what is considered "normal" in human life.

New powers to prevent the birth of babies with disabilities or conditions of many kinds, leading to the power to "customize" children on the basis of parental preferences.

THE POSITION STATEMENT

The position statement developed is entitled "Fearfully and Wonderfully Made: The National Council of Churches Policy Statement on Human Biotechnologies." It included three sections: Our Theological Self Understanding, The Church's Calling, and Key Challenges for Church Engagement. Disability became one of the lens through which the Task Force explored and defined issues. The following are the portions of the Position Paper relating specifically to disability:

I. Our Theological Self Understanding

(Lines 21-26) Our humility must extend as well to our own limited knowledge of God's infinite design. Human frailties have allowed us too often to define too readily what constitutes "normal" or "whole" or "able-bodied" life. In so doing we relegate many of our sisters and brothers to the status of "other", seeing only their differences, which we call "disabilities," rather than seeing them as those who manifest, like us, reflections of the imago dei (Image of God).

(Lines 46-59) The potential impact of biotechnology on people with disabilities raises profound philosophical and theological questions. Many people living with disabilities have meaningful, productive lives, and would state that the major suffering in their lives comes from the environment and social context: the physical, attitudinal, and social barriers that limit them much more than their disability. Disability is increasingly understood as contextual and as simply one part, not the whole, of a person's identity.

As such, disability then raises questions about what it means to be human: whether disability is seen as defect, disease, or simply a difference in the diversity of humankind, and what it means to be a community that welcomes and supports everyone. Because "disability" can so easily and frequently be a place where we encounter the human capacity to make "one of us" into "the other," it calls for deep commitment to include the voices and perspectives of people with disabilities and their families in the dialogue and decisions about the use of biotechnology in personal, clinical, social, and political contexts.

(Lines 77-84)Thus, in our biblical understanding, our highest dignity as human beings is not individuality in an individualistic sense. It is rather the paradox of sharing with all humans that we are each created uniquely in the image of God: "So God created humankind in his image, in the image of God he created them; male and female he created them" (Genesis 1:27). The belief that every person, no matter what race, nationality, gender, disability, or "genetic makeup" embodies the image of God is a profound declaration of the goodness God intends for all creation

II. The Church's Calling

C. Pastoral Care

Lines 223-261) Individuals and families are faced with ever-increasing possibilities to shape life through use of genetics and biotechnologies. This challenges pastors to adapt traditional roles and skills to a growing variety of places and times where people might struggle with the questions of faith that may arise, or with how to apply their own faith and belief to the decisions they face. Those roles include, but are not limited to:

Pastoral presence at times of decision and crisis, including marriage when issues of genetics arise, decisions about pregnancy and the implications of testing, guilt or blame in relation to those decisions, response to a birth of a child with a genetic condition, support at the times of onset of a genetic disease, and end of life issues related to terminal care.

Pastoral assistance in determining new forms of family and selfhood in relation to new forms of conception and medical treatment as individuals and families struggle to understand the personal, spiritual, and theological questions that are raised.

Pastoral advocacy in the role of assisting individuals and families to acquire needed services or supports, or serving as an interpreter and bridge between the worlds of families, faith, and healthcare. That bridging role can be two ways, helping families to understand the language and perspective of health care professionals and, vice versa, helping health care professionals to understand the questions and feelings of families, particularly in relation to their issues of faith.

Pastoral supports through a community of faith that can be called and empowered to support individuals and families at times of decision, loss, and need. The pastoral role of equipping and empowering a community of faith can be both proactive, through roles of preaching and education, and reactive, in response to particular individuals and families. Chaplains, genetic counselors, and even hospital ethics committees can become part of the larger equipment of the community of faith.

The pastoral role and challenge is thus both large and complex. It is also paradoxical, for it calls upon clergy to know enough about the world of genetics and biotechnology to be alert and proactive, but also humble enough to know what they don't know. The same is true for health care professionals, who are called to know enough about the spiritual and religious implications of their work to be helpful, but also to recognize the complexity and diversity of religious practices and understandings. With humility and mutual respect we look forward to more appreciative collaboration and more effective support between clergy and health professionals.

III. Key Challenges for Church Engagement

(Lines 272-280) Of the many matters we could have chosen, we selected four areas that have been the subject of much current debate. We hold up these four key challenges in light of our understanding of the crux of the matter: (A) stem cell research, (B) disabilities, (C) the conduct of the biotechnology industry, (D) new genetics or old eugenics, and (E) concern for the fabric of the commonweal.

(Lines 301-304) Effective germ line could offer tremendous potential for eliminating genetic disease, bu tit would raise difficult distinctions about "normal" human conditions that would support discrimination against people with disabilities

(Lines 402-437) Perception of Disability

The promise and danger of biotechnology is perhaps nowhere more obvious than the ways it affects people with disabilities and their families. There is no one "disability" perspective on the use of biotechnology, for people with disabilities and their families are first of all people, with different values, theologies, and understandings about the purpose of life and God's call to care for one another. The use of tools and processes declared to be neutral and value free, and designed to relieve suffering, holds great promise when they can support the lives of people with disabilities or alleviate unnecessary pain or suffering. But biotechnology becomes profoundly disquieting to many with disabilities when disabling conditions or predictions are equated with life long suffering, imperfection, or disease. When those personal and social values are combined with the power of technology to prevent the birth of a child with a disability or defect, the possibility of a new eugenics fueled by social values, market forces, and personal choice, rather than official policy, becomes quite real.

Our reflection causes us to challenge the assumptions that everything needs to be "fixed" or "improved" and that we know how best to do this; and that just because something <u>can</u> be done does not mean it <u>ought</u> to be done. Science cannot save us from finitude. The pre-supposition for life and appreciation of the whole human person as an entity argue for society to offer no disincentives to reproduction by and of persons with disabilities, in the absence of deliberate cruelty and undue hardship.

Among the principles that have been identified by those with disabilities which ought to guide application of biotechnologies, and which we affirm are:

(a)   The use of new human genetic discoveries, techniques and practices should be strictly regulated to avoid discrimination and protect fully, and in all circumstances, the human rights of people with disabilities.

(b)   Genetic counseling that is non-directive and rights based should be widely available and reflect the real experience of disability,

(c)   Parents should not be formally or informally pressured by medical, insurance or governmental policy to take prenatal tests or undergo "therapeutic" terminations,

(d)   Organizations of disabled people must be represented on all advisory and regulatory bodies dealing with human genetics,

(e)   The human rights of disabled people who are unable to consent are not violated through medical interventions

IV. New Eugenics or Old Eugenics

(Lines 547-563)Along with consideration of racial and ethnic bias the issue of social class and economics location must be considered. Emerging biotechnologies could become a forceful means of social division with the poor, or near poor, denied the health benefits such technologies may offer others with greater financial means.

As in the case of disability, bias based on race, ethnicity and class have been historically compounded within American society in ways that thwart democracy and scandalize

Christian morality. Left unchecked and unregulated event the bright promise of biotechnologies could be dimmed by their application in ways that foment human misery and social injustice. Such a bleak outcome would lead us as a human race not into an age of new genetics but a return toward a lamentable old eugenics.

The social fabric can be rent or more closely woven by the ways in which our societies meet the challenge of emerging biotechnologies. We believe that it is our Christian duty to address these issues on behalf of the least, lost, and marginalized of our world.

NOTE

The Position Statement can be found on the web and downloaded in its entirety at http://www.ncccusa.org/pdfs/adoptedpolicy.pdf. Other material related to it is at is at: http://www.ncccusa.org/biotechnology. Feedback or comments are welcome and will be passed on to the National Council of Churches.

Chapter 55

Signs of the Times: Interpreting Developments in Spiritual Supports for People with ID through a Theological Lens

W.C. Gaventa

The Elizabeth M. Boggs Center on Developmental Disabilites, UMDNJ, New Brunswick, NJ USA

Introduction

There is a growing awareness of the importance of spirituality in the lives of people with ID and their families and the services which support them. At the heart of the values that shape many services and supports, particularly in the West, are fundamental values that reflect answers to core spiritual questions:

The core question of identity, "Who am I?," is reflected in the value of independence and the changing images of disability from deficit to diversity.

The question of purpose, "Why am I?," is reflected in the values of employment, productivity and contribution.

The question of community and belonging, "Whose am I?," is reflected in the values of inclusion and integration.

The question of power and capacity, "What control do I have?," is in the values of choice and self determination.

It has not been easy for professional service providers to integrate spiritual needs, desires, and services in their work for a number of reasons. For decades, professional identity has assumed a separation from one's own belief or faith system, a separation based with good cause on fear of proselytizing. But there is a growing awareness of the need for professionals to be value clear, not value free, and of the role of spirituality in motivation, calling, and vocation as well as in fundamental ethical and philosophical questions which one encounters in relationships and services with people with ID. Professionals have also been reluctant to integrate spiritual and religious needs of the people with whom they work because of the bewildering array of practices and beliefs. The power of religious perspectives to harm as well as help has also contributed to a tendency to avoid spiritual concerns and supports.

That is changing as people recognize the ways in which many people value their own faith and the role of what they consider to be sacred in their lives. Whether or not one is religious, spirituality is also the way by which many find meaning to cope with struggles and questions. In an era of self determination, professionals are also called to support the choices of individuals and families in terms of what is important to them. Services which profess to be culturally competent also have to take into account the profound role of spirituality in many cultural practices. There is also increasing research demonstrating connections between spirituality and quality of life on the one hand and spirituality and commitment/vocation on the part of caregivers on the other.

In the United States, there are numerous developments indicating increased awareness of the role of faith and spirituality in the lives of people with ID and their families. Growing numbers of religious congregations are developing "inclusive ministries" and focusing on accessibility and welcome. Written resources and organized networks are dramatically increasing in numbers. Congregations are making connections between ministries with people with disabilities and those who are elderly. The needs are often similar. New films like Praying with Lior (www.prayingwithlior.com) capture the growing awareness of the importance of congregational welcome and participation and the role of faith based rites of transition and membership in shaping community. Many religious and ecumenical networks have developed policy statements on disability, and resource offices to support congregations. The Association of Theological Schools has just passed a voluntary policy on disability for its member seminaries.

Not all of the "signs" are good ones. Spirituality is often still viewed as a private, individual affair that should not be discussed in services or supports. Organizations who receive public funding sometimes misunderstand "church/state separation" to mean that spiritual needs and supports should not be discussed or be part of the planning. Mistrust between "scientific" and "religious" perspectives often shape the capacity to collaborate. Faith is sometimes equated with the ability to reason and understand, leading to reluctance by faith communities to address intellectual disability in particular. There are also ways in which people with profound disabilities become the focal points around which ethical questions in health and human services get raised.

But there are also growing numbers of theological writings and perspectives on disability. In the stories of inclusion and the rationales for expanding spiritual supports, faith communities are also discovering or re-discovering core spiritual and theological themes at the heart of inclusive faith supports. The lessons being learned are not just about "disability" but about core beliefs and practices at the heart of spiritual traditions. Some of them are:

Hospitality to the stranger. At the heart of Christianity, Judaism, and Islam is a belief in the importance of hospitality to the one who is a stranger. Congregations are re-discovering this value as they work on welcoming those who are assumed to be "different" because of disability.

Re-membering the body. Every major faith tradition has an understanding of community, of God's people, the "body of Christ," etc. Inclusive supports are helping people with disabilities get re-connected, to become members again.

Restoring the sanctuary. For some, this is making worship space accessible, but in a much more profound way, it is making worship and faith life safe for people with disabilities, recognizing that questions and equations of sin with disability or lack of cure with lack of faith have often made religious life very unsafe.

Redeeming the gifts. This is learning to see people with disabilities as people with gifts, with their own capacity. The theological understanding of "redemption" is helping a people enslaved to become free, or a worthless people become valued.

Reversing the call. People with disabilities, like everyone, are called to use their gifts in service to others and to God. So the question is not just how faith communities give to people with disabilities, but how they, too, can feel invited and respect to use their gifts in valued roles that serve others and the community. It is helping people with disabilities, like everyone, be givers and not simply receivers

Recovering the senses. As faith communities include people with different kinds of disabilities, new forms of communication and interaction, utilizing all of the human senses, movement, signing, spontaneity, visual cues, and more, become a way of helping everyone express their faith in creative, diverse ways.

In the last several years, there have been a growing number of theological voices exploring the role of faith and spirituality in the lives of people with ID, and using lessons like these and others to re-explore and re-frame theological assumptions and traditions. They include Hans Reinders, Amos Yong, Thomas Reynolds, Frances Young, Stanley Hauerwas, John Swinton, Erik Carter and others. The Journal of Religion, Disability and Health published by Taylor and Francis is one arena where a number of people and networks involved are connected. Other publishers, such as Exceptional Parent Magazine, are developing regular series of articles on spiritual supports. The Religion and Spirituality Division of the AAIDD is no longer the only network at work in the United States.

There is much to be done. Advocates in faith communities for full spiritual supports need the support of researchers and professionals to explore the role of spirituality and faith in the lives of people with ID just as faith communities work to listen to, welcome, and respect the needs and gifts of people with ID, and find new ways to work in partnership with service providers of all kinds.

NOTE

Expansion of this text is published by the author in two publications:

Gaventa, W. (2006) "Signs of the Times: Theological Themes in the Changing Forms of Ministries and Spiritual Supports with People with Disabilities." *DSQ (Disability Studies Quarterly)*, Fall, 2006. 26.4.

Gaventa, W., "Defining and Assessing Spirituality and Spiritual Supports: Moving from Benediction to Invocation." In Switzky, H. and Greenspan, S. (2006) *What is mental retardation? Ideas for an evolving disability in the 21st century*. Washington, D.C.: AAMR. Pp. 149-164.

Chapter 56

SPIRITUALITY AT THE END OF LIFE: CHALLENGES AND OPPORTUNITIES

W.C. Gaventa

The Elizabeth M. Boggs Center on Developmental Disabilites, UMDNJ, New Brunswick, NJ USA

CHALLENGES

Dealing with aging, death, grief, and end of life issues with people with ID is a growing challenge in services and supports. It is a challenge brought on, in some ways, by success in terms of effective health supports, in that people with ID are living longer into old age. But the challenges are many:

Dealing with decline and death seems like the antithesis to the values of growth and development, i.e., independence, productivity, inclusion and self determination, that are at the core of so many services and supports.

Loss of ability and decline to death may seem like a "double injustice" to staff and caregivers, adding the "Why?" of death to the "Why"" of disability in the first place. For younger staff without personal life experience with death and loss, this can be even harder, and for all staff and carers, may feel like "failure" in their responsibility. That can be compounded in systems where normal deaths get investigated as if they were a "critical incident" or evidence of abuse or neglect.

As in any relational system, intense feelings about responsibility and care can be part of the mix between people with disabilities, their friends, their families or relatives, and professional caregivers.

Until recently, there has been little attention to the ways that people with ID experience and process grief and loss, a paradox given the amount of loss that they have to deal with in so many areas of their life, including staff and caregiver turnover. People worry about their capacity "to understand," yet rather than taking more time and attention to help that happen, the pressure is to move on quickly. There is pressure in agencies to fill the empty beds, to get back to the programs and plans, rather than recognizing the power of relationships.

OPPORTUNITIES

Those same challenges present opportunities:

To revision the end of life not as decline but as journey, and to give people as much choice and control as possible in the final stages of life.

To focus on the importance of relationships, and remember connections to the past, present, and future relationships. "Remember" is about connections with important relationships, and "re-membering" can be about helping people get connected again to relationships and communities of which they have been a member.

To build new communities of caregiving and meaning around a person in the latter stages of life.

To pay attention to the importance of spirituality in people's lives, what is most important to them, the cultural and religious rituals that are part of old age and death, and the opportunities to participate in and practice spiritual connections.

To revision the core values of independence from "Who am I?" to "Who have I been?", of productivity from "Why am I'" to "What difference have I made with my life?" and inclusion from "Whose am I?" to "Whose have I been? Who will remember me, and how will I be remembered?"

ADAPTING THE TASKS OF AGING TO PEOPLE WITH INTELLECTUAL DISABILITIES

In a resource manual called *The Challenges of Aging: Retrieving Spiritual Traditions*, the Park Ridge Center in Chicago identified five tasks of aging that were common to all major spiritual traditions:

1. Reaffirm covenant obligations to community
2. Blessing…how have you been a blessing and given your blessing?
3. Honor, respect and appreciation for aging and the elder.
4. Maintaining and growing faith in face of loss
5. Reconciliation of discordant experiences, e.g., letting go, reunion, forgiving.

As we think about adapting those tasks to and with adults with ID, here are some ways we might do so.

REAFFIRMING COVENANT OBLIGATIONS TO COMMUNITY

What communities has someone been part of? What has been important to them about those communities? What might they want to do in those communities? So, for example, would people like to revisit places they have lived in their lives? Would they like to volunteer somewhere? Make photo album of places and people that have been important to them? If they have never had the chance to join a desired community, could this now happen? For example, there are powerful stories in the state where I live, New Jersey, of people with ID being able to have the bar or bat mitzvah they never had, or having the chance to be confirmed or baptized.

GIVING AND RECEIVING BLESSING

Service providers have gotten better at identifying the key strengths and gifts of individuals with ID as well as their needs or deficits. This is a time to focus on those gifts and strengths. How can we celebrate and honor them for those gifts? Could they give them to others, such as by writing or telling their life stories to younger professionals or others. Could we help individuals think about what they want others to have when they die, i.e., make a will, and think about who would like valued possessions as a keepsake, something to remember them by?

In New Jersey, a chaplain at a small residential facility started a practice of identifying key strengths in each person, and then developing of "Certificate of Appreciation" for that person and their gifts that was presented to each individual and their family at the annual plan review. Not only did those certificates start ending up in frames and on their walls, but they changed the ways that others saw the people with whom they worked.

RESTORING HONOR TO AGING

Many cultures see the elderly as those to be honored, in stark contrast to some modern culture that sees aging as curse. As people with ID age, how might professionals and caregivers do the same? We could ask for their blessing, in a variety of ways. We can help turn records and charts into life stories. We can revision "consumers" as "survivors and veterans" of endlessly changing service systems, and honor them as we would any veterans. We can also do so by restoring mutuality to the relationship between professional and "client" by finding ways to tell and thank them for what "they" have meant to us, and how they have helped us. Professionals all know people with ID who touch deep parts of their own lives and values, and have provided part of their own sense of calling and vocation. We need to share that appreciation with others as they age, as we would with other elders who have been our teachers or mentors.

Maintaining Faith in the Face of Loss

How do we help people prepare for and deal with the losses they have, losses of relationships and losses of their own health or vitality? Can we help people participate in rituals of loss and mourning, or develop new ones in service systems where grief and loss has often been unacknowledged or recognized? Many elderly people get more involved with religious communities. Can we help that happen, and build supports that will be there at the end of life? And, can we find new and creative ways to help people express their own grief and develop their own form of understanding? The *"Books Beyond Words"* Series from the Royal College of Psychiatrists in the UK (www.rcpsych.ac.uk/bbw) is one example of creative ways to help people understand both facts and feelings, loss and mourning.

Reconciliation

Are their old relationships that need to be renewed as people get older? Or connections with families, old friends, or former staff that need to be "re-membered?" For the rest of us, "reunions" become more important in old age. Can we work with people with ID to see if there are people they want to see, or need to see? Many old institutions where people lived were terrible places and times; so is war. But people who survived and went their separate ways to better lives often choose and seek the opportunity to have reunions, or to revisit those places and relationshps that shaped their lives?

Support and service agencies can develop their own creative ways to address these "tasks of aging." Resources like Jeffrey Kauffman's book, *Helping Adults with Mental Retardation Mourn*, also outline policies and practices that agencies can develop to provide safe, shared ways to address grief, loss, and end of life experiences. The challenges can indeed become opportunities.

Note

The ideas and resources are more fully developed in a chapter entitled "Spirituality Issues and Strategies in Facing End of Life Journeys with People with Intellectual Disabilities, their Caregivers, and Friends. Or, Crisis and Opportunity" in an upcoming book on end of life issues published by the AAIDD (American Association on Intellectual and Developmental Disabilities)

PART IX. POPULATIONS AND SERVICE SYSTEMS

Internationally, there are a wide range of policy and service delivery systems caring for people with intellectual disabilities (ID). They range from wholly state funded to privately lead. The continuing disparity of health care for people with ID necessitates a significant improvement in the existing systems. Future services need to be target the specific needs of people with ID. *O'Hara and Bacon* highlight the differing issues of service delivery and policy implementations. *Riches* emphasizes that those caring for people with ID still require further ongoing training and support. The delivery of a specific care service is reported on by *Arentz and colleagues*. They review the association between ID and visual impairment and discuss the publication *Care with Vision* which provides a step model in how to provide a high quality service.

Access to community services remains an ongoing issue. Factors in successful de-institutionalisation are considered by *Parlalis,* whilst *Barelds and colleagues* highlight the issues of care pathways/trajectories. Within the UN convention, the issue of citizens with or without disability having equal rights and being seen as citizens of the world is discussed by *Towell.* Equality does depend on greater empowerment and greater participation within the community of individuals with ID. Both *Sirkkola* and *del Carmen Malbran* discuss how this can be better achieved. Future service developments, include   better access to systemic family therapy (*Smyly and colleagues),* Walk-In Centers (highlighted by *Godsell and Scarborough*) and 'evaluation capacity building' programs as discussed by *Issacs and Clark.*

Chapter 57

ENHANCING SELF-DETERMINATION IN HEALTH CARE AND IMPROVING HEALTH OUTCOMES: FOR INDIVIDUALS WITH INTELLECTUAL DISABILITIES

D. O'Hara[1] and A. Bacon[1]

[1]Westchester Institute for Human Development, Valhalla, New York, USA

INTRODUCTION

Three issues stand between individuals with intellectual disabilities (ID) and improvements in their health. The first is the problem of persistent health disparities among this group of people. Second is the problem of adapting known and effective models of chronic disease care to accommodate to different abilities in health literacy and communication skills. And third is the need to modify existing approaches to health literacy by adopting more functional definitions and alternative communication and information access strategies.

PERSISTENT HEALTH DISPARITIES/INEQUALITIES

People with ID have increased risk for secondary health conditions (cardiovascular disease, diabetes, high blood pressure, obesity, osteoporosis; are less likely to routinely exercise; have generally poor health outcomes and reduced life expectancy (Scheepers et al, 2005).

They have untreated, yet treatable, simple medical conditions as well as untreated chronic health problems related to their individual disabilities and in general do not participate in generic health promotion or preventive health screening programs (Lennox and Kerr, 1997) .

DEVELOPING EFFECTIVE MODELS OF HEALTH CARE DELIVERY

The combination of simple yet untreated medical problems combined as well as persistent chronic health problems for individuals with ID presents a challenge for the integration of generic and specialist health care services which to date has been difficult to meet. It requires close collaboration between generic and specialist health care practitioners as well as strategies that promote active patient participation in preventive health and health promotion activities.

Perhaps the most successful model for effective chronic disease care comes from the work of Wagner and colleagues (1996). Two key elements in this approach are the creation of individualized health care plans and the use of self-management education programs. Their model also stresses the importance of the use of an electronic health record to promote effective care coordination among the medical care team; use of strategies that promote remote care management; and, the importance of close communication between patients and their health care team.

IMPROVING HEALTH LITERACY AND HEALTH EDUCATION

However current self-management health education and health promotion programs are not targeted or adapted for people with ID. They do not address difficulties in developing an understanding of the effects of their behavior on their health for these individuals. Also, few include education of health care professionals to work collaboratively with people with ID and their caregivers in community-based health programs.

SHIFTING THE FOCUS FOR IMPROVING HEALTH OUTCOMES – ENHANCING SELF-DETERMINATION FOR INDIVIDUALS WITH INTELLECTUAL DISABILITIES

A shift in the strategy for improving health outcomes by innovation in the promotion of self-determination in health care builds on the voices and experiences of those directly involved.

"Perhaps the greatest lesson is that as a society we have not really been listening and paying attention to {people with ID}. We have been too likely to expect others to speak their needs. We have found it too easy to ignore even their most obvious and common health conditions. Just as important, we have not found ways to empower them to improve and protect their own health" (Closing the Gap, 2002).

The work of a new Center on Disability, Health and Technology at the Westchester Institute for Human Development (WIHD) is designed to address all these issues. Its mandate for the promotion of health and well-being among people with ID includes: develop effective health promotion interventions; examine risk factors and measures of health, functioning, and disability; evaluate the potential of existing and emerging information, communication, assistive and smart technologies to enhance the health of people with disabilities.

It builds on three areas of technological innovation to create accessible health care supports. The first is the development of an online health education training curriculum designed to be fully accessible by people with different cognitive and communication abilities. This curriculum "My Health, My Choice, My Responsibility" can be accessed using the touch screen potential of many current personal computer technologies from full size desk top or small ultramobile computers as well as the new smart cellular phones. The curriculum is incorporated into a customized patient/ provider portal "Desktop Discovery" developed by the WIHD accessible information and communication technology partner AbleLink Technologies. The image below shows the icon for this curriculum on the touch screen of an ultramobile pc (Figure 1). Touching the image produces a verbal description of what the icon represents with the instruction to touch the image again to run the application. Other images represent other elements of a custom interface for an individual patient.

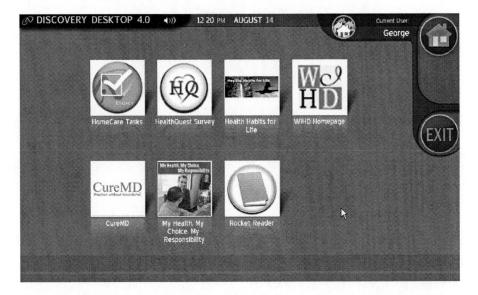

Figure 1.

Figure 2 shows the screen display for the online curriculum "My Health, My Choice, My Responsibility" which is designed to integrate with the electronic health record system used by WIHD and provided by its EHR record provider CureMD.

This training program on health self-advocacy curriculum "My Health, My Choice, My Responsibility" covers a range of topics over an 8-session program. It can be used in small groups facilitated by health education and self-advocate trainers or as an independent online resource. Session topics include such areas as:

Take charge of your health
    o   Healthy lifestyles – Not being sick doesn't make you well
    o   Setting goals, getting support, following through
Develop a health plan
    o   Knowing your health history
    o   Understanding your own health and wellness needs
Be a health self-advocate

- o Preparing for medical appointments
- o Speaking up for good health

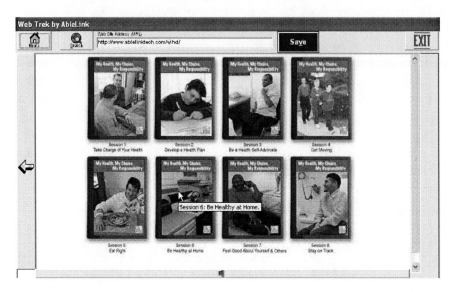

Figure 2.

Online resources in this curriculum include tools for collecting health and health management information and the development of a personal health care self-management plan.

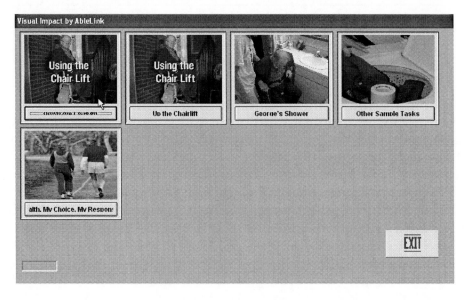

Figure 3.

The Home Care icon in Figure 1 leads to a customized set of self-management or home care tasks that can be customized to meet the health care needs of the individual. In the example shown in Figure 3 for an individual with physical disabilities this display contains links to video clips showing personal care assistants the appropriate ways to help with mobility or personal care issues.

For another individual the personal computer display might change during the day to prompt and coach someone through a critical health care task (Figure 4). So, for example, this technology has been used on individual smart phones to remind and coach dental patients with very poor oral hygiene practices through an effective oral hygiene program (O'Hara et al, 2008).

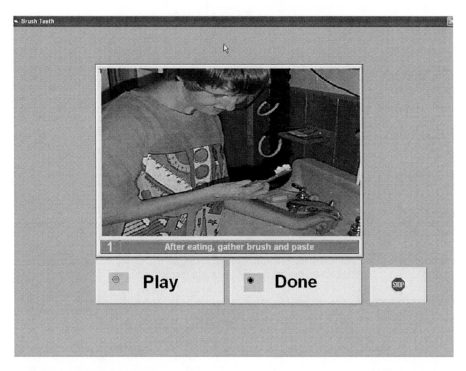

Figure 4. "Janice after you eat every meal you need to go brush your teeth and you need to get your brush and your toothpaste and go to the bathroom."

Almost any other aspect of self-management support can be made available to an individual through customized information or the use of tools for nutrition management (Figure 5) or patient self-report on symptoms or care compliance using and online survey "Health Quest" (Figure 6).

All these accessible technologies are designed so that customization can easily be accomplished using built-in software applications located on the individuals computer. Or they can be "pushed" out to a patient using the resources built in to the electronic health record (EHR) used by WIHD. This application produced by WIHD's EHR technology partner CureMD contains the full complement of EHR resources as well as a custom patient/caregiver/ health care provider portal designed for WIHD. This customization provides the ability for the generation of targeted health records and health information which can be accessed electronically or printed out.

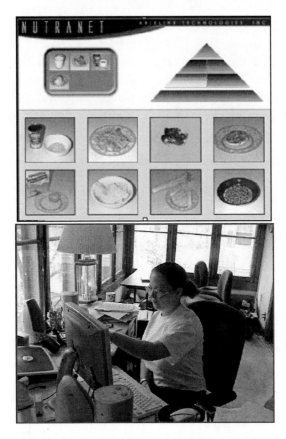

Figure 5. Nutranet – a self-directed picture-based meal planning program to facilitate independent living and nutrition education.

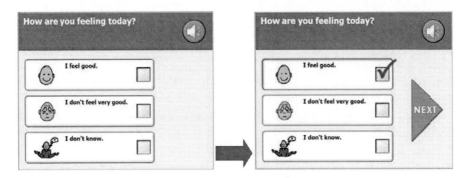

Figure 6. Halth Quest: An accessible survey tools to enable individuals with intellectual disabilities to become active participants in their own health and wellness.

WIHD now has the opportunity to put to the test the promise of these accessible electronic health technologies for improving health outcomes through enhanced self-determination in health care for individuals with ID. It has been awarded a two year grant from the New York State Department of Health to demonstrate how the use of Telemedicine strategies can enhance primary care access for individuals with ID, reduce the inappropriate use of emergency rooms, and improve chronic disease care.

REFERENCES

Scheepers, M., Kerr, M., O'Hara, D, Bainbridge, D., Cooper, S-A., Davis, R., Fujiura, G., Heller, T., Holland, A., Krahn, G., Lennox, N., Meaney, J., & Wehmeyer, M. (September/December 2005). Reducing health disparity in people with learning disabilities: A Report from the health issues special interest research group of the International Association for the Scientific Study of Intellectual Disabilities. *Journal of Policy and Practice in Intellectual Disabilities*, 2(3/4), 249-2550.

Lennox and Kerr, 1997. Primary Health Care and people with an intellectual disability: the evidence base. *Journal of Intellectual Disability Research*, 41, (5), 365-371.

E.H. Wagner, B. Austin, and M. Von Korff, "Improving Outcomes in Chronic Illness," *Managed Care Quarterly* 4, no. 2 (1996): 12–25.

O'Hara, D., Seagriff-Curtin, P., Levitz, M., Davies, D., & Stock, S. (2008). Using personal digital assistants to improve self-care in oral health. *Journal of Telemedicine and Telecare*, 14: 150-151.

U.S. Public Health Service. Closing the Gap: A National Blueprint for Improving the Health of Individuals with Mental Retardation. Report of the Surgeon General's Conference on Health Disparities and Mental Retardation. February 2001. Washington, D.C.

Chapter 58

SUPPORTING STAFF WHO SUPPORT CLIENTS WITH INTELLECTUAL DISABILITIES

V.C. Riches

Center for Disability Studies affiliated with The University of
Sydney, Australia

INTRODUCTION

Disability support professionals who work in accommodation settings supporting individuals who have an intellectual disabilities (ID) and high and complex needs are expected to be well trained and competent, understand their roles and responsibilities, and have clear boundaries (Coleman, 1992; Day & Howells, 2002; Riches & Stancliffe, 2003; Thompson & Brown, 1997). These direct care staff also need to be valued and supported. Although their jobs can be very rewarding, they face many challenges.

But what are the most effective and efficient strategies for providing support to front line staff? Who do staff turn to when things get tough? What support functions do they need and value most? And what contributes to staff satisfaction and resistance?

Disability Services Queensland's Accommodation Support and Respite Services recognized there was a need to provide additional support to staff who were working in settings that provided services to clients with high and complex support needs (Disability Services Queensland, 2005). A program was initiated that aimed to support direct care staff and consequently enhance the quality and effectiveness of service delivery to clients who were living in community based group home settings. The Center for Disability Studies (CDS) was engaged to undertake an external evaluation over an 18 month period, to ascertain whether the functions of the support position did improve outcomes for clients, staff, and the organization itself, as well as inform the development of future policy and program responses.

METHODOLOGY

Four support personnel were appointed who were each assigned to work across three group homes located in south east Queensland, using a team management approach. The position was seen as a leadership position but had no line authority. Each of the 12 group homes housed four to six clients with ID and high and complex needs. Houses were staffed on a 24 hour roster basis, with an average of six direct care staff involved per house per week in permanent and casual positions.

Staff who were working in 12 group homes that received support from the specially appointed support officers were invited to complete the *Staff Support and Satisfaction Questionnaire (3SQ) Version 2* (Harris & Rose, 2002) after 18 months. The *3SQ* yields a Total Score and five sub-scales: Role Clarity, Coping Resources, Risk Factors, Supportive People and Job Satisfaction. Permission was gained from the authors to modify the Supportive People sub-scale to include two additional items relating specifically to the role of the support position. Thirty two staff completed the *3SQ*, 24 of whom were female (75%). All were aged 25 years and over, with the majority were aged between 35 to 55 years. Most worked full time (84%) and had been working in the group home before the support role was introduced. *Semi structured interviews* were also conducted with 24 direct care staff in these houses, in relation to the functions provided by support staff.

RESULTS AND DISCUSSION

Overall, a high level of satisfaction was recorded on the *3SQ* Total Scale (M = 91/115, SD = 12.54) and on each of the five sub-scales (Table 1). There were no significant differences according to gender, age or length of time employed.

Table 1. Staff Support & Satisfaction Scales (3SQ) summary results (n=32)

	Role Clarity	Coping Resources	Risk Factors	Supportive People	Job Satisfaction	Total Score
Mean	16.8	16.9	15.4	22.9	18.9	91.0
Std Dev	2.46	3.21	3.67	3.41	3.83	12.54
Median	17	17.5	15.5	24	19	95
Actual Range	11-20	10-20	8-20	16-30	7-25	67-109
Possible range	4-20	4-20	4-20	6-30	5-25	23-115

On the Supportive People sub-scale, staff indicated there were supportive people in their workplace (M = 22.9/30, SD = 3.41). However, mixed patterns were evident regarding just who was considered supportive. Staff who turned to their direct line manager for support when experiencing difficulties at work were found to be significantly more likely to seek help from the support officer rather than colleagues (r = 0.42, p= .02), and were more satisfied with this support over support from their colleagues (r =0.49, p = .01). Conversely, those staff who turned to colleagues for support were less likely to turn to either their manager or the support officer. These staff were significantly more satisfied with the support from their colleagues ($r = 0.49$, $p = .00$) and less satisfied with the support officer position ($r = -0.37$, $p = .04$). Comments from these direct care staff indicated a culture in certain houses where (experienced) staff turned to one another for support and did not welcome outside involvement, nor trust the support person.

Interviews revealed most staff were extremely positive about the position and its functions, and reported a number of improved outcomes for staff and clients. Apart from expected functions related to support for behavior (54%), health needs (50%) and aging (21%), surprisingly, over half the respondents appreciated support for administrative activities (58%), such as organising household files, updating the house routine folder and individual planning files, and helping staff learn about record keeping and budgeting. Several experienced staff (30%) commented that emotional support and debriefing were particularly valuable for newer and less experienced staff (including casuals), whereas experienced staff felt they did not really need this kind of support. Team building (21%) and mediation between staff and management (8%) were also valued and appeared critical in cases where the team had been highly conflicted.

However, there was marked resistance to the support position from staff in 3 of the 12 houses (25%), despite various attempts by support officers to build rapport, gain entry to the houses and break down barriers. Some experienced staff felt that they knew best and were reluctant to accept advice, and this was compounded by the reluctance of some support officers to train or coach experienced staff. Overall, 30% of staff stated they felt the role made no difference to the house in which they worked, and there had been no impact for their clients. These individuals held negative attitudes towards the leadership person and/or the position, lacked trust, were sceptical of the role and were resistant to outside involvement. In these houses, colleagues supported colleagues.

The seemingly contradictory responses obtained for the same individuals illustrate several issues: establishing trust is vital and support personnel require excellent interpersonal skills to achieve trust; individual staff and staff teams can prevent a support officer from working effectively in a house; support officers who do not consult can alienate staff and contribute to staff resistance; and different staff can express widely differing views about the same support officer and their contribution, views that may reflect local circumstances and 'politics' within a house.

The support position was a leadership position that relied on the use of social power, particularly expert and referent power (French & Raven, 1959). Expert, referent and reward powers are significantly related to high employee performance (Carson et al, 2002), and results indicated high satisfaction and improved outcomes for most staff and houses. However, there was also resistance. It is not uncommon for there to be resistance to change, since change is an unknown and therefore presents a threat to those affected, change can challenge the status quo and may be resisted because of powerful vested interests in maintaining the current equilibrium position, and change often means extra workloads for those affected by it (King & Anderson, 2002).

CONCLUSION

Supporting staff who support clients with ID and complex needs is an important role. However, a range of skills, competencies and personal qualities emerged as critical for building trust and influence. People in leading support roles also require skills in understanding social power and dealing with resistance.

AUTHOR NOTE

This research project was conducted with funding from Disability Services Queensland, AS&RS Branch. The views expressed in this paper are those of the author. There are no conflicts of interest.

REFERENCES

Carson, P.P., Carson, K.D., & Pence, P.L. (2002). Supervisory power and its influence on staff members and their customers. *Hospital Topics*, 80(3), 11-15.

Coleman, E. (1992). Working with sex offenders: A therapist's survival guide. *SIECCA Newsletter, 27* (2), 11-12.

Day, A. & Howells, K. (2002). Psychological treatments for rehabilitating offenders Evidence-based practice comes of age. *Australian Psychologist, 37* (1), 39-47.

Disability Services Queensland (2005). Consultancy Service: Evaluation of the Pilot of Support Officer (004) Positions within Accommodation Support and Respite Services. Queensland Government.

French, J.R.P., & Raven, B. (1959). The bases of social power. In D.Cartwright (Ed.), Studies in Social Power, 150-167. Ann Arbor: University of Michigan.

Harris, P. & Rose, J. (2002). Measuring staff support in services for people with intellectual disability: the Staff Support and Satisfaction Questionnaire, Version 2. Journal of Intellectual Disability Research, 46, 151-157.

King, M. & Anderson, N. (2002). *Managing innovation and change.* Sydney: Thompson Learning.

Riches, V.C., & Stancliffe, R.J. (2003). *Specialist Support Services Unit Final Report.* Prepared for the Department of Ageing, Disability, and Home Care. Sydney: Center for Developmental Disability Studies.

Thompson, D. & Brown, H. (1997). Men with intellectual disabilities who sexually abuse: A review of the literature. *Journal of Applied Research in Intellectual Disabilities, 10*, 140-158.

Chapter 59

FIVE COMPONENTS TOWARDS A SUCCESSFUL DE-INSTITUTIONALISATION

S.K. Parlalis
Elm Row, Edinburgh, Scotland

BACKGROUND

Various reasons impeded regular movement from the institution to the community in theUK. Professional and cultural differences, disparate organisational structures, divergent service objectives between professionals (Field and Peck, 2003; Sharples *et al.* 2002), the lack of a formal national policy and the lack of communication in multi-disciplinary teams (Cannaby *et al.* 2003; Watts *et al.* 2000) have been observed as barriers in discharge programmes. Also, fiscal difficulties (Stalker and Hunter, 1999; Watts *et al.* 2000), the simultaneous operation of dual systems (i.e. institutional and community care) (Baldwin, 1993; Rees *et al.* 2004), the lack of appropriate accommodation in the community (Watts *et al.* 2000; May and Hogg, 2000; Poole *et al.* 2006), the concurrent reorganisation of local government (Dalrymple, 1999) and also the fact that local authorities were in a low state of readiness (Todd *et al.* 2000) created further difficulties in the way of people's discharges. Continuity of care during the move from the hospital to the community setting (Dukkers van Emden *et al.* 1999) and the fact that most professionals had been prepared for working in center-based services were also barriers in discharges (Mendis, 1995, as cited in O'Toole and McConkey, 1998).

The current study explored the development of a discharge programme in a learning disability institution in Scotland. The main aim was to identify what lessons could be learnt from this programme, in order to make the findings available for countries whose welfare systems may be less well developed compared to Scotland.

This was a qualitative study, in which a case study was employed. Data was collected by means of interviews and structured schedules were used. A purposive sample was formed and 28 professionals were interviewed. A grounded theory approach was employed for the analysis of the data and "NUD*IST" was used as a technical tool.

FINDINGS

The study revealed that professionals varied in their conceptualisations of de-institutionalisation. Two diverse conceptualisations were identified; the *"close down approach"* and the *"community relocation approach"* (Template 1). The "close down approach" refers to a conceptualisation of de-institutionalisation in which the ultimate target is the closure of the institution, emphasising on person's physical movement from the institution. The "community relocation approach" is a conceptualisation of de-institutionalisation which also aims to the closure of the institution but it is governed by the values of normalisation and the recognition of individuals' rights.

Through the years, due to a mixture of conceptual understanding over the programme, a hybrid model was created, which contained mixed characteristics[9]; this model was developing in parallel lines, between the two fundamental conceptual approaches. Each approach affected the programme towards opposing directions preventing it from achieving a stable progress. The existence of conflicting approaches constituted a major barrier for its progress. The study concluded that the theoretical conceptualisation which drives de-institutionalisation is closely linked with the quality of services provided in the community.

The "community relocation approach" was considered more appropriate for the promotion and implementation of a discharge programme. This approach focuses on person-centerd practices and refers to the need to see the whole programme holistically and not just as a *change of locus*. The study concluded to five components which encode specific policies, practices and attitudes, in order to enrich the conceptualisation of a discharge programme as a unity and to describe how barriers of the past could be overcome. These components were:

1. 1. The creation of a unified discharge programme, meaning the need for central government to establish an official and legally binding agreement between the stakeholders from the outset of the programme,
2. 2. The formation a template regarding how discharges could be advanced. The study stressed the need to a) plan a *full* individual care package before discharging service users, b) proceed with the discharge of all patients *the same time* and c) move service users to *single tenancies*.
3. 3. The creation of a model of management which could advance the discharge programme. The characteristics that should be incorporated in such a model were the existence of a small, joint dedicated team, led and managed by a joint manager, to whom all professionals are accountable.
4. 4. The creation of a framework for the promotion and improvement of joint working. The establishment of joint leadership, collaborative decision-making and co-location of the discharge team were issues that had to be considered.
5. 5. The adoption of methods to support professionals during the transition. The study suggested methods such as creating a multi-professional team, providing special training, mentoring, secondments or re-deployment of professionals.

---

[9] E.g.: Did not place service users' desires in first place (close down approach), set up a framework for promoting joint working (community relocation approach).

DISCUSSION

The relevance and potential applicability of the identified components in the international context are discussed here.

The creation of a consortium with centralized authority is supported by some organisations through the creation of joint services and the establishment of numerous strategic and policy commitments (Disability Rights Commission 2006) or through "encouraging agencies to develop flexible responses" (NHS, National Library for Health 2007). At European level, the literature underlines the importance of empowering stakeholders in order for partnerships to be formed between public, non-governmental and private sectors (European Coalition for Community Living 2007). These policies reflect the need for "integration" at all levels, from strategic planning through to practice, such structures could allow coordination between all different policy fields in the process of de-institutionalisation (European Commission, Unit of Integration of People with Disabilities 2003).

The policy of establishing a formal process finds application in some countries, since the need for "concerted action" between partnerships has been recognised (NHS, National Library for Health 2007) and the positive outcomes for individuals and the enhancement of their quality of life has been considered (Newton *et al.* 2000).

The benefits of employing a management structure similar to the one described in this study are reported in the literature, in cases such as in Scotland, where the Disability Rights Commission stressed the need to create a political and organisational structure (2006) or in the Czech Republic, where it has been recognised that the current legal and political structures stands as a major barrier to the development of de-institutionalisation (Vann and Siska 2006).

The proposals regarding discharge practices also have wider applications. The need to form full individual care packages prior to discharges is recognised in Australia through the Mental Health Council (2003) and AHURI (2001), which stressed the need for detailed transition plans to be developed. Moreover, the proposal that discharge plans should incorporate people moving into single tenancies - in preference to any other kind of accommodation - does feature in other studies, which indicate that individuals in supported living setting would have greater inclusion than in small group homes or residential homes (McConkey, 2007) or tenants of small houses will have more independence to those in other settings (Wing, 1989; Canadian Center for Justice Statistics, 2003).

Due to the mental health reforms, the workforce has to undergo substantial redeployment and reconfiguration (Health Canada 2002). Particular consideration has to be given to staffing arrangements because the quality of outcomes in community-based services depends to a great extent to the quality of the staff (European Commission, Unit of Integration of People with Disabilities 2003). Incentives have to be given to new workers (European Foundation for the Improvement of Living and Working Conditions, 2006). Proposals which could encourage professionals to adapt to their new roles have been made; training programmes and lifelong learning schemes have been introduced in the EU (Commission of the European Communities, 2007) and courses in Canada (Health Council of Canada, 2007), introducing the new skills the professionals need (Bauduin, 2001).

CONCLUSION

This study aimed to give a multi-faceted and holistic picture of the discharge process from the outset to its completion and to transfer the knowledge gained in Scotland to countries with less developed welfare systems.

The findings could find application in two different settings. In the first place, in countries with welfare systems that are less developed compared to the Scottish one, in which policies and practices relating to de-institutionalisation are in an early phase. Countries such as those in South East Europe[10] or the Baltic countries[11] are still in the early stages of promoting and implementing discharge policies and the progress of de-institutionalisation is subject to idiosyncratic conditions, due to a number of political, economical and social reasons (e.g. war in the countries of the former Yugoslavia).

The second context in which the policies could be applied is in those countries already implementing discharge policies. They could find application for example in the reprovision of established large group community residences which have existed in parallel with other developments in the community, like hostels, which could be considered as mini institutions. These proposals could constitute the foundation on which policies and practices for individuals' movement to more person-centerd housing could be enhanced.

Nevertheless, as Claire (1988) has pointed out, it has to be understood that mental retardation is not only an intrinsic function of the people with disabilities but it is also a function of social beliefs. This means that communities need to be educated (Eilbert & Lafronza, 2005) and people's rights have to be emphasised (Johnson, 1998), since "the right to independent living is still a dream rather than a reality" (Disability Rights Commission, 2004).

REFERENCES

Australian Housing and Urban Research Institute (2001) *Deinstitutionalisation and housing futures: final report*, Australia: AHURI.

Baldwin, Steve (1993) *The Myth of Community Care*. London: Chapman & Hall.

Bauduin, Dorine (2001) *Ethical aspects of deinstitutionalisation in mental health care*. The Netherlands: Netherlands Institute of Mental Health and Addiction.

Canadian Center for Justice Statistics (2003) *Special Study on Mentally Disordered Accused and the Criminal Justice System*. Prepared by Steller. Ontario: Statistics Canada.

Cannaby, Ann-Marie; Parker, Stuart Graeme and Baker, Richard (2003) *Identifying barriers to improving the process of discharging patients from hospital*. Primary Health Care Research and Development, vol.4, pp.49-56.

Claire, Lindsay St. (1988) *Mental Retardation: impairment or handicap?* Disability, Handicap & Society, vol.1, no.3, pp.233-243.

Commission of the European Communities (2007) *Joint Report on Social Protection and Social Inclusion*. Luxembourg: Office for Official Publications of the European Communities.

---

10 Serbia, Albania, FYROM, Bosnia and Herzegovina
11 Lithuania, Latvia

Dalrymple, John (1999) *Deinstitutionalisation and Community Services in Greater Glasgow.* Tizard *Learning Disability* Review, vol.4, no.1.

Disability Rights Commission (2004) *Independent Living and the Human Rights Act 1998.* A paper commissioned by the Disability Rights Commission, The Social Care Institute for Excellence and the National Center for Independent Living from Camilla Parker, Legal & Policy Consultant.

Disability Rights Commission (2006) *Independent Living in Scotland. Executive Summary.*

Dukkers van Emden, Dorothea M.; Wynand, Ros J.G. and Berns, Mary P.H. (1999) *Transition of care: an evaluation of the role of the discharge liaison nurse in the Netherlands.* Journal of Advance Nursing, vol.30, no.5, pp.1186-1194.

Eilbert, Kay W. and Lafronza, Vincent (2005) *Working together for community health – a model and case studies.* Evaluation and Program Planning, vol.28, pp.185-199.

European Coalition for Community Living (2007) *Report from the User Involvement Seminar. Involving people with disabilities in the development, provision and evaluation of quality community-based services.* Zagreb, Croatia, 20-21 April 2007. Brussels: European Coalition for Community Living.

European Commission, Unit of Integration of People with Disabilities (2003) *Included in Society.* Results and Recommendations of the European Research

European Foundation for the Improvement of Living and Working Conditions (2006) *Employment initiatives for an ageing workforce in the EU15.* Luxembourg: Office for the Official Publications of the European Communities.

Initiative on Community-Based Residential Alternatives for Disabled People. Brussels: European Commission.

Field, Janet and Peck, Edward (2003) *Mergers and Acquisitions in the Private Sector: What are the Lessons for Health and Social Services?* Social Policy & Administration, vol.37, no.7, pp.742-755.

Health Canada (2002) *The Health Transition Fund.* Ontario: Health Canada.

Health Council of Canada (2007) *Health Care Renewal in Canada: Measuring Up?* Toronto: Health Council of Canada.

Johnson, Kelley (1998) Deinstitutionalisation: the management of rights. *Disability & Society*, vol.13, no.3, pp.375-387.

May, David and Hogg, James (2000) Continuity and change in the use of residential services by adults with intellectual disability: the Aberdeen cohort at mid-life. *Journal of Intellectual Disability Research*, vol.44, part 1, pp. 68-80.

McConkey, Roy (2007) Variations in the social inclusion of people with intellectual disabilities in supported living schemes and residential settings. *Journal of Intellectual Disabilities Research,* vol.51, no.3, pp.207-217.

Mental Health Council of Australia (2003) *'Out of Hospital. Out of Mind! A report detailing mental health services in Australia in 2002 and community priorities for national health policy for 2003-2008.* Canberra: Mental Health Council of Australia.

Newton, Lesley; Rosen, Alan; Tennant, Chris; Hobbs, Coletta; Lapsley, Helen M. and Tribe, Kate (2000) *Deinstitutionalisation for long-term mental illness: an ethnographic study.* Australian and New Zealand Journal of Psychiatry, vol.34, no.3, pp.484-490.

NHS, National Library for Health (2007) *Delayed hospital discharge: the social care perspective.* Emergency Care Specialist Library: Management Briefing. Originally compiles by Glasby, Jon and last updated by Fowler, Susan in May 2007.

O'Toole, Brian and McConkey, Roy (1998) A training strategy for personnel working in developing countries. International Journal of Rehabilitation Research, vol.21, pp.311-321.

Poole, Dennis L.; Duvall, Deborah and Wofford, Bethany (2006) Concept mapping keyelements and performance measures in a state nursing home-to-community transition project. *Evaluation and Program Planning*, vol.29, pp.10-22.

Rees, Gwyneth; Huby, Guro; McDade, Lian and McKechnie, Lorraine (2004) Joint Working in Community Mental Health Teams: Implementation of an Integrated Care Pathway. *Health and Social Care in the Community*, vol.12, no.6, pp.527-536.

Sharples, Ann; Gibson, Sarah and Cathleen, Galvin (2002) "Floating support": implications for interprofessional working. *Journal of interprofessional care*, vol.16, no.4, pp.311-322.

Stalker, Kirsten and Hunter, Susan (1999) To close or not close? The future of disability hospitals in Scotland. *Critical Social Policy*, vol.19, no.2, pp.177-194.

Todd, Stuart; Felce, David; Beyer, Stefan; Shearn, Julia; Perry, Christopher J. and Kilsby, Mark (2000) Strategic planning and progress under the All Wales Strategy: reflecting the perceptions of stakeholders. *Journal of Intellectual Disability Research*, vol.44, no.1, pp.31.

Vann, Barbara H. and Siska, Jan (2006) From 'cage beds' to inclusion: the long road for individuals with intellectual disability in the Czech Republic. *Disability & Society*, vol.21, no.5, pp.425-439.

Watts, R.V.; Richold, Pam and Berney, Thomas P. (2000) Delay in the discharge of psychiatric in-patients with learning disabilities. *Psychiatric Bulletin*, vol.24, pp.179-181.

Wing, Lorna (1989) *Hospital Closure and the Resettlement of Residents*. Avebury: Aldershot.

Template 1. Diverse conceptualisations of de-institutionalisation: The "Close Down Approach" and the "Community Relocation Approach"

"Close Down Approach"	Themes under consideration	"CommunityRelocation Approach"
1. Discharge programme is operating in a contingent environment		
Key persons' willingness	Political Will	National Political Agenda
Individual (local) attempts	Financial Issues	Central Financial Planning
Limited organisations	Quasi-market	Many stakeholders in the programme
2. Discharges were not always developed according to professionals' plans or service users' needs		
Scandals, pressure from society, reducing beds in institutions	Promoting Factors	Normalisation, person-centerd approach
Arranged and taken care of by others (professionals, voluntary organizations, families)	Service Users' Rights	"Sitting in the driving seat"
3. Lack of a unified approach for supporting professionals under transition		
Basic training was provided	Support provided to professionals in transition	More liberal approach to training provision
Policies for re-deployment were promoted	Re-deployment	Employees are free to decide their future career
4. Ambiguous model of management during the implementation of the discharge programme		
Fragmented approaches by each organization (mainly social work side)	Model of Management	Joint Approach between main stakeholders was promoted
5. Lack of interest for the promotion of joint working		
Limited joint working between stakeholders	Joint Working	Recognised the need for joint working. Framework for its promotion

Chapter 60

CARE FOR PEOPLE WITH LEARNING DIFFICULTIES AND WITH A VISUAL IMPAIRMENT: A TRAIN THE TRAINERS PROGRAM

G.M.H.J. Arentz[1], P.S. Sterkenburg[2] and J. Stolk[3]
[1]Bartiméus, Marga Klompélaan 6, 6836 BH Arnhem, The Netherlands.
[2]Bartimeus, 3940AB, Doorn, The Netherlands & VU University, Van der Boechorststraat 1, 1081 BT, Amsterdam, The Netherlands
[3]VU University, Van der Boechorststraat 1, 1081 BT, Amsterdam, The Netherlands

INTRODUCTION

Visual (and hearing) impairments are a common problem in people with learning difficulties, but are often underestimated or even not recognised. A study in the Netherlands (Van Splunder, 2003) teaches us that about 20% of the people with intellectual disabilities (ID) also have a visual impairment. The more severe the ID, the more often they are at risk of a visual impairment, even up to over 70% in profound ID and in cerebral palsy. Furthermore, a hearing impairment is also present in about 20% of the people with an ID and deaf-blindness in about 5%. These figures are quite impressing.

Visual disabilities make people with learning difficulties even more dependent and their behavior is often not understood. The cognitive and social development is more difficult for children with an ID than for children without a learning difficulty, but a visual (or hearing) problem may even further delay the development. In addition, the development of secure attachment is a difficult process and calls for special attention, as the combination of disabilities may present a higher risk for insecure attachment. Highly insecure or even failed attachment to parent's, presents an important risk factor for psychological stress and the development of psychopathology, especially in cases when children are unable to cope with life's stress on their own (Schuengel & Janssen, 2006). On the other hand, an acquired visual impairment may also lead to psychological stress and psychopathology as the loss of activities and hobbies may result in depression or even behavioral problems.

These facts call for action. From 1996 up to 2007 the authors, in cooperation with the National Council for the Blind in South Africa in Pretoria and the Athlone School for the Blind in Cape Town organised several workshops on visual impairment in people with learning difficulties. Students (parents, teachers, care-givers, psychologists, occupational therapists, etc.) from different Southern African countries participated in the courses. The aim of the courses was to teach people who work or live with children and adults with learning difficulties about the prevalence and impact of a visual impairment. The impact for the disabled person but also for the parents, caregivers and teachers are highlighted. Next to sharing knowledge concerning the assessment of visual disabilities among persons with learning difficulties the courses focused on careful elaboration of a psychological evolution. During the assessment the goal is to gain information concerning the problem presented by the child or the child's parents/caregivers/teachers, concerning the child's disabilities, possibilities, and environment. By assembling the information and interpreting in a systematic way the most adequate intervention can be advised. This process is meant to give a well-considered answer to the client, parent, caregiver or teacher. This method of psychological evaluation is described in a 'Step-by-Step' model.

Over time the course material was developed, based on co-operation with many highly motivated caregivers and teachers, who were anxious to improve the quality of their work as fully committed professionals. The idea was that caregivers and teachers who participated in the course would pass on their newly attained knowledge and skills to colleagues, based on a 'train-the-trainer' principle. In other words we focused on training professionals in such a way that they themselves could train their colleagues. To assist them with this task, the participants in the courses received the content of the course in print supported with DVD's.

Because the method we use can be applicable all over the world we decided to expand the course material. The course material and fragments from the DVD's are combined in a publication *Care with Vision. Care with Vision* is divided in two parts: In part 1 the focus is on information on visual disabilities among persons with learning difficulties. The goal is to share (background) knowledge on the basic concepts of a visual disability. The prevalence of visual disabilities among persons with learning difficulties is mentioned and information is given on the most common eye abnormalities and eye-diseases known in the care for persons with learning difficulties. Also, information is given on the possible causes for eye-problems and on Cerebral Visual Impairment (CVI). Furthermore, information is given on signaling a visual impairment during daily care for persons with learning difficulties and to try to understand the impact of the visual disability on the way of living and functioning of persons with learning difficulties. In Part 2 the use of the 'Step-by-Step' model is described using case studies. Specific ways in which the client can be supported are described and special attention is given to understand and help parents in need of support.

Care with Vision has a threefold goal based on the 'train the trainers' principle. The first goal is to share knowledge concerning visual disabilities among persons with learning difficulties and to provide the 'Step-by-Step' model as a resource to improve the process of diagnostic evaluation of professionals themselves. The second goal is to provide material that can be used to share the knowledge with colleagues concerning visual disabilities among persons with learning difficulties and the 'Step-by-Step' model. The third goal is to provide material that can be used during a course on visual disabilities in persons with learning difficulties and the process of psychological evaluation: the 'Step-by-Step' model.

Care with Vision and the added DVD-material covers a full curriculum of a course or teaching programme for professionals which starts with training themselves and may result in training colleagues and giving regional courses for parents of, and professionals working with, people with visual and learning difficulties.

REFERENCES

Van Splunder, J. (2003). *Prevalence and causes of visual impairment in adults with intellectual disabilities*. Utrecht: Utrecht University.

Schuengel, C., & Janssen, C.G.C. (2006). People with mental retardation and psychopathology. Stress, affect regulation and attachment. A review. *International Review of Research in Mental Retardation, 32,* 229-260.

Chapter 61

CARE AND SERVICE TRAJECTORIES FOR PEOPLE WITH INTELLECTUAL DISABILITIES: QUALITY ASPECTS FROM THE CLIENT'S PERSPECTIVE

A. Barelds[1], L.A.M. van de Goor[1] , G.L.M. van Heck[1], and J.M.G.A. Schols[1]

[1]Tilburg University/Tranzo,Room T502,P.O. Box 90153,5000 LE Tilburg

INTRODUCTION

People with intellectual disabilities (ID) mostly need long-term support in multiple domains of everyday life (e.g., with respect to living, care, education and leisure time) for which they are dependent on care and service providers from different sectors. Before the needed support can actually be received, people with ID and their families generally have to go through a 'care and service trajectory'. Care and service trajectories are routes within the health care delivery system that consist of five distinct phases (Barelds et al., 2009a):

1. The client and/or his parents or relatives become aware that care and services are needed and express the related requests for help.
2. In collaboration with professionals, these requests for help will be clarified. Subsequently, it is determined how provision of care and/or services could answer these requests.
3. In order to get funded the needed care and services, an assessment-based recommendation is often applied for by a so-called 'indication agency'. The questions as to whether it is necessary to apply for such an assessment-based recommendation and (in case of an affirmative answer) which indication agency has to provide it, depend on the type of requests for help and on the particular life domains the questions refer to. Frequently, more than one assessment-based recommendation may be required.
4. When the care and services applied for are not immediately available, a waiting period or a period of intermediate bridging care follows.

5. The care and/or services needed and applied for are delivered.

People with ID are mostly incapable of going through trajectories completely by themselves. Therefore, they receive help from diverse care institutes. Besides, their parents/relatives mostly are closely involved in their trajectories and regularly act as their representatives.

COLLABORATIVE ARRANGEMENTS

Care and service trajectories take place during transitions from childhood services to adult services, but also during transitions to other subsequent stages in life (e.g., the transition from primary to secondary education). Transitions can occur over the lifespan and in multiple areas, such as in health, education, employment, living, and financing (Betz & Redcay, 2005; Lotstein et al, 2005). Moreover, trajectories are often confronted with problems in more life domains at the same time and with the involvement of multiple care and service providers. Trajectories can be difficult and challenging, especially for people with ID and their families (Rous et al., 2005; Stainton et al., 2006). Therefore, the arrangement of collaborative relationships between care providers is very important during trajectories (Betz & Redcay, 2005; Rous et al., 2005). Providers from different sectors increasingly institute collaborative relationships with the intention to formulate an adequate supply of care and services in response to the requests for help from their clients (Van der Aa et al., 2002).

QUALITY ASPECTS OF CARE AND SERVICE TRAJECTORIES

Various failure and success factors influence the quality of trajectories. It is possible to discuss the quality aspects of care and service delivery on the basis of the literature. First, departing from the phenomenon of 'integrated care', the quality of trajectories is determined by the degree of continuity, accessibility, availability and flexibility of care and services, and by the ease of transition between care events (e.g. Haggerty et al., 2003). However, these aspects are addressed mostly by professionals and not by the reports of service users. Second, the structure-process-outcome model of Donabedian (1980) and the SERVQUAL skeleton of Parasuraman et al (1988) can be used for quality assessment from the client's perspective. However, these models are concerned with service delivery in general rather than with specific care trajectories. So, the literature in fact reveals that specific knowledge on the quality of care and service delivery that is both *user*-orientated and concerned with the quality of *care and service trajectories* is lacking. Therefore, our research aims to identify the quality aspects of *trajectories* that are considered important by people with ID and their parents/relatives *themselves*.

Focus Group Discussions

In order to identify the quality aspects of trajectories that are considered to be important by people with ID and their parents/relatives, eight focus group discussions have been organized: four with people with ID and four with parents/relatives. In total, 25 people with ID and 21 parents/relatives were recruited to discuss the quality of trajectories. The study has been described more in detail and published in a scientific journal (Barelds et al., 2009b).

Results

In summary, the quality aspects presented by the people with ID are particularly related to the *content* of the daily care and services they receive. For example, 'keeping appointments' (degree to which personal care providers keep appointments with their clients), and 'taking wishes and competencies seriously' (degree to which personal care providers take into consideration the wishes and competencies of their clients). The quality aspects presented by parents/relatives did not only refer to the content of the care and services, but also to broader *organisational issues*, such as 'access to support' (the accessibility of supporting services that provide help in following individual paths), and 'problems with placement' (the obstacles that have to be overcome before appropriate care and services actually can be provided) (Barelds et al., 2009b).

Relationship with Existing Knowledge

The focus group quality aspects can be related only to a limited extent to the quality determinants of integrated care. For instance, the focus group participants seemed to pay little attention to the continuity of trajectories; in general, they related their experiences to separate care events and not to trajectories as a whole, as they generally are viewed in the case of integrated care. Furthermore, their experiences were related mainly to events in which they themselves were involved and to bilateral relations between them and their care providers. This might indicate that people with ID and their parents/relatives have minimal insight into the coherence of the separate care events. The focus group quality aspects fit closely into the different categories of the structure-process-outcome model and the SERVQUAL skeleton. This observation is comprehensible: the aspects mentioned by the focus group participants are primarily related to the content of care and services and to the direct interaction between client and care provider in specific care events. This exactly is the primary focus of both models; the models are minimally concerned with issues like continuity and coherence (Barelds et al., 2009b).

Conclusion

Several insights can be gained from the main results. First, trajectories can only become more user-orientated if people with ID and their parents/relatives have formulated their quality aspects themselves and also have the possibility to judge the quality of trajectories themselves. Second, people with ID and their parents/relatives have to be approached separately during (the preparations for) quality assessments, because they value different quality aspects of trajectories. Third, it also seems important to include the quality determinants related to integrated care in quality assessments. People with ID and their parents/relatives appear to have difficulties getting an overview of the coherence of trajectories. Therefore, it is important that their attention is drawn to these issues and that they are encouraged to assess them, because, based upon their stories during the focus groups, it is reasonable to conclude that these issues do play an important role during trajectories (Barelds et al., 2009b).

On the basis of the focus group discussions, a measurement instrument will be developed that provides people with ID and their parents/relatives the possibility to judge the quality of their trajectories from their own perspectives. The instrument will exist of a written questionnaire for parents/relatives and an oral interview for people with ID.

REFERENCES

Barelds, A., Van de Goor, I., Bos, M., Van Heck, G., & Schols, J. (2009a). Care and service trajectories for people with intellectual disabilities: Defining course and quality determinants from the client's perspective. *Journal of Policy and Practice in Intellectual Disabilities,* in press.

Barelds, A., Van de Goor, I., Van Heck, G., & Schols, J. (2009b). Quality of care and service trajectories for people with intellectual disabilities: defining the aspects of quality from the client's perspective. *Scandinavian Journal of Caring Sciences,* in press.

Betz, C.L., & Redcay, G. (2005). Dimensions of the transition service coordinator role. *Journal for Specialists in Pediatric Nursing, 10,* 49-59.

Donabedian, A. (1980). *Explorations in quality assessment and monitoring: The definition of quality and approaches to its assessment.* Ann Harbor, MI: Health Administration Press.

Haggerty, J.L., Reid, R.J., Freeman, G.K., Starfield, B.H., Adair, C.E., & McKendry, R. (2003). Continuity of care: A multidisciplinary review. *British Medical Journal, 327,* 1219-1221.

Lotstein, D.S., McPherson, M., Strickland, B., & Newacheck, P.W. (2005). Transition planning for youth with special health care needs: Results from the national survey of children with special health care needs. *Pediatrics,115,* 1562-1568.

Parasuraman, A., Zeithaml, V.A., & Berry, L.L. (1988). SERVQUAL: A multiple item scale for measuring consumer perception of service quality. *Journal of Retailing, 64,* 12-37.

Rous, B., Hallam, R., Harbin, G., McCormick, K., & Jung, L. (2005). The transition process for young children with disabilities: A conceptual framework. Human Development Institute: University of Kentucky. RetrievedOctober6,2008,from http://www.ihdi. uky.edu/nectc/Documents/technicalReports/Updated_Tech_Reps/Conceptual%20Framework%20Web.pdf

Stainton, T., Hole, R., Yodanis, C., Powell, S., & crawford, C. (2006). Young adults with developmental disabilities: Transition from high school to adult life. Vancouver, BC: School of Social Work and Family Studies: The University of British Columbia.

Van der Aa, A., Beemer, F., Konijn, T., Van Roost, M., De Ruigh, H., & Van Twist, M. (2002). *Naar een methodisch kader voor ketenregie in het openbaar bestuur [To a methodological framework for chain control in public administration]*. Den Haag, The Netherlands: Bestuur en Management Consultants, de Verbinding en Berenschot Procesmanagement.

Chapter 62

ACHIEVING EQUAL CITIZENSHIP: MEETING THE CHALLENGES OF THE UN CONVENTION ON THE RIGHTS OF PERSONS WITH DISABILITIES

D. Towell

Center for Inclusive Futures, 47 Highbury Hill, London, United Kingdom

INTRODUCTION

In the economically rich countries of the 'North', it is more than sixty years since the first national family associations emerged to campaign for better lives for intellectually disabled people and their families. As our aspirations have risen in this long history of struggle, we have continually faced the challenge of how best to express these in a language which is both right in itself and can build support among our allies in government, the professions, universities and indeed in the wider society.

In the last thirty years, these efforts have increasingly tried to ensure that both policy and practice are clearly focused on outcomes in people's lives. The work for which I am best known coined the slogan 'An Ordinary Life' (Towell, 1987) to capture the goal of our agenda for social change. We, like many others, found useful the early specification of desired outcomes in John O'Brien's 'five accomplishments' (O'Brien, 1986) and there has since been a huge growth in the 'quality of life' literature (see, for example Shalock 2005), usually identifying a limited number of 'domains' (concerned for example with self-determination, well-being, relationships and inclusion) in which to measure success. Public policy has increasingly reflected these trends, as we can see, for example in England, in the White Paper 'Valuing People' (DH, 2001) and its recent updating in 'Valuing People Now' (DH, 2009).

Now in the new 'United Nations (UN) Convention on the Rights of Persons with Disabilities' (this Convention was adopted by the UN General Assembly on 13 December, 2006 and entered into force as a global human rights instrument on 3 May, 2008. However it only gains real power when ratified nationally, which at March 2009 had been agreed by 50 countries), we have a powerful fresh statement of outcome objectives to shape our work as advocates, policy-makers, professionals and scientists for the 21st Century.

TOWARDS EQUAL CITIZENSHIP: THE UNITED NATIONS CONVENTION ON THE RIGHTS OF PERSONS WITH DISABILITIES

This Convention (UN 2008) is a global response to the recognition that, taking a wide view of disability, some 10% of the world's population are affected and their human rights have often been overlooked in implementing existing UN Conventions addressed to all of humankind. Thus the new Convention doesn't so much create new rights but rather sets out explicitly the legal obligations on governments in relation to all disabled people. The appeal of this Convention is six-fold:

Of course, it has the important imprimatur of the United Nations and the support of government's from more than 130 countries.

It was negotiated with the active participation of disabled people and their allies from across the world, including the global network of family associations supporting intellectually disabled people, now represented by Inclusion International.(More information at www.inclusion-international.org)

In adopting the 'social model' of disability (i.e. that disability results from the interaction between people with impairments and the barriers which hinder their full participation in society) it represents a radical shift in attitudes to a view of disabled people as equal to others in their human rights, capable of deciding about the life they want to lead and play their part as active members of society.

It is commendably broad-ranging: the Convention contains 28 Articles addressed to substantive outcomes.

It grounds its provisions in the fundamental commitment to universal human rights on which the UN is based.

And when ratified at the country level, it has the force of law.

Article 1 establishes the purpose of this Convention as to:

'promote, protect and ensure the full and equal enjoyment of all human rights and fundamental freedoms by all persons with disabilities, and to promote respect for their inherent dignity'

I summarise this broad aspiration as a commitment to promoting **equal citizenship**. Other articles define these rights in more detail to include:

Having legal capacity on an equal basis with other citizens, individual autonomy and freedom to make one's own choices.

Being supported to grow up in families and enjoy family life.

Fully developing one's potential through inclusive education and other means.

Getting the personal support required to live independently and be included in the community.

Being employed.

Enjoying the highest attainable standard of health.

Being protected from discrimination and having good access to information, services and the wider environment.

Participating in public life.

Of course these rights are relevant to all disabled people. In negotiating the convention, representatives of intellectually disabled people had to put their case for the importance of family support in promoting these rights and for investment in supported decision-making as a route to ensuring everyone is recognized as having legal capacity. Moreover in arguing for real inclusion, for example, in education, these representatives sought recognition of the fundamental nature of the changes to existing systems required to ensure that people with intellectual disabilities are 'part of the everyone'.

For intellectually disabled people as for all disabled people, this is clearly a bold vision. The immediate priority is to secure meaningful national ratification, the creation of an implementation focus for the Convention within governments and independent monitoring arrangements which include disabled people. Beyond formal ratification, we know of course that even in the richest countries with strong democratic traditions and substantial investment in public services, there typically remains a large gap between the current experience of most intellectually disabled people and these aspirations.

What have we learnt in countries like the United Kingdom about the strategies required to close this gap?

STRATEGIES FOR EQUAL CITIZENSHIP

The Convention itself of course is not just a statement of rights: it is also a broad route map for government leadership in implementation (accepting that all these goals need to be adapted to different national contexts).

Taking Article 19 on living independently and being included in the community as an example, the Convention envisages a multi-dimensional set of interventions which include:

Ensuring disabled people have an equal right with other citizens to choose their place of residence and where and with whom they live;

Making community services for the general population available on an equal basis to disabled people; and Providing the services including personal assistance necessary to support living as part of the wider community.

Similarly in relation to education (Article 24), action is prescribed to:

Establish equal opportunities to education like other people;

Develop an inclusive system of education at all levels with reasonable accommodation of individual requirements; and

Provide the support required to facilitate each person's effective education.

And in relation to employment (Article 27), governments are required to:

Ensure that there is support to individuals to develop their skills and express their
    aspirations;
Introduce legislation and policies to prohibit discrimination, raise awareness, improve
    access and widen opportunities; and
Invest in vocational services which provide the link between personal aspirations and
    these wider opportunities.

The detail of course varies, but similar patterns of intervention are identified in other
sectors of life, concerned with maintaining good health, participating in leisure and sport, etc.

Looking across these sectors and expressing these interventions more generally, we can
identify three main building blocks for advancing equal citizenship (Figure 1). (This analysis
is developed further in O'Brien and Towell, 2003.) We need to take action to promote:

Self determination: 'I can say what matters to me and how I want to live'.
Inclusion: 'I'm valued for the contribution I make in my community and benefit from the
    services everyone uses'.
Personalized support: 'I get the assistance I need to live as I want'.

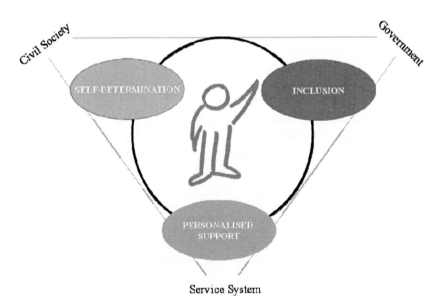

Figure 1.

In turn, these three requirements provide a useful framework around which to array the
key elements in national strategies for positive change which have been 'tested' in many rich
countries over recent decades (See, for example, Felce and Grant, 1998). For the purposes of
this analysis, I have summarized these under twelve headings.

NATIONAL STRATEGIES: 12 KEYS

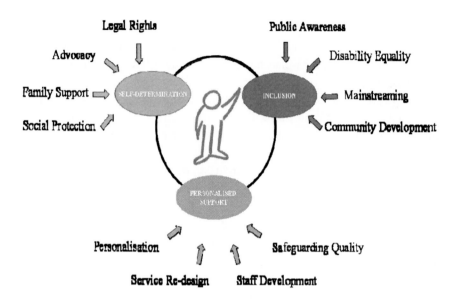

Figure 2.

In promoting self-determination, we have invested in:

Establishing **legal rights**, for example to define legal capacity and institute arrangements
for supported decision-making.

Encouraging **advocacy**, for example through support to disabled peoples' organizations
and the independent provision of information, advice and peer support.

Supporting families, for example through both self-help initiatives and addressing the
needs of unpaid carers, so that everyone gets the chance to grow up in a family with
high
expectations.

Providing **cash support**, for example through social protection schemes which recognize
the extra costs of disability and so seek to reduce the poverty of people and families.

In promoting inclusion, we have invested in:

Raising **public awareness**, for example through sharing positive images of inclusion in
the mass media, so as to foster respect for intellectually disabled people and what they
can contribute.

Strengthening **disability equality**, for example through anti-discrimination legislation
and monitoring arrangements.

Ensuring access to **mainstream** provision, for example by removing barriers to access,
encouraging universal design and including intellectually disabled people in the services
everyone uses.

Fostering **community development**, for example through investing in local 'connectors' who help potentially marginalized individuals widen their social networks.

And in promoting personalised support, we have invested in:

Introducing greater **personalization**, for example by adopting person-centerd approaches to assist each individual to plan for their own future with the help of their circle of friends and increasingly to take control of a budget for their own support.

Re-designing services to better deliver quality outcomes, for example through replacing traditional congregate provision with individualized support in ordinary settings.

Developing staff with the values and skills to deliver personalised support, for example rough relevant training.

Safeguarding quality, for example through strengthening commissioning, regulating provision and instituting multi-faceted quality assurance.

CRAFTING STRATEGY

Clearly this simple framework is neither comprehensive nor detailed. However if our goal is to meet the call for deep change required by the UN Convention and to promote equal citizenship not just for the few but for the many, it does suggest four important propositions about achieving future progress.

First, while the UN Convention naturally focuses on the duties of governments, the pursuit of equal citizenship is fundamentally a political process requiring the active engagement of disabled people and their allies. Moreover the changes we seek in the every-day lives of people in our communities cannot be delivered only from the 'top' down and through administrative means. Rather we require an active partnership between at least three main sets of stakeholders which I characterize here (Figure 1) as civil society, government and the current service system. Critically, intellectually disabled people need to know about the importance of this Convention and the rights it offers them, once ratified. They also need to know how they can get involved in checking whether its promises are being delivered.

Managers and other professional staff working in the service system therefore have an important function in helping to link the aspirations of disabled people and families to the opportunities potentially available in the mainstream of life so as to advance this agenda for equal citizenship (Giraud-Saunders and Towell, 2007).

Second, our efforts need to address the three key building blocks of self-determination, inclusion and personalized support: indeed because we can't do everything at once, effective strategies will balance investments across these three areas, through the variety of means identified in Figure 2, so that progress on each helps to strengthen the others. Applying this principle and using the 12 elements of strategy in Figure 2 as a check-list, we can see that in past national strategies we have often put too many of our eggs in the third basket, engaging professionals and improving services, to the relative neglect of efforts both to strengthen the voices of disabled people and their allies and secure mainstream inclusion. Third, in national strategies, we have to take appropriate action in these three areas at (at least) three different levels: around every individual, to help them pursue their aspirations; locally, to listen to people's experiences, open up opportunities and personalize services; and nationally to create the conditions in law, policy and investment required for local success. Effective strategies require therefore that we find good ways of both linking action at these three levels and learning from what unfolds.

Fourth and most importantly therefore, our framework in Figure 2 requires a thirteenth element in national strategies: an investment in developing the capacity for **whole system leadership** (Towell and Beardshaw, 1991) required precisely to build effective partnerships, link action at different levels and craft together the other 12 elements of strategy so as to create a virtuous spiral of positive change and continuously update this in the light of experience. Public policy cannot deliver real change without engaging civil society, but at the same time progress towards equal citizenship requires effective government, both nationally and locally. (See for further discussion, Green, 2008).

Ratification of the UN Convention offers a great opportunity to advance the interests of intellectually disabled people and their families. Looking forward, both nationally and across similar countries, one priority in the coming years is that we develop and share our understanding of the leadership and organizational processes required to shape effective strategies for equal citizenship, as efforts to secure Convention implementation proceed. In a lengthy period of global crisis, where there is a major economic down-turn and public loss of confidence in governing institutions, slow progress in addressing global poverty and major failure in coming to terms with the even larger challenges of climate change, it will be essential to ensure this agenda for disability equality is an important part of these larger challenges, not submerged by them. All past experience tells us that this struggle will be a long one!

NOTE

An earlier version of this presentation was published in the *Tizard Learning Disability Review* Vol 14, Issue 2, 4-9, April 2009, copyright Pavilion Publishing (Brighton) Ltd.

REFERENCES

Department of Health (2001) *Valuing People: A New Strategy for Learning Disability for the 21st Century* Norwich, The Stationery Office Department of Health (2009) *Valuing People Now: A New Three-Year Strategy for people with learning disabilities* London, Department of Health.

Felce, D. and Grant, G. (1998) *Towards a full life. Researching policy innovation for people with learning disabilities* Oxford, Butterworth-Heinemann.

Giraud-Saunders, A. and Towell, D. (2007) *Including people with learning disabilities* Indexed at www.idea.gov.uk

Green, D. (2008) *From Poverty To Power: How active citizens and effective states can change the world* Oxford, Oxfam.

O'Brien, J. (1986) A guide to personal futures planning. In Bellamy G.T. and Wilcox B. *A comprehensive guide to the activities catalog: an alternative curriculum for youth and adults with severe disabilities.* Baltimore, Paul H. Brookes.

O'Brien, J. and Towell, D. (2003) *Person Centerd Planning In It's Strategic Context: Towards a framework for reflection in action.* London, Center for Inclusive Futures.

Shalock, R.L. (2005) Special issue on quality of life: introduction and overview *Journal of Intellectual Disability Research* Oct. 49 (Part 10) 695-8.

Towell, D. (1987) *An Ordinary Life in Practice* London, King's Fund.

Towell, D. and Beardshaw, V (1991) *Enabling Community Integration* London, King's Fund.

United Nations (2008) *Convention on the Rights of Persons with Disabilities* New York, United.

Nations. (Available together with updates on national ratification etc. at the UN's own website: www.un.org/disability/ For an easy-to-read guide to human rights and the Convention, see *We have human rights* at http://hpod.pmhclients.com/pdf/we-have-human-rights.pdf)

Chapter 63

INCREASING PARTICIPATION AND EMPOWERMENT OF PEOPLE WITH INTELLECTUAL DISABILITIES THROUGH SOCIOCULTURAL MULTISENSORY WORK

M. Sirkkola

HAMK, University of Applied Sceinces, Hameenlinna, Finland

INTRODUCTION

Modern Finnish research and research projects in special education and social care often combine theories of participation with theories of empowerment (Siitonen, 1999; Malmet al, 2004; Vehmas, 2006). These developments echo the participation principle of '*nothing about us without us*' (Ball, 2005, 81), the traditions of the universal concept of participation (UN, 1983) and especially one of the Convention's guiding principles called '*Full and effective participation and inclusion in society*' (UN, 2006). Also empowerment theories refer to processes of enabling individuals and groups to take part in collective actions (Daly & Cobb, 1994).Furthermore, Siitonen (1999) uses empowerment as a synonym for '*internal feelings of power*' and claims that through active participation individuals undertake responsibility over their own activities of life and get empowered by these initiatives. Both participation and empowerment have connections to subjective feelings of well-being and quality of life (Vittersö, 2003).

The emerging concept of sociocultural multisensory work combines social pedagogy (Freire, 1968/2001; Hämäläinen & Kurki, 1997; Kurki, 2000; Hämäläinen, 2003) with multisensory media. These include Snoezelen® (Hulsegge & Verheul, 1986/1987), Sensory Integration (Ayres, 1979), and Multisensory Environment (Pagliano, 1999), and are used in combinations with other creative activities which facilitate multisensory experiences like gardening, music, visual art and body expressions. The media of Multisensory Environment (Pagliano, 1999; 2001; 2007), known all over the world (Vlaskamp et al, 2003), is most often used in education, therapy and leisure of people with disabilities. Multisensory Environment (MSE) has influenced the Finnish Sociocultural Multisensory work in a fundamental way.

Sociocultural Multisensory Work has similar goals as social pedagogy, but it aims more clearly towards emotional well-being (joy, happiness and flow) and empowerment through multisensory activities. One reason why multisensory media has become popular in Finland is staff education at HAMK (University of Applied Sciences in Hämeenlinna, Finland) since the year 2000. These studies have led to numerous local developmental projects and to an increasing number of evidence based practises (Ala-Opas & Sirkkola, 2006).

The emerging concept of Sociocultural Multisensory Work offers a four level framework, called 'Happiness Capital', that allows situations for the sociocultural context of the individual (micro level as immediate environment, e.g. the MSE), local community (meso levels as connections between two immediate environments), extended community (exosystem as expanded connections with indirect environment) and larger society (macro level of sociocultural context) to be taken into account when multisensory activities are provided (compare to Bronfenbrenner, 1979; Bourdieu, 1979/1984; Putnam, 1993; Coleman, 1988). Its aim is to increase inclusion and prevent isolation of cultural activities.

There is a lack of scientific evidence how participation in multisensory activities influences the lives of people with disabilities. Practitioners want to know the most efficient ways to improve their everyday practices and this is the obvious and simple reason for continuing further research on this area.

The new science of positive psychology (Csikszentmihalyi, 1990; 2002; Seligman, 2002) examines how people can use their own minds to create happier lives for them and their clients. Neuroscience is reporting on the connection between training the mind to be more positive and on actual changes in the structure of the brain. These fields hold the exciting view that happiness can be enhanced by training and education in Multisensory Environments.

BACKGROUND

Before the main study began, three pilot projects (2004-2006), were carried out. They were MSE experiments combining creative methods; empowering photography (Savolainen, 2008), 'pop idols' - type of music groups and applications of colour therapy (Gimbel, 2002). These pilots were carried out by seven students at HAMK's Degree Programme in Social Services (Ala-Opas & Sirkkola, 2006) together with 21 adolescents or adults with disabilities.

After the pilot projects, three focus group interviews of interdisciplinary multisensory teams with 12 practitioners at communal services for adults with profound and multiple disabilities (2006-2007), and eight developmental projects in southern and north-western parts of Finland were conducted (2008).

Furthermore, eight MSE developmental projects were conducted as part of an international 'Professional Specializing Studies in Multisensory Work' with eleven Finnish students. A cautious estimation about the number of people with intellectual disabilities who were participants in these eleven projects in Finland is 180.

AIMS

Sackett et al. (2000) defined evidence-based practice in medicine as: "... the integration of best research evidence with clinical expertise, and patient values." Since "without practice based evidence, there is no evidence based practice" (Gilroy, 2006). Theories on participation and empowering individuals (Wallerstein & Bernstein 1988; Wallerstein, 1992; Lord & Hutchison, 1993; Siitonen, 1999) encouraged me and my further education students to conduct research projects on these topics. Applied participatory action research strategies (applied PAR) were used in projects to "do research with and for people" (Reason, 1988) and to find out possibilities of participation in multisensory activities (compare to Kemmis & McTaggart, 2000; White, Suchowierska & Campbell, 2004).

METHODS

Data for this research were collected in Finland during the years 2004-2008, from three creative multisensory pilot projects at HAMK (Ala-Opas & Sirkkola, 2006), three focus group interviews of multidisciplinary teams, and eight local developmental multisensory projects using evidence based practices (Sackett et al, 1996; Gilroy, 2006). Applied PAR (White et al, 2004) was used as an overall research strategy. Main data collecting methods were; participatory observation, participant and staff interviews, reflective discussions, digital videos and pictures, and diaries. Any other data, which helped to generate the concept, were used; dialogues at experts' meetings, research articles, taking part at international conferences and national symposiums. To include and combine all results research bricolage was used (Denzin & Lincoln, 2000; Kincheloe & Berry, 2004). The three focus group interviews following Patton's (1990) advice were performed halfway of the research process, to make sure that the emerging concept was valid and consisted of practitioners' experiences of client participation and empowerment.

EMERGING RESULTS

The three pilot projects gave evidence about the usefulness of collecting digital visual data. These offered valuable information especially at the end of the process when we started to understand the complexity of the contents of sociocultural multisensory work at various four levels of 'Happiness Capital'.

The eight multidisciplinary developmental projects created accessible environments at extended community level; practitioners developed multisensory environments like Finnish sauna and multisensory reminiscence environments for elderly with dementia and for people with disabilities. Also novel sensory equipments and accessible wellness technology were developed (echoing microphones causing other multisensory events in a sensory room, thread mills with interactive videos, games combining touch, light and colour).

All students defined their local working methods according to their goals, environments and possibilities of developing their work. Eight articles, one thesis paper, two project reports and eight international symposium presentations about project findings were produced (Ala-Opas & Sirkkola, 2005; Sirkkola et al, 2008).

Results offer practical evidence about the usefulness and effectiveness of participatory and empowering working methods. They inform about appropriate data collection methods (applied PAR, visual data collecting, participatory observation and focus group interviews) and recent practices of socio cultural multisensory work at four levels. The importance of interplay between all levels of 'Happiness Capital' is essential.

SOCIOCULTURAL MULTISENSORY WORK

The main goal of socio cultural multisensory work is to empower people with disabilities to achieve happiness through multisensory experiences. This is achieved by increasing happiness through pleasant sensory experiences and feelings of togetherness in creative multisensory activities like music, dance and art. Staff members, families and friends are needed to contribute their competences to the development of a better society supporting its citizens in achieving happiness.

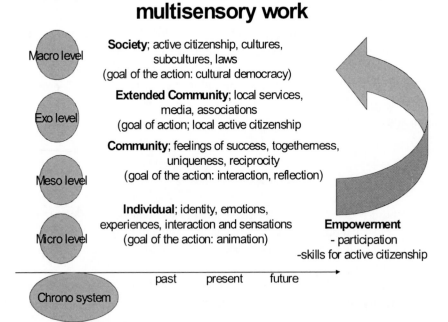

Levels of Happiness Capital in sociocultural multisensory work

Macro level — **Society**; active citizenship, cultures, subcultures, laws (goal of the action: cultural democracy)

Exo level — **Extended Community**; local services, media, associations (goal of action; local active citizenship

Meso level — **Community**; feelings of success, togetherness, uniqueness, reciprocity (goal of the action: interaction, reflection)

Micro level — **Individual**; identity, emotions, experiences, interaction and sensations (goal of the action: animation)

Empowerment - participation -skills for active citizenship

Chrono system — past   present   future

Compare to Bourdieu, 1979/1984 Bronfenbrenner, 1979; 2006; Coleman, 1988 Putnam, 1993; Sirkkola, Veikkola & Pagliano.

Figure1. 'Levels of Happiness Capital in sociocultural multisensory work' desc ribes the emerging concept of sociocultural multisensory work.

Chrono system describes socio historical patterns over the lifetime. It takes into account the person's transitions in life like marriage, work and studies. People with disabilities have several transitions in their lives; between schools, day activity centers, housing and friendships. Bourdieu's ideas of 'habitus' and cultural capital (1979/1984) are combined with Coleman's (1988) and Putnam's ideas of social capital (1993).

Micro level of sociocultural MSW focuses on an individual's primary contacts which link emotional development and identity, experiences and senses. The focus at this level is between the enabler and the individual. The working method at this level is sociocultural animation, which supports individuals' participation to community.

At **meso level** the various micro levels are connected together and they form a community. The idea of work is to promote individuals' feelings of success, community's togetherness and persons' uniqueness within the community. The action within this level is characterized by reciprocity of empowerment (clients and staff members' interaction and sharing of multisensory experiences). The goal of action is to promote interaction and reflection.

At **exo level** individuals have active roles within the community. Exo level describes the importance of extended families, neighbours and local communities. It includes building inclusive and accessible environments for example to city parks, libraries and theatres. These environments have influence both at micro and meso levels, where inclusion joins the local decision making processes and individual learning experiences.

Macro level describes ideologies and attitudes of culture, in which persons live. Sociocultural multisensory work offers tools for cultural democratization which is a civil right for everyone. Individuals and groups with disabilities are facilitated to choose where they prefer to carry out their daily activities; in MSEs built in schools, homes and institutions or at communities' adjustable, but ordinary facilities. The goal of action is to promote cultural democracy (Kurki, 2000), which in this case means building inclusive, adjustable environments, easy access contents and offering enough personal assistance.

Levels of happiness capital can be seen as pedagogy which aims to achieve active citizenship. Since culture is born within the society, both culture and society are closely linked to each other. Individual's and communities' choices develop a culture and society within time and space. Their future expectations and goals define a qualitative change in the life of culture and society. In sociocultural multisensory work the qualitative change can be understood in a way that each individual is creating culture together with others. An example of this is creating a sensory theatre, where creativity, primary senses and interaction with each other are facilitated. Modern digital video technique and other adjustable wellness technology and staff members' developing abilities to use these techniques are part of this cultural process.

CONCLUSION

Sociocultural multisensory work is culturally sensitive and socially transformative; it aims to create positive changes in society. It is therefore important that clients together with their carers become active and critical. Together with their advocates individuals with disabilities are facilitated to participate to local and national political decision making processes. In other words, staff members help their clients to become active citizens.

It is worth while to campaign for accessible MSEs built into ordinary environments and it is worth while demanding 'design for all'- types of equipments and 'easy to use' - technology. There are also other service users who benefit from this development (elderly, individuals with sensory impairments and families with children). The process of cultural democracy promotes for better laws and legislation and hence to better activities and environments.

REFERENCES

Ala-Opas, T., & Sirkkola, M. (Eds.).(2006). *Sosiokulttuurinen multisensorinen työ – kokemuksia vammaistyöstä.* (In English: Sociocultural multisensory work – Experiences from disability work). Hämeen Ammattikorkeakoulu, University of Applied Sciences. HAMKin julkaisuja 7/2005. Finland, Saarijärvi: Saarijärven Offset Oy.

Ayres, A.J. (1979). Sensory *integration and the child.* Los Angeles: Western Psychological Services.

Ball, J. (2005). Restorative research partnerships in indigenous communities. In A. Farrell (Ed.), *Ethical research with children* (pp. 81-96). Berkshire, England: Open University Press.

Bronfenbrenner, U. (1979). The ecology of human development: Experiments by nature and design. Cambridge, MA: Harvard University Press.

Bourdieu, P. (1979/1984). *Distinction. A social Critique of the Judgement off Taste* (first published in French as *La Distinction, Critique sociale du jugement,* in 1979). Massachusetts: Harvard University Press.

Coleman, J.S. (1988). Social capital in the creation of human capital. *American Journal of Sociology,* 94, 95-120.

Csikszentmihalyi, M. (1990). *FLOW – The psychology of optimal experience.* New York: Harper & Row.

Csikszentmihalyi, M. (2002). *FLOW – The classic work on how to achieve happiness.* London: Rider.

Farrell, A. (Ed.).(2005). *Ethical research with children.* Berkshire, England: Open University Press.

Freire, P. (in Portuguese 1968 / 2001). 30th English edition by Myra Bergman Ramos. *Pedagogy of the Oppressed.* New York: Continuum.

Fröhlich, A., Heinen, N., & Lamers, W. (Eds.) (2001). Schwere Behinderung in Praxis und Theorie- ein Blick zurück nach vorn. Texte zur Körper- und Mehrfachbehinderung. Düsseldorf: Selbstbestimmtes Leben.

Glaser, B., & Strauss, A. (1964). *The discovery of grounded theory: Strategies for qualitative research.* New York: Aldine.

Gilroy, A. (2006). *Art therapy, research and evidence-based practice.* London: Sage Publications.

Gimbel, T. (1994). Healing with Colour. Singapore: Gaia Books Limited.

HAMK, University of Applied Sciences, Hämeenlinna, Finland. Retrieved September5,2008,from
http://portal.hamk.fi/portal/page/portal/HAMK/In_English/Hakijalle.

Hulsegge, J., & Verheul, A. (1986 original Dutch edition; 1987 English translation by R.Alink). *Snoezelen: Another world. A practical book of sensory experience environments for mentally handicapped.* Chesterfield, UK: Rompa.

Hämäläinen, J. (2003). The Concept of social Pedagogy in the Field of Social Work. *Journal of Social Work,* 3, 69-80.

Hämäläinen, J., & Kurki, L. (1997). *Sosiaalipedagogiikka.* (Social pedagogy). Porvoo, Finland: WSOY.

Kincheloe, J.L. & Berry, K.S. (2004). *Rigour and complexity in educational research: Conceptualizing the bricolage.* Series: Conducting educational research. Bodmin, Cornwall, GB: MPG Books Ltd.

Kincheloe, J.L. (2005). On to the next level: Continuing the conceptualization of the bricolage. *Qualitative Inquiry,* 11, 323-350.

Kurki, L. (2000). *Sosiokulttuurinen innostaminen,* (In English: Sociocultural animation). Tampere, Finland: Vastapaino, Tammer-Paino Oy.

Lord, J. & Hutchison, P. (1993). The process of empowerment: Implications for theory and practice. *Canadian Journal of Community Mental Health,*12, 5-22.

Malm, M., Matero, M., Repo, M., & Talvela E-L. (2004). *Esteistä mahdollisuuksiin - Vammaistyön perusteet* (In English: From barriers to possibilities – Basics of disability work). Porvoo: WSOY.

Pagliano, P.J. (1999). *Multisensory Environments.* London: David Fulton Publishers.

Pagliano, P.J. (2001). *Using a Multisensory Environment: A practical guide for teachers.* London: David Fulton Publishers.

Pagliano, P.J. (2007). Multisensory Environments and their use in education with children with profound multiple disabilities. Sensory Conference: *Come to your Senses.* Opening the Sensory World to Children & Adults with Complex Disabilities. Toronto, Canada.

Patton, M.Q. (1990). *Qualitative evaluation and research methods.* (2nd ed.). London: Sage.

Putnam, R. D. (1993) *Making Democracy Work: Civic Traditions in Modern Italy.* Princeton: Princeton University Press.

Reason, P. (1988). *Human inquiry in action: Developments in new paradigm research.* London: Sage Publications.

Sackett, D. L., Rosenberg, W.M., Gray, J.A., Haynes, R.B., & Richardson, W.S. (1996). Evidence-based medicine: What it is and what it isn't. *British Medical Journal,* 312, 71-72.

Sackett, D.L., Richardson, W.S., Rosenberg, W.M.C., & Haynes, R.B. (2000). *Evidence-Based medicine: how to practice and teach EBM.* 2nd Ed. London: Churchill Livingstone.

Savolainen, M.(2008). *The loveliest girl in the world.* (Originally in Finnish: Maailman ihanin tyttö), Retrieved September 8, 2008, from http://www.voimauttavavalokuva. net/english/kuvakirja.htm

Seligman, M.E.P. (2002). *Authentic happiness: Using the new positive psychology to realize your potential for lasting fulfilment.* New York: Free Press

Sirkkola, M., & Veikkola P., & Pagliano, P. (*2007*). *Happiness capital and empowerment in the multisensory environment (snoezelen)*. Workshop at ISNA 's 5Th Congress in Montreal, Canada.

Sirkkola, M., Veikkola P., & Ala-Opas, T. (Eds.) (2008b). *Multisensory Work - Interdisciplinary approach to multisensory methods*. HAMK julkaisut, 7/2008. HAMK, University of Applied Sciences, Finland. Retrieved January3,2009.from (http://portal.hamk.fi/portal/page/portal/HAMK/Yleisopalvelut/Julkaisut/Kirjat/kasvatus_kielet_ja_kulttuuri_-_e-kirjat)

Teittinen, A. (Ed.) (2006). *Vammaisuuden Tutkimus* (In English: Research of disabilities). Helsinki: Yliopistopaino.

United Nations (1982). *The world programme of action for people with disabilities*. New York.

United Nations (2006). *Convention of the rights of persons with disabilities*. New York.

Vehmas, S. (2006). *Kehitysvammaisuus, etiikka ja sosiaalinen vammaistutkimus* (In English: Intellectual disability, ethics and social research of disabilities). In A. Teittinen (Ed.), Vammaisuuden Tutkimus (In English: Research of disabilities), (pp. 211-236), Helsinki: Yliopistopaino.

Wallerstein, N. (1992). Powerlessness, empowerment and health: Implications for health promotion programs. *American Journal of Health Promotion, 6*, 197-205.

Wallerstein, N., & Bernstein, E. (1988). Empowerment Education: Freire's Ideas Adapted to Health Education. *Health Education & Behavior, 4*, 379-394.

White, G.W., Suchowierska, M., & Campbell, M. (2004). Developing and systematically implementing participatory action research. *Archives of Physical Medicine and Rehabilitation, 85*, 3-12.

Chapter 64

DIGITAL SUPPORTS FOR MULTIPLE DISABLED PERSONS

M. del Carmen Malbrán
University of Buenos Aires, Argentina

INTRODUCTION

Digital supports are changing the vision about multiple disability, opening paths for expressing needs, expectancies and interests building and enriching communication. Oral and written language may be complemented and even replaced by visuo – spatial and auditives codes –pictures, icons, sounds and words mediated by the computer. Lack of motor control is not an unsurmountable obstacle when the response can be given on a digital keyboard.

The accessibility of these devices needs training in relatives, institutional staff, teachers, peers, friends and persons with disabilties.The development of new digital tools grows rapidly demanding a continuous effort for adaptation to particular situations.Examples were taken from the literature, the mass media and the author`s experience.Collected information shows the relevance of digital resources for improving the quality of life and questions predictions about the real abilities of persons with multiple disabilities. The introduction of digital communication supports combined with an approach centered on the person opens a more promising future for persons with multiple disabilites.

Disability may be seen as a set of barriers coming from the individual traits and to the physical and social context. Persons with multiple and intellectual disabilities (PMID) are subjected to a dual vulnerability: biological and environmental, running risks of social deprivation and experience of failure.

THE ACCESS OF DIGITAL CULTURE FOR PMID MAY BE JUDGED AS A MATTER OF HUMAN RIGHTS

A number of important issues are determining the presence of intellectual disabilities (ID), to give digital assistance according to the different requirements of supported technology, and to reduce limitations to a   minimum. The availability of digital and the training of human resources must also be taken into account. Complex layout and structure may be an obstacle to implement adequate supports both for the person and the human mediator.

Digital technology is going to change our current views about disability. Diagnostic criteria such as the IQ and the social competence is being replaced or complemented by the determination of the kind, extent and length of digital supports. The diagnostic base line focuses the selection of tools respecting the cognitive status in terms of the previous knowledge, the extent of understanding symbols, signs and pictures, the functional capabilities – body, hands, leg and mouth, and facial movement as eye blinks and wispers that determines the kind, amount and continuity of support. Designing digital supports must pay attention to the cultural relevance of symbols, number of exposure, guarantee of its continuous use, association between pictures and icons , part – whole perception, directionality and familiarity. The aim is to produce positive behavioral, cognitive and emotional outcomes.

To do so professionals, caregivers and support persons have to be trained on:

- the potentialities of diferent digital devices;
- the availability of digital resources in the context;
- the criteria of selection according to particular needs;
- the abilities for making adaptations or for transforming resources;
- the use of creativity for introducing innnovations;
- the enriched knowledge for nonconventional ways of communication.

Examples of existing means are:
- domestic robots, that can do the household and serves for security and control;
- special alphabet, supporting with images and pictorial symbols;
- magnetic ring consisting of an equipment that receives the sounds amplifying them and sending to a wire. Persons who use earphones with phone bobbin can access the magnetic space;
- eye mouse where the computer can be operated and controlled by visual movement. The screen verbalizes the text lines, paragraphs, words and letters;
- bionic prothesis such as arms, legs, hands and eyes ;
- Braille computer keyboard;
- video console for people who have suffered brain accidents;
- wrist finder for enhancing free and secure environmental movement.

Areas of application of digital means are mobility, domestic living, communication, and social interaction in formal and informal environments.

Digital technology centered on the person is aimed at

- enhancing communication;
- reducing dependence;
- diminishing obstacles and barriers;
- increasing self - confidence and self - determination;

- avoiding isolation;
- respecting human rights;
- improving the quality of life;
- helping empowerment;
- expressing preferences and choices in meaningful ways;
- widening inclusion;
- making decisions;
- active participation;
- communicating expectancies, motives, interests, needs, likes and dislikes, and moods - happiness; sadness, fears, anger; temper outbursts;
- expanding the body;
- supporting everyday life:
- providing alternative and augmentative communication.

PARADIGMATIC CASES

Stephen Hawking born in 1942 with amiotrophic lateral sclerosis (ALS) called Lou Gehrig Disease, is a widely known astrophysic, author of the theory of the black holes. He neither speaks nor moves his hands and legs. He only does slight facial expressions with the muscles around his eyes, eyebrows, cheeks and mouth. He speaks through a computer selecting the words presented on a screen with a sensor placed on a helmet that detects his cheek movements.He obtained a PhD in Cambridge University where he is a Professor of Mathematics.

He has received many important distinctions and honoris causa doctorates from many universities all over the world. His latest production includes a text "The theory of all" (2008) and a book for children "George`s secret key to the universe" written with his daugther. The book tries to explain the main secrets of the cosmos in plain language. In 2007 he had the experience of floating in an environment free from gravity in a flight of the Zero Gravity Corporation.

Jean Dominique Bauby, born in 1952, died in 1997, suffered the Locked in Syndrome. He was the editor of Elle magazine. At 44 he was the victim of a cerebral vascular accident (CVA) surviving for two years. The only way of communication was by blinking his left eye. The language therapist modified the alphabet order putting in the first places the most frequently used French letters. She told Jean the letters in a loud voice and he indicated yes (one eye blink) or no (two eye blink). Doing so he was able to dictate words and sentences. The strategy allowed him to write a book entitled "Le scaphandre et le papillon" (The diving bell and the butterfly) working with an assistant in a three hours daily. The book reflects his experience. He called himself an exiled in is own body, a shipwrecked, trapped in a diving bell.

The situation would have been different if Jean had had a digital aid giving orders to the computer using the eye blink. He would have been more autonomous avoiding emptiness, boredom and solitude.

CASES FROM ARGENTINA

Juan C. Aged 17 years. Multiple disbliliites. Seizure episodes. He cannot walk or speak. Reduced facial expression. Digestive troubles due to the motor restriction. He only eats mashed food. Initially diagnosed as profoundly intellectual disabled, but later as having autism. Late in his infancy he went to special schools changing for one school to another without evident progress. His mother seeked training in the United Kingdom. There she learned to use digital means to meet the challenge. An individual digital system was designed. Using a special keyboard connected to a computer Juan translates words on the screen. He learnt to read and write, and completed elementary and secondary education.

In 2007 he went to Washington participating in an international meeting, was interviewed in a TV program and wrote a letter published in Disability Tribune about the denied rights of multiple disabled people.

Clara P. Aged 25 years. Right cortical hemiatrophy. Quadriparesia. Severe intellectual disability. She does not speak, walk or move her hands and legs and has to be fed. She understands very simple orders if they are accompanied with gestures and movements from the speaker. Evident difficulties in expressing needs and pains. Her first encounter with the computer was at 20 . The software showed hippos of different size displayed on the screen. The size migth be enlarged with a straw in her mouth while she whispered. As a result she begun to show increased interest smiling and moving her body. Her mother and the caregiver informed a cognitive advance when Clara realized that she could make changes in the environment due to her action.

Both cases show:

- very collaborative mothers;
- suitability of digital resources;
- cognitive and emotional progress;
- improve of communication;
- loss of time for effective action.

REFERENCES

Articles from the press and magazines: The New York Times, Argentine Newspapers (Clarín, La Nación, Perfil).

Brown,U. & Percy,M. Eds. (2007). *A Comprehensive Guide to Intellectual & Developmental Disabilities*. Baltimore: Paul H. Brookes Publishing Co.

People with Intellectual Disabilities: Citizens in the World. *Journal of Intellectual Disabilities Research (JIDR),*vol. 52, parts eight & nine. August 2008.

Mayer, R. E. Ed. (2005). *The Cambridge Handbook of Multimedia Learning*. New York: Cambridge University Press.

Wikipedia

IMPROVING ACCESS TO BRISTOL NHS WALK-IN CENTERS FOR PEOPLE WITH INTELLECTUAL DISABILITIES

M. Godsell[1] and K. Scarborough[1]
[1]University of the West of England, Bristol , UK

DESIGN

The aim of this study was to examine the impact of teaching and learning related to the health needs of people with learning disabilities involving staff from Bristol NHS Walk – in Centers. A baseline measurement of knowledge, skills and attitudes related to the health needs of people with learning disabilities was established prior to participants' engagement with teaching and learning and another set of measurements was taken after teaching and learning had occurred.

DATA COLLECTION

Measurements were taken using questionnaires. Participants were also asked to evaluate the event. Questionnaires combined multiple choice responses with rating scales and yes/no/true/false answers. There were also some open questions. There were 22 participants. Two sets of data were produced. One set from a group that had input from a facilitator with learning disabilities (Group A) and one set from a group that had a session with a facilitator without learning disabilities (Group B).

FINDINGS

Question 1 - What is a Learning Disability? List 3 Things that are Included in Most Definitions.

In the pre-workshop questionnaires respondents from Groups A and B:

Produced definitions using words or phrases that were similar to the ones in the question e.g. "difficulty in learning", "learning difficulties and understanding"
Referred to "brain damage", "a genetic condition" and "dementia".
> In the post-workshop questionnaire 21/22 respondents changed their responses. The differences between the pre and post-workshop questionnaires indicated a better understanding of some of the key concepts (e.g. social skills, communication) and the terminology used to describe people with learning disabilities.
3 respondents from Group A changed their responses so that they indicated a wider range of abilities and needs (i.e. mild, moderate, severe and profound levels of impairment).
3 respondents in Group A and 7 respondents in Group B changed their responses to indicate that learning disabilities had an impact throughout the lifespan
4 respondents in Group A dropped direct references to dementia and made more references to social skills, comprehension and learning.
5 respondents in Group B stated that having learning disabilities made it hard for someone to cope independently.

Question 2 – People with Learning Disabilities that Have Long Standing Illnesses and Impairments are Likely to Have (Arranged in Rank Order so that 1= The Most Frequent, 5= The Least Frequent)

Pre-workshop questionnaires		Post-workshop questionnaires	
Group A	**Group B**	**Group A**	**Group B**
1. Physical disability	Difficulty speaking	Epilepsy	Epilepsy
2. Epilepsy	Epilepsy	Difficulty seeing	Difficulty speaking
3. Difficulty speaking	Physical disability	Difficulty Speaking	Mental health
4. Mental health	Mental health	Mental health	Difficulty seeing
5. Difficulty seeing	Difficulty seeing	Physical disability	Physical disability

Question 3 – People with learning disabilities do not receive good health care because (complete the sentence)

In the pre and post-workshop questionnaires respondents identified a range of factors that were barriers to good health care for people with learning disabilities. Respondents mentioned:

Communication
Understanding, recognising and reporting illness
Travelling to appointments (i.e. using/paying for transport)
>   The differences between the pre and post-workshop questionnaires indicated a broader understanding of the communication process. In the pre-workshop questionnaire a majority of respondents in both groups had focussed on the individual with learning disabilities e.g. a person with learning disabilities would not be able to say what was wrong with them. In the post-workshop questionnaire respondents from both groups made more frequent references to other factors that might contribute to poor communication e.g. health care professionals and carers found it difficult to interpret non-verbal communication, poor attitudes/prejudice led to low levels of engagement between people with learning disabilities and health professionals.

Question 4 – List 3 Things that Have an Impact on Communication between Health Care Providers and People with Learning Disabilities

In the pre and post-workshop questionnaires respondents identified a range of factors that had an impact on communication between health care providers and people with learning disabilities. Respondents mentioned:

Not having enough time to explain or listen
Additional impairments that impeded the communication process (physical and/or sensory impairments as well as cognitive impairments)
Limited vocabulary
>   The differences between pre and post-workshop questionnaires indicated that the language and ideas used by one of the lecturers were reflected in some of the responses:
2 respondents from Group A included responses in the post-workshop questionnaires that replicated the language and ideas that had been used by the presenter with learning disabilities i.e. "talking about them not to them", "talk to the person not the carer", "use pictures/photographs", "use large font and clear white background".
3 respondents from Group A referred to aids for improving communication in their post-workshop questionnaires e.g. signage, pictures.

Question 5 – Pre and Post Worshop Questionnaire

Question 5 a, b, c Pre workshop questionnaire

	True responses		False responses	
a - Everyone with a learning disability uses makaton or another sign language to express their basic needs	Group A Group B Total (A+B)	0 0 0	Group A Group B Total (A+B)	10 9 19
b – People with learning disabilities can not give their consent to medical treatment	Group A Group B Total (A+ B)	0 0 0	Group A Group B Total (A+B)	10 9 19
c – People with learning disabilities need help from carers to get access to health services	Group A Group B Total (A+B)	3 5 8	Group A Group B Total (A+B)	7 4 11

Question 5 a, b, c Post workshop questionnaire

	True responses		False responses	
a - Everyone with a learning disability uses makaton or another sign language to express their basic needs	Group A Group B Total (A+B)	0 1 1	Group A Group B Total (A+B)	10 8 18
b – People with learning disabilities can not give their consent to medical treatment	Group A Group B Total (A+ B)	0 0 0	Group A Group B Total (A+B)	10 9 19
c – People with learning disabilities need help from carers to get access to health services	Group A Group B Total (A+B)	2 4 6	Group A Group B Total (A+B)	8 5 13

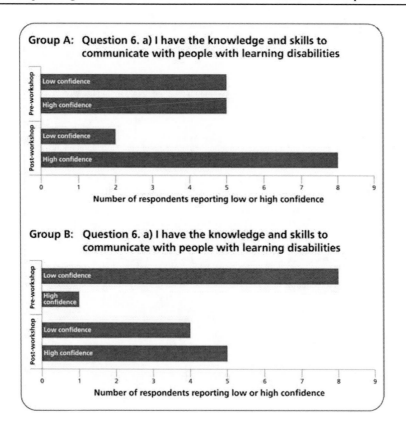

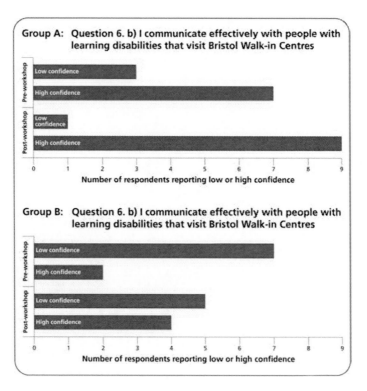

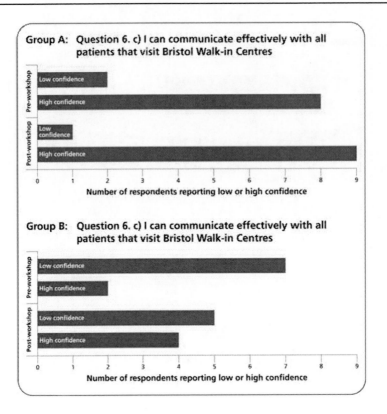

Chapter 66

EMERGING EVIDENCE FOR THE USE OF SYSTEMIC FAMILY THERAPY

S.R. Smyly[1], H. Lynggaard[2] and S. Baum[3]

[1]Department of Psychology, Ridgeway Partnership Learning Disability NHS Trust, Headington, Oxford, UK

[2]Camden and Islington Mental Health Trust, London, UK

[3]Newham Primary Care Trust, Romford Road, London, UK

INTRODUCTION

We introduce this topic by setting the scene for the relevance and potential helpfulness on drawing on systemic conceptualization in working with people who are affected by intellectual disabilities (ID). We argued that people identified with ID often have life long dependency on others, and many live within complex networks consisting of family, carers and professionals. As they seldom initiate their own referrals, problems can readily be located within them without reference to the contributions of the wider system. Systemic models consider the individual within their relational context. Considering what is a problem to whom and incorporating the many and different views (multiple perspectives) that any particular network, including the client themselves, in addition to family, carers and professionals, may have of the client and the presenting problem and how these may be different in different contexts, can give a fuller and often more helpful perspective on what may be happening. From these considerations a view of the client emerges which respects multiple perspectives and which widens the ways in which any particular "problem" situation may be perceived and therefore re-solved.

Many referrals to psychology are often at times of change or transition for families. Life cycle transitions, such as birth of a child, going to school, leaving home, family illness and death, may create stressors within a given system or family as individuals reorganise and negotiate change. Transitions can upset family interaction because they often demand a change in how family members interact and may disturb previous pattern of behavior. How families/people cope at different stages will depend on what life cycle issues each member faces at that time. For example, an adult with ID may want to move home to become more independent at the very time that a parent wants companionship, perhaps because of widowhood. A family member may become 'symptomatic' if the family cannot adapt or negotiate this new transition. Systemic family therapy offers a way in which these wider issues can be discussed with the whole family in a safe setting.

We now go on*to* discuss our experience of developing an evaluation tool for the family therapy work with this client group. The participants involved in this research included 9 families who took part in family therapy, offered by the psychology team working as part of a multidisciplinary ID team. Each family had a family member who had an identified ID. The sessions included one lead therapist and two additional psychologists who formed a reflecting team. Methods of evaluating the impact of family therapy for adults with ID and their families are still in the early stage of development.

Our own tools were developed for evaluating outcome based on goals identified at the first session of therapy and the achievement of these at the end of therapy. The goals were identified through focusing on specific questions in the initial session by clarifying the presenting problem from the perspectives of the carer, different family members, lead therapist and the reflecting team. Goals were identified by two different therapists and fed back to the family for verification. Similarly the outcome tool used at the end of the final session focused on finding out family members views about whether goals were achieved, any changes they had noted in their relationships and communication, any symptom reduction and their views about the most useful and least useful aspects of therapy. In addition routine data was collected throughout the sessions, which identified emerging themes for these families. These included; transitions from childhood to adulthood, illness and bereavement related issues, marital difficulties and sibling relationships, fear of violence and parents feeling 'captive or captivated'. Interrater reliability for these evaluation tools was found to be high and further projects to use these outcome evaluation tools are being planned.

Our work also focused on participants' views of being part of a systemic consultation meeting, which included a lead therapist and a reflecting therapist. The majority of referrals to the psychology team in this study related to "challenging behavior" within group home settings. The participants (N=64) included staff members, multidisciplinary team colleagues, family members and clients. The largest category were staff members N=39 followed by colleagues N=20. Sixty four retrospective, telephone interviews were conducted with the participants to find out their views about what aspects of these sessions had been found to be more or less helpful.

The overwhelming majority (86%) had found the sessions to be overall positive. The most common themes emerging from the replies related particularly to the helpfulness and usefulness of the reflecting conversations and how these had helped to broaden perspectives and helped to give new ideas. Participants also felt that the format of the meetings enabled people to be heard and express their views. Some colleagues said that they felt uncomfortable with the unfamiliar structure of the meetings and other commented on feeling unprepared for meetings. In conclusion, offering an initial systemic consultation session was reported as helpful by staff team members as this seemed to help promote alternative views about clients and broadened staff views on presenting problems.

REFERENCES

Baum, S. (2006). Evaluating the impact of family therapy for adults with learning disabilities and their families. *Learning Disability Review,* 11, 1, 8 – 18.

Baum, S.& Lynggaard, H. (Eds) (2006) *Intellectual Disabilities. A Systemic Approach.* London: Karnac Books.

Rikberg Smyly, S., Elsworth, J., Mann, J., & Coates, E. (2008) Working Systemically in a Learning Disability Service: What do Colleagues and Carers Think? *Learning Disability Review,* 13, 2, 15-24.

Chapter 67

EVALUATION CAPACITY BUILDING IN A COMMUNITY BASED AGENCY

B.J. Isaacs[1] and C. Clark[1]
[1]Surrey Place Center, Toronto, ON Canada

INTRODUCTION

Government funded and non-profit agencies are facing growing demands from funders and other stakeholders to demonstrate accountability (Chaytor et al, 2002). Most community based agencies, however, are mandated to deliver services to their target populations but not specifically to carry out program evaluations to meet these accountability demands. These agencies lack important resources, such as staff with the necessary skills and knowledge to adequately design and carry out evaluation (Bozzo, 2002). For such agencies Evaluation Capacity Building (ECB) is a necessary step to enable meaningful program evaluation.

ECB focuses on the development of knowledge, and skills and resources within organizations so that they can carry out useful program evaluation activities as part of their regular and on-going practice and effectively utilize evaluation results (Bozzo, 2002; Cousins et al, 2004; Preskill & Boyle, 2008; Stockdill et al, 2002). Preskill & Boyle (2008) outlined a comprehensive model that accounts for an array of factors and processes that should be considered in ECB. Broadly these factors can be spit into two categories: 1) contextual (organizational leadership, culture, motivations and structure), and 2) the actual characteristics of the ECB initiative, including the goals, expectations and assumptions, overall design and the specific strategies employed.

King (2007) discusses contextual factors both external and internal to organizations undertaking ECB. External factors include accountability demands of funders or legislation and supports funders may provide for evaluation. This support may come directly from operating dollars specifically slated for evaluation or in the form of grant programs. Internally: 1) program evaluation must be seen as viable approach to organizational improvement (Preskill & Boyle, 2008); 2) an organization must be open to learning and change (Cousins et al, 2004); and 3) management must support program evaluation (King, 2007).

Preskill & Boyle (2008) identify three target areas for teaching strategies in ECB: 1) *knowledge* about evaluation concepts, methods and issue, 2) skill development in various aspects of evaluation and 3) affective (beliefs) about the value of program evaluation. Teaching activities can range from formalized workshops (Stevenson et al, 2002) to a less structured but still intentional "learning while doing" approach (Forss et al, 2006; King, 2007). Other needed elements for successful ECB include evaluation champions, an evaluation specialist as a facilitator, and an ECB structure and process (King, 2007).

The following chapter describes an evaluation of an ECB initiative at a community based agency in Toronto serving persons with ID. In a recent review, (Cousins et al, 2004) identified only four structured and six descriptive of evaluations of ECB initiatives. The evaluation reported here combines both the structured and descriptive approaches.

DESCRIPTION OF THE EVALUATION CAPACITY BUILDING INITIATIVE

Surrey Place Center (SPC) is a government funded developmental service agency in Toronto, Canada serving individuals with intellectual disabilities of all ages and their families. It is a multidisciplinary setting that serves clients and families over the lifespan. A Research and Evaluation Unit was established at the Center in 2004. At that time the context within the center was, and continues to be, favourable to ECB. There is organization support at the management and board levels for program evaluation as a valuable activity, staff enthusiasm for evaluation, and a sector push for accountability. There are, however, limited resources for undertaking evaluation; Evaluation needs, opportunities, and challenges vary across service provider groups within the Center; Staff time and competing priorities are also constraints, in that client service is a higher priority compared to evaluation, particularly with a subset of clients presenting with urgent client needs and requiring immediate service and another subset facing wait times for some services. The agency has, however, committed specific resources to program evaluation.

One of the first tasks of the Research and Evaluation Unit was to develop an ECB plan through consultation with staff. The resulting ECB model is shown in Figure 1. The activities in the model stress the collaboration between clinical and evaluation staff, the use of logic models to teach about, guide and plan evaluation, and clinical staff engagement in the evaluation process as capacity building strategies. The collaborative strategy is based on the assumption that education is needed but facilitation is necessary for application of evaluation knowledge (King, 2007).

The process of developing and using logic models is viewed as central to the ECB plan. Logic models have been identified as useful tools that can be applied for ECB in any government funded and non-profit service setting (Bozzo, 2002; Chaytor et al., 2002). A logic model is a pictorial representation of a program in which key components, activities, and expected outcomes are listed and connected (Cooksy et al, 2001; Dwyer & Makins, 1997; Hernandez, 2000; Porteous et al, 2002; Rush & Ogbourne, 1991; Schalock & Bonham, 2003). A completed model is a tool that can be used in evaluation planning to develop evaluation questions and place those questions within the context of the larger program. Including staff in the development and use of such models to plan evaluation serves several ECB functions:

1. It clarifies and builds consensus among program staff about what a program does and intends to achieve and as such readies a program for evaluation
2. It orients staff to four basic issues within which program evaluation can be grounded: Who is being served? What is being done in the program? What are the outcomes? How are these program elements connected?
3. Fosters buy-in to evaluation by allowing input into the process
4. Assists staff in seeing evaluations within the larger context of the overall service they provide
5. Helps staff plan a series of evaluations in which each successive project builds on its predecessor
6. Provides information for picking clinically relevant outcome measures

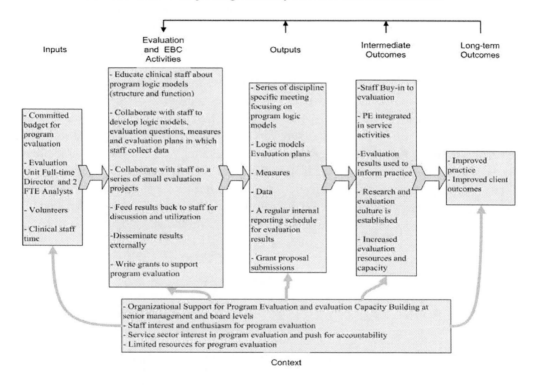

Figure 1. Evaluation Capacity Building Model.

All activities in the plan are based in a model that uses the evaluation specialist as a facilitator, but specific roles have developed for the various participants. Research and Evaluation Unit staff work together with clinicians to develop: logic models, evaluation plans, evaluation methods/procedures, and measures. Clinical staff are expected to take a lead role in data collection, but evaluators are responsible for activities that require research skills as data analysis and reporting. Dissemination and grant writing activities are usually undertaken collaboratively. Together the ECB activities are intended to lead to an overall increase in evaluation capacity by enhancing staff buy-in to evaluation and integrating it into clinical practice such that a research ad evaluation culture is established at the Center.

EVALUATION OF THE ECB INITIATIVE

An assessment of both the outputs and outcomes of the ECB process as depicted in the model was undertaken. Outputs were counted through a review of activities in the years following the establishment of the ECB plan, 2005 – 2008. During that time period evaluation projects were initiated in 7 clinical services. A logic model for each of these seven services was developed. Forty-six clinical staff were involved in logic model development, evaluation planning and/or data collection. Data collection for all evaluations covered 221 clients. Reporting of data back to clinicians is unstructured, occurring as needed for each project. Although there are limited funding opportunities to support program evaluation in community based agencies 5 grant proposals were submitted and 2 were funded.

Information about the outcomes of the ECB initiative was obtained through a survey sent to 35 of the 46 clinicians who had participated in program evaluation at the center. Three of the original 46 had either left the center or were on leave and several others were only involved in logic model development. These latter individuals were excluded as much of the survey referred to the aspects of the evaluation process in which they were not involved. Survey was comprised of quantitative and qualitative questions. In 3 separate questions clinicians were asked to rate on a 5 point semantic differential scale, the degree to which program evaluation was important to their work, integrated into their work and influenced their work. Prompts for qualitative explanations of the ratings were included. In addition 4 open ended questions asking about the factors that make program evaluation easy or difficulty to carry out, suggestions for how evaluation staff could further support clinicians in program evaluation, and things clinicians have learned from program evaluation were included. Ten surveys were returned. Results for the quantitative ratings are shown in Figures 2 – 4.

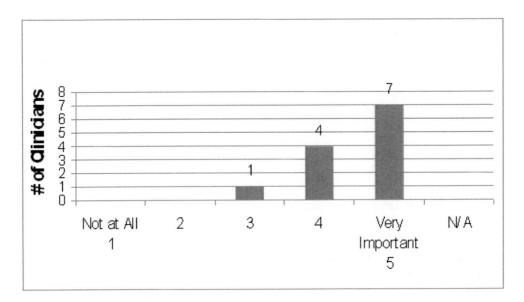

Figure 2. Importance of program evaluation?

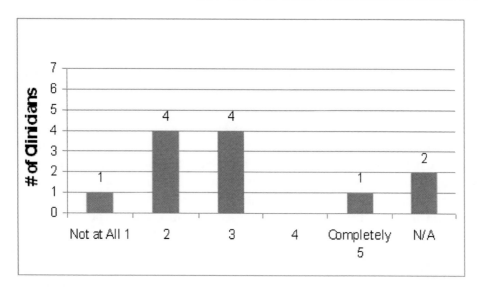

Figure 3. Integration of program evaluation into regular work?

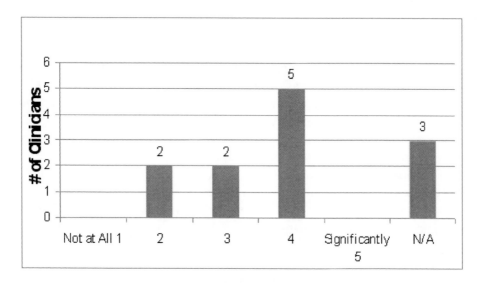

Figure 4. Influence of program evaluation on work?

The qualitative data provided further elaboration of these results and several themes emerged. While program evaluation is considered important, it is currently not well integrated into clinical practice. It is perceived by several clinicians as adding more work to their already busy jobs. Barriers to implementation include lack of relevant and user friendly measures, language barriers (a large percentage of clients for whom English is a second language), lack of structure to the evaluation process and not enough management involvement. Most clinicians were still struggling to use evaluation results, but some had indicated that they had been able to do so. The support provided by the Research and Evaluation Unit was valued and appreciated. Two major areas of improvement were identified. Clinicians expressed the need for more structure to the evaluation process. Currently evaluation staff meet with clinicians on an as needed basis. Clinicians would like to increase the frequency of and regularity of meetings. Second, clinical staff would like management to become more involved in evaluation.

The results represent only a preliminary evaluation of the ECB initiative at Surrey Place Center. Unfortunately, no pre-initiative baseline data are available. Several observations about the state of program evaluation within the Center before as compared to after the ECB initiative, however, can be made. Prior to 2005 evaluation had been occurring at the center, but only one logic model had been constructed. While the relative merits of using logic models have not been demonstrated by the data presented in this chapter there are a number of advantages to, and a sizable literature on the merits of, using such an approach that are referred to above. Also, before the ECB initiative program evaluation was organized on an age program basis i.e. the Infancy and Early Childhood, Children and Youth, and Adult Services programs in the Center each undertook evaluation separately. Under the new initiative 4 evaluations spanned more than one age program. Thus, evaluations are now able to cover services for a wider range of clients. It can also be argued that the new approach fosters cross program collaboration and understanding that would contribute to smoother transitions for clients from one age program to the next. Thus, except in the case of logic models, the data cannot demonstrate an increase in program evaluation outputs, but the new approach to program evaluation taken under the ECB initiative does seem to have some advantages over the previous model taken in the Center.

While the results can only be viewed as preliminary, they are consistent with what has been generally observed by the program evaluation staff. The value placed on evaluation by the clinicians is encouraging, but as expected barriers to the integration of program evaluation into clinical work were identified and the use of evaluation results is to this point limited. To begin addressing these issues the Research and Evaluation Unit will set-up meeting schedules with the various clinical teams in an effort to bring more structure to the process. A more formal role for management in the evaluation process will also be developed.

The work presented in this chapter is the first stage in evaluating the ECB initiative. While the data is limited due to low response rates it can serve as a useful baseline. The same data will be compiled on a 2 year cycle to assess growth in evaluation activities, integration of evaluation into clinical work and use of results.

REFERENCES

Bozzo, S. L. (2002). Evaluation capacity building in the voluntary/ nonprofit sector. *The Canadian Journal of Program Evaluation, 17*(3), 75-92.

Chaytor, K., MacDonald, G., & Melvin, D. (2002). Preparing nonprofits for new accountability demands. *The Canadian Journal of Program Evaluation, 17*(3), 93-112.

Cooksy, L. J., Gill, P., & Kelly, A. (2001). The program logic model as an integrative framework for a multimethod evaluation. *Evaluation and Program Planning, 24*, 119-128.

Cousins, B. J., & Goh, S.C., Clark, S.H., Lee, L.E. (2004). Integrative evaluative inquiry into the organizational culture: A review and synthesis of the knowledge base. *The Canadian Journal of Program Evaluation, 19*, 99-141.

Dwyer, J. J. M., & Makins, S. (1997). Using a program logic model that focuses on performance measurement to develop a program. *Canadian Journal of Public Health, 88*, 421-425.

Forss, K., S-E. Kruse, S. Taut, & E. Tenden. (2006). Chasing a ghost? an essay on participatory evaluation and capacity development. *Evaluation, 12*(1), 128-144.

Hernandez, M. (2000). Using logic models and program theory to build outcome accountability. *Education and Treatment of Children, 23*, 24-40.

King, J. A. (2007). Making sense of participatory evaluation. *New Directions for Evaluation, 2007*(114), 83-105.

Porteous, N. L., Sheldrick, B. J., & Stewart, P. J. (2002). Introducing program teams to logic models: Facilitating the learning process. *Canadian Journal of Program Evaluation, 17*(3), 113-141.

Preskill, H., & Boyle, S. (2008). A multidisciplinary model of evaluation capacity building. *American Journal of Evaluation, 29*(4), 443-459.

Rush, B., & Ogbourne, A. (1991). Program logic models: Expanding their role and structure for program planning and evaluation. *The Canadian Journal of Program Evaluation, 6*, 95-106.

Schalock, R. L., & Bonham, G. S. (2003). Measuring outcomes and managing results. *Evaluation and Program Planning, 26*(3), 229-235.

Stevenson, J. S., Florin, P., Mills, D. S., & Andrade, M. (2002). Building evaluation capacity in human service organizations: A case study. *Evaluation and Program Planning, 25*, 233-243.

Stockdill, S. H., Baizerman, M., & Compton, D. W. (2002). Toward a definition of the ECB process: A conversation with the ECB literature. *New Directions for Evaluation, 93*, 7-26.

INDEX

A

B

D

depression, 3, 4, 6, 8, 10, 30, 34, 55, 58, 60, 61, 70, 76, 104, 105, 134, 145, 231, 239, 240, 242, 243, 244, 246, 268, 269, 371
depressive symptoms, 55, 244, 245
deprivation, 397
desensitization, 10
destruction, 4, 153
detection, 17, 91, 99, 189
determinism, 199
developed countries, 69
developed nations, 204
developing countries, 168, 169, 368
developmental disorder, 21, 153, 244, 245, 246
deviation, 216
diabetes, 98, 138, 247, 248, 251, 253, 351
Diagnostic and Statistical Manual of Mental Disorders, 11, 160
diagnostic criteria, 1, 7, 8, 9, 10, 19, 98, 104, 127
dialogues, 391
dichotomy, 250
diet, 92
differential diagnosis, 8, 10, 58, 152, 154, 167
digital communication, 397
dignity, 296, 336, 382
direct measure, 258
direct observation, 7
directionality, 398
discharges, 363, 364, 365
discomfort, 28, 36, 77, 205
discourse, 202, 206, 213
discrimination, 39, 132, 133, 134, 210, 320, 328, 338, 383, 384, 385
diseases, 22, 97, 98, 99, 372
disorder, 4, 9, 16, 20, 21, 34, 39, 51, 103, 106, 107, 124, 157, 161, 163, 189, 244, 245, 247, 328
displacement, 154
distress, 77, 80, 153, 154, 157, 159, 246
diversity, 88, 335, 336, 337, 341
division, 24, 172, 339
DNA, 106, 222
doctors, 20, 93
domestic violence, 40, 41, 111, 112
dominance, 151, 153, 154, 156
dopamine, 112, 160, 162
dopamine antagonists, 160
dopaminergic, 188
Down syndrome, 1, 27, 30, 31, 45, 53, 56, 60, 61, 63, 69, 72, 92, 94, 95, 96, 101, 113, 117, 183, 199, 231, 239, 244, 245, 246, 273, 277, 333
draft, 315, 316

drawing, 175, 192, 409
dream, 366
Drosophila, 108
drug safety, 25
drug use, 26, 158, 159, 160
drugs, 1, 20, 22, 24, 25, 70, 140
DSM, 7, 8, 11, 12, 34, 157, 160, 167, 241
DSM-IV, 7, 8, 11, 157, 160, 167, 241
dualism, 330
duality, 265, 268
duration, 16, 17, 143
duties, 97, 302, 386
dynamics, 51, 193, 195, 201, 210, 237, 269
dyslexia, 132
dysphagia, 176
dysphoria, 158

E

eating, 12, 33, 34
eating disorders, 33, 34
echoing, 391
ecology, 151, 154, 394
economic disadvantage, 302
economic growth, 295
economics, 339
education, 12, 79, 113, 118, 191, 196, 213, 215, 218, 225, 247, 254, 332, 352, 396, 419
educational programs, 106
educational research, 395
educational services, 204
EEG, 160
elaboration, 372, 417
elderly, 53, 58, 59, 60, 72, 85, 276, 286, 342, 347, 348, 391, 394
elders, 347
electrolyte, 27
emotion, 147, 149, 155, 270
emotional distress, 41
emotional exhaustion, 144
emotional health, 310
emotional intelligence, 146
emotional reactions, 143, 145, 146, 147, 149, 153
emotional responses, 185
emotional state, 144, 184
emotional well-being, 236, 390
emotions, 49, 53, 76, 78, 148, 240
empathy, 163, 227
employment, 41, 305, 313, 317, 341, 376, 383
employment status, 317

F

J

K

L

O

P

Q

R

S

T